Handbook of Orthopedic Surgical Procedures

Handbook of Orthopedic Surgical Procedures

Editor: Markus Wagner

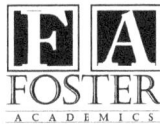

FA FOSTER
ACADEMICS

www.fosteracademics.com

www.fosteracademics.com

FA
FOSTER
ACADEMICS

Cataloging-in-Publication Data

Handbook of orthopedic surgical procedures / edited by Markus Wagner.
    p. cm.
Includes bibliographical references and index.
ISBN 978-1-63242-582-9
1. Orthopedic surgery. 2. Orthopedics. I. Wagner, Markus.
RD731 .H35 2019
61747--dc23

Foster Academics,
118-35 Queens Blvd., Suite 400,
Forest Hills, NY 11375, USA

ISBN 978-1-63242-582-9 (Hardback)

Contents

Permissions

List of Contributors

Index

Preface

This book has been an outcome of determined endeavour from a group of educationists in the field. The primary objective was to involve a broad spectrum of professionals from diverse cultural background involved in the field for developing new researches. The book not only targets students but also scholars pursuing higher research for further enhancement of the theoretical and practical applications of the subject.

Orthopedic surgical procedures are used for treating musculoskeletal trauma, injuries, degenerative diseases and tumors. Arthroscopy and arthroplasty are the principal surgical procedures in this field. Arthroplasty is a procedure in orthopedic surgery, which involves the replacement, realignment or remodeling of the articular surface of a musculoskeletal joint. It is done to relieve pain due to arthritis and restore function to the joint. Joint replacement, interpositional arthroplasty, silicone replacement arthroplasty, etc. are some of the different types of arthroplasty. Arthroscopy is a minimally invasive surgical procedure that is done on a joint. It is done by inserting an arthroscope into the joint through a small incision. It is a great alternative to traditional surgery as it reduces recovery time and trauma. The objective of this book is to give a general view of the different types of orthopedic surgical procedures and their clinical advances. It presents the complex subject of orthopedic surgery in the most comprehensible and easy to understand language. It will help the readers in keeping pace with the rapid changes in this field.

It was an honour to edit such a profound book and also a challenging task to compile and examine all the relevant data for accuracy and originality. I wish to acknowledge the efforts of the contributors for submitting such brilliant and diverse chapters in the field and for endlessly working for the completion of the book. Last, but not the least; I thank my family for being a constant source of support in all my research endeavours.

Editor

Is combined use of intravenous and intraarticular tranexamic acid superior to intravenous or intraarticular tranexamic acid alone in total knee arthroplasty?

Bobin Mi[1], Guohui Liu[1*], Huijuan Lv[2], Yi Liu[1], Kun Zha[1], Qipeng Wu[1] and Jing Liu[1]

Abstract

Background: Tranexamic acid (TXA) has been proven to be effective in reducing blood loss and transfusion rate after total knee arthroplasty (TKA) without increasing the risk of deep vein thrombosis (DVT) and pulmonary embolism (PE). Recently, an increasing number of studies have been interested in applying combined intravenous (IV) with intraarticular (IA) tranexamic acid in total knee arthroplasty. The purpose of this meta-analysis was to compare the blood loss and complications of combined TXA with IV TXA or IA TXA on TKA.

Methods: Systematic search of literatures were conducted to identify related articles that were published in PubMed, MEDLINE, Embase, the Cochrane Library, SpringerLink, ClinicalTrials.gov, and Ovid from their inception to September 2016. All studies that compare blood loss and complications of combined TXA and IV TXA or IA TXA on TKA were included. Main outcomes were collected and analyzed by the Review Manager 5.3.

Results: Five studies were included in the present meta-analysis. There was significant difference in total blood loss and blood volume of drainage when compared combined TXA group with IV TXA group or IA TXA group ($P < 0.05$). There was no difference in transfusion rate and thromboembolic complications when comparing combined TXA with IV TXA or IA TXA alone ($P > 0.05$).

Conclusions: Compared with administration of IA TXA or IV TXA alone on TKA, combined use of TXA has advantages in reducing total blood loss and blood volume of drainage without increasing the incidence of thromboembolic complications. We recommend combined TXA as the preferred option for patients undergoing TKA.

Keywords: Tranexamic acid, Combined, Intravenous, Intraarticular, Total knee arthroplasty

* Correspondence: liuguohui@medmail.com.cn
[1]Department of Orthopedics, Union Hospital, Tongji Medical College, Huazhong University of Science and Technology, 1277, Jiefang Avenue, Wuhan, China
Full list of author information is available at the end of the article

Background

As the number of patients who were afflicted with osteoarthritis (OA) is steadily increasing, the surgical volume of primary total knee arthroplasty (TKA) is increasing as well [1]. However, primary TKA is closely associated with the increase of total blood loss and transfusion rate. Some studies reported that the total blood loss can reach to 1500 mL and 60% of patients need allogeneic blood transfusion [2, 3]. Massive blood transfusion requirements in TKA increased the risks of allergic reaction, immune response, cost, and infection [4, 5]. Various blood-conserving techniques have been used to reduce blood transfusion, including controlled hypertension, tourniquet, and tranexamic acid (TXA) [6–8].

It has been widely accepted that patients undergoing TKA have an increased risk of perioperative bleeding [9]. TXA is an antifibrinolytic drug that inhibits the activation of plasminogen so as to decrease the amount of blood loss [10]. TXA can be applied by the intravenous (IV) or the intraarticular (IA) route. However, to achieve the maximum plasma concentration, TXA takes about 5–15 min for IV administration and 30 min for IA administration. Thus, IV administration is a rapid route for patients to increase the therapeutic concentration of TXA. Then, an increasing number of studies began to pay close attention on the effect of IV TXA on TKA [11, 12]. It was reported that IV TXA decreased perioperative bleeding and caused a reduction in total blood loss by up to 32%. Compared with IV TXA, the IA TXA has some advantages, such as easy administration, providing a maximum concentration of TXA at the bleeding site and inhibiting local activation of fibrinolysis [13]. Recent studies have confirmed that the administration of TXA, which is used directly into the surgical wound, reduced postoperative bleeding from 20 to 25% [13].

Recently, more and more studies tended to use combined TXA instead of using IV or IA TXA alone [14, 15]. It was shown that this method (combined TXA) can effectively reduce the amount of bleeding after TKA. Nevertheless, these studies reported inconsistent results of comparing combined TXA with IV or IA TXA alone on TKA [15–17]. Therefore, this meta-analysis was designed to compare the effectiveness and safety of combined TXA with IV TXA or IA TXA for patients undergoing primary TKA through evaluating the total blood loss, blood volume of drainage, transfusion rate, and thromboembolic complications.

Methods

Search strategy

Articles were searched in the following databases from their inception to September 2016: PubMed, MEDLINE, Embase, the Cochrane Library, SpringerLink, Clinical-Trials.gov, and Ovid. The following search terms were used: tranexamic acid or TXA or topical tranexamic acid or topical TXA or intraarticular tranexamic acid or IA TXA or intravenous tranexamic acid or IV TXA or total knee arthroplasty or TKA or total knee replacement or TKR.

Data selection

To evaluate eligibility for inclusion, two investigators screened the title and abstracts of the articles independently. Any disagreements were resolved by discussion among the authors. A third researcher was the adjudicator when there were debates between two investigators. Articles should meet the following criteria: (1) the studies should be designed as RCTs, (2) the participants should be at least 18 years old, (3) the articles should be comparing the combined TXA with IV or IA TXA, and (4) the articles were restricted to English language.

Data extraction

Two authors independently extracted the following data from each eligible study: study design, type of study population, age, number of participants, and interventions. Discrepancies were resolved by a third investigator.

Quality and risk of bias assessments

The modified Jadad scale was used to assess the methodological quality of each study. A score of ≥4 indicates high quality. The Cochrane Handbook for Reviews of Interventions (RevMan Version 5.3) was used to assess the risk of bias. Two authors subjectively reviewed all articles and assigned a value of "high," "low," or "unclear" based on the following: selection bias, performance bias, detection bias, attrition bias, reporting bias, and other bias. Any disagreements were resolved by discussion and consensus. In order to improve accuracy, a third investigator was consulted when any disagreement emerged.

Statistical analysis

RevMan software was used to analyze the data from included studies. For binary data, risk ratio (RR) and 95% confidence interval (CI) were assessed ($\alpha = 0.05$ for the inspection standards). For continuous data, means and standard deviations were pooled to a weighted mean difference (WMD) and 95% confidence internal (CI) in the meta-analysis. Heterogeneity was tested using the I^2 statistic. Studies with an I^2 statistic of 25 to 50% were considered to have low heterogeneity. Those with an I^2 statistic of 50 to 75% were considered to have moderate heterogeneity. Those with an I^2 statistic >75% were considered to have high heterogeneity. When the I^2 statistic was >50%, sensitivity analyses were performed to identify the potential sources of heterogeneity [18]. Statistical significance was indicated by a P value <0.05.

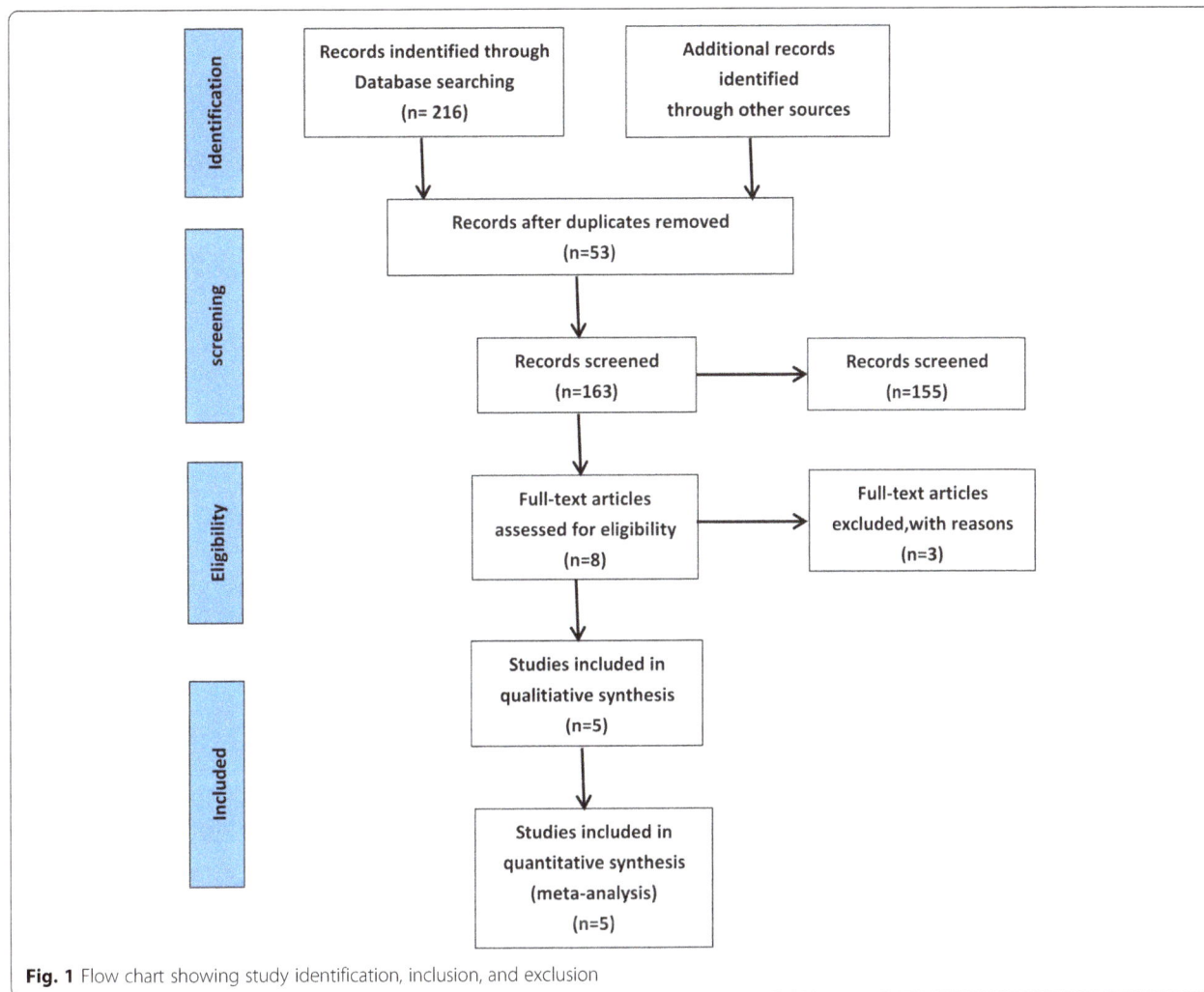

Fig. 1 Flow chart showing study identification, inclusion, and exclusion

Results

Description of studies and demographic characteristics

As shown in Fig. 1, a total of 216 articles were identified as potentially relevant studies. According to the agreed criteria, subsequent scrutiny leads to the exclusion of 208 citations. Full publications were obtained for eight citations: these were assessed and three further citations were excluded, leaving five trials included in the meta-analysis. The demographic characteristics were summarized in Tables 1 and 2. Among them, three trials

[15, 17, 19] compared the effect of the combined TXA group with the IV TXA group, one trial [16] compared the combined TXA group with the IA TXA group, one trial [20] compared the combined TXA group with both the IA TXA group and the IA TXA group, respectively.

Risk of bias in included studies

The assessment of risk of bias was presented in the "Risk of bias assessment of included studies" (Fig. 2). All trials were described as randomized trial design. One trial [15]

Table 1 The characteristics of included studies

Study	Year	Country	Patients (n)			Age (years)			Study design	Diagnosis	Quality score
			C	IA	IV	C	IA	IV			
Huang ZY	2014	China	92		92	65.4 ± 8.7		64.7 ± 9.5	RCT	OA	4
Jain NP	2016	India	59		60	68.2 ± 8.66		70.0 ± 6.56	RCT	OA	5
Lin SY	2015	Taiwan	40	40		70.7 ± 8.2	71.0 ± 7.2		RCT	OA	4
Nielsen CS	2016	Denmark	30		30	65.5 ± 7.8		63.2 ± 8.6	RCT	OA	7
Song EK	2016	Korea	50	50	50	70.8 ± 6.8	69.8 ± 6.8	69.2 ± 6.4	RCT	OA	7

Table 2 Characteristics of the five trials selected showing general intervention information

Study	Combine		IA	IV	Transfusion criteria	Pneumatic tourniquet	Thromboprophylaxis	DVT screening method
	IA	IV						
Huang ZY	1.5 g TXA 50 mL NS after implantation of the components	1.5 g TXA before inflation of the tourniquet		3 g TXA before inflation of the tourniquet	7.0 g/dL < HB < 10 g/dL + symptomatic anemia HB < 7.0 g/dL	Yes	LMWH	Doppler ultrasound
Jain NP	2 g TXA 30 mL NS 5 min before closure of arthrotomy	15 mg/kg TXA 30 min before skin incision 10 mg/kg TXA 3 and 6 h after surgery		15 mg/kg TXA 30 min before skin incision 10 mg/kg TXA 3 and 6 h after surgery	7.0 g/dL < HB < 8.0 g/dL + symptoms HB < 7.0 g/dL	No	Aspirin	Ultrasonographic + clinical symptom
Lin SY	1 g TXA after joint capsule closure	1 g TXA 15 min before skin incision	1 g TXA 20 mL NS after joint capsule closure		HB < 8.0 g/dL HB < 9.0 g/dL +symptoms	Yes	Rivaroxaban	Clinical symptom
Nielsen CS	3 g TXA 100 mL NS after closure of the capsule	1 g TXA preoperative		1 g of TXA	HB < 7.5 g/dL HB < 10 g/dL +symptoms postoperative Hb level was reduced >25% + symptoms	No	Rivaroxaban	NS
Song EK	1.5 g TXA 50 mL NS after wound close	10 mg/kg 20 min before tourniquet application 10 mg/kg 3 h after the second dose	1.5 g TXA 50 mL NS after wound closure	10 mg/kg 20 min before tourniquet application 10 mg/kg 15 min before deflation of the tourniquet 10 mg/kg 3 h after the second dose	HB < 8 g/dL	Yes	LMWH	Clinical symptom + Doppler ultrasonography and CT angiography

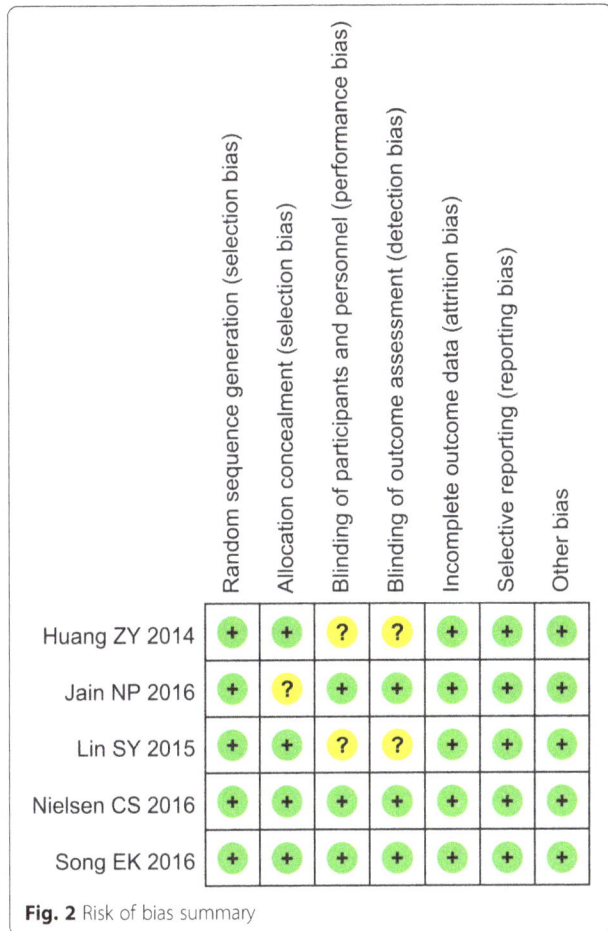

Fig. 2 Risk of bias summary

did not show detailed information of random sequence generation, and one trial [19] did not describe the methods of allocation concealment. Blinding of participants and personal (performance bias) were considered to be unclear in two trials [15, 16].

Sensitivity and heterogeneity analysis

There was significant heterogeneity for the impact of IV TXA application on total blood loss. The leave-one-out analysis showed that the key contributor to this high heterogeneity was one study conducted by Jain et al. [19]. After excluding it, heterogeneity was reduced to $I^2 = 73\%$ for total blood loss. But significance of the pooled changes was not altered, which demonstrated that the results were robust.

Total blood loss

All of the studies provided the data of total blood loss. Three studies [15, 17, 19] reported data of the combined group compared with the IV group, one study [16] reported data of the combined group compared with the IA group, and one study [20] reported data of the combined group compared with both the IV group and the IA group respectively. There was significant difference in terms of reducing total blood loss when comparing the combined group with the IV group (chi^2 = 18.44, I^2 = 84%, P < 0.05) or the IA group (chi^2 = 1.35, I^2 = 26%, P < 0.05) (Fig. 3).

Blood volume of drainage

Three studies [15, 16, 20] provided data on blood volume of drainage. The result of the blood volume of drainage illustrated significant difference in the combined group when compared with the IV group (MD –38.19, 95% CI –63.31 to –13.08, P < 0.05, I^2 = 0%). There was significant difference in blood volume of drainage between the combined group and the IA group (MD –42.34, 95% CI –62.39 to –22.30, P < 0.05); however, this result should be interpreted with caution due to the presence of statistical heterogeneity (chi^2 = 7.17, I^2 = 86%) (Fig. 4).

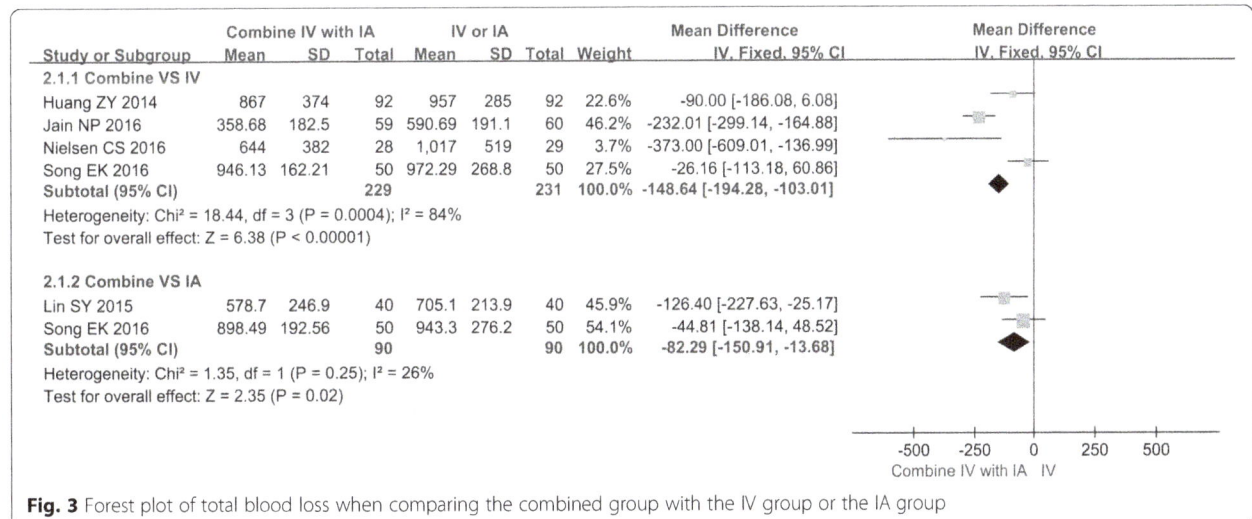

Fig. 3 Forest plot of total blood loss when comparing the combined group with the IV group or the IA group

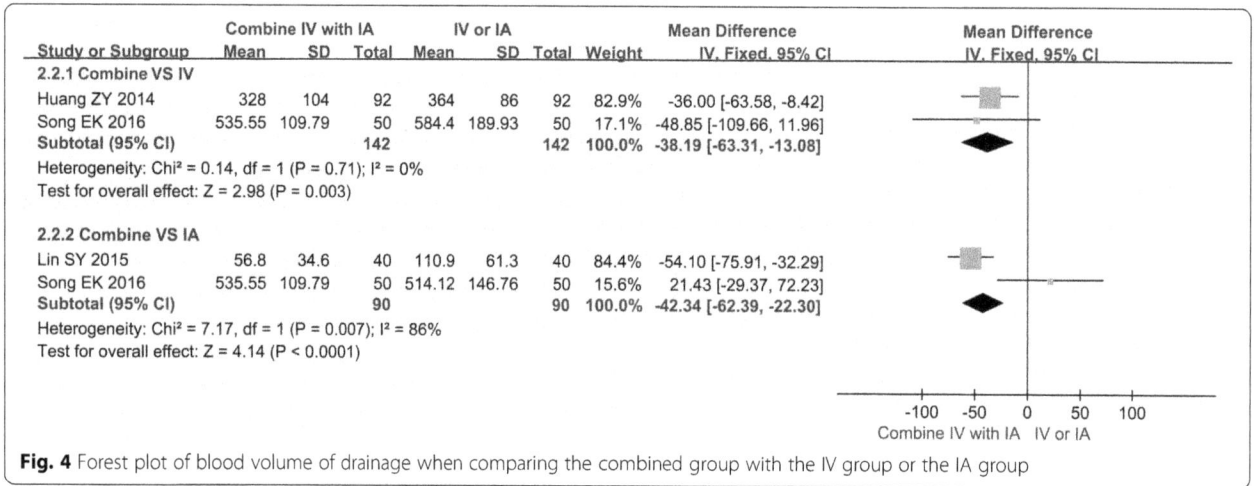

Fig. 4 Forest plot of blood volume of drainage when comparing the combined group with the IV group or the IA group

Transfusion rate

The data of transfusion rate was provided from all of the studies. There was no significant difference in transfusion rate when comparing the combined group with the IV or the IA group (chi^2 = 0.74, I^2 = 0%, $P > 0.05$; chi^2 = 0, I^2 = 0%, $P > 0.05$) (Fig. 5).

Thromboembolic complications

All of the studies provided data of thromboembolic complications. There was no significant difference in thromboembolic complications when comparing the combined group with the IV or the IA group. There was only one study that reported one case of DVT in the IV group [15]. Song [20] reported that there were three patients from the IV group and two patients from the combined group and one patient from the IA group had

clinical suspicion of DVT based on calf swelling and tenderness. One case of clinical suspicion of DVT in the IV group was reported by Jain et al. [19] (Fig. 6).

Discussion

TXA is an antifibrinolytic agent which has been widely used today. Several studies have reported that IV administration of TXA can effectively reduce total blood on TKA [21]. Compared with IV TXA, the IA administration of TXA has the advantage of reaching to a maximum concentration of TXA at the bleeding site, and it is associated with low systemic absorption [22]. Considering the advantages of both IV TXA and IA TXA, it is logical to suggest that combined use of IV TXA and IA TXA is a more efficient method of reducing total blood loss. Karaaslan et al. [23] reported that combined use of

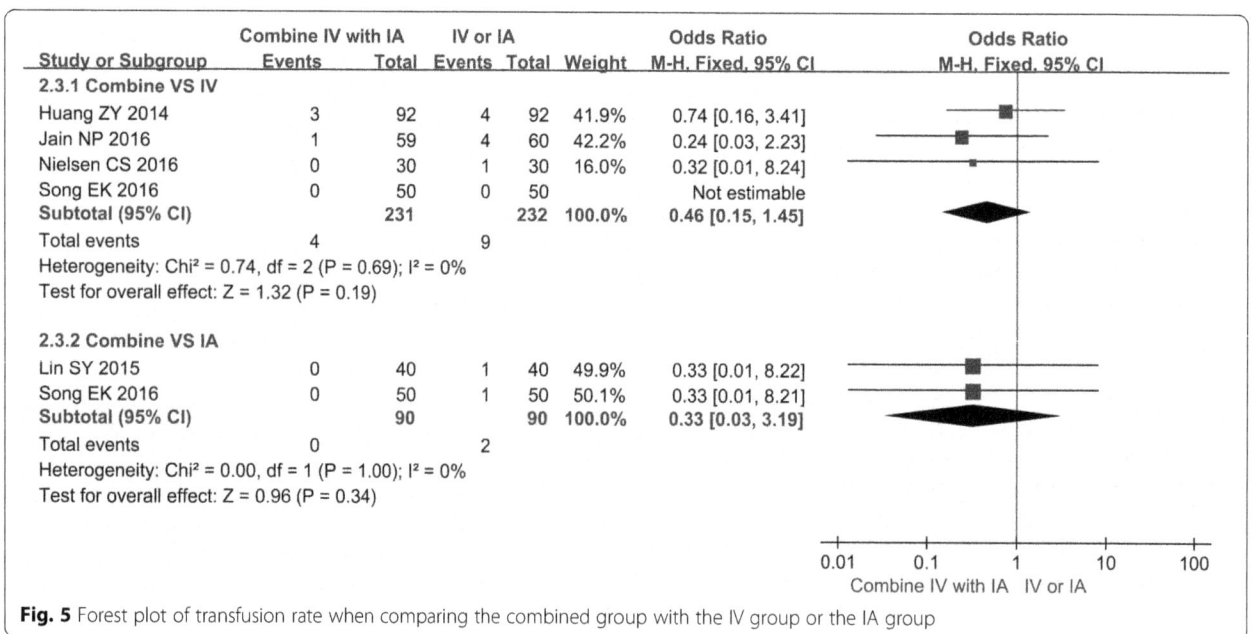

Fig. 5 Forest plot of transfusion rate when comparing the combined group with the IV group or the IA group

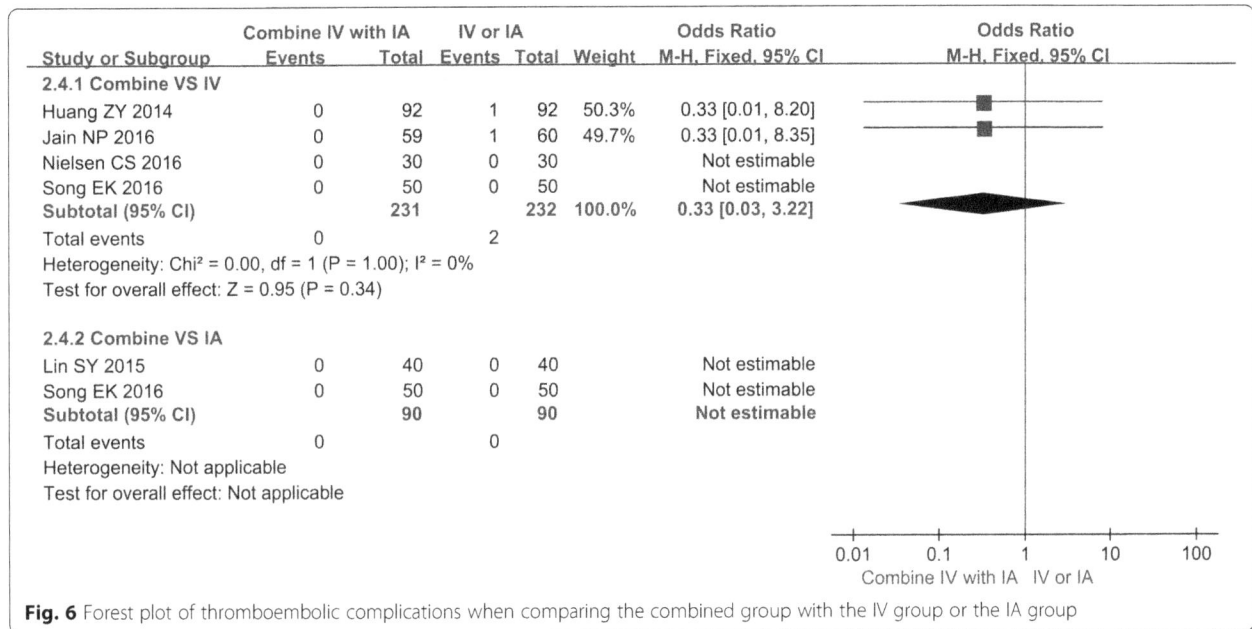

Study or Subgroup	Combine IV with IA Events	Total	IV or IA Events	Total	Weight	Odds Ratio M-H, Fixed, 95% CI	Odds Ratio M-H, Fixed, 95% CI
2.4.1 Combine VS IV							
Huang ZY 2014	0	92	1	92	50.3%	0.33 [0.01, 8.20]	
Jain NP 2016	0	59	1	60	49.7%	0.33 [0.01, 8.35]	
Nielsen CS 2016	0	30	0	30		Not estimable	
Song EK 2016	0	50	0	50		Not estimable	
Subtotal (95% CI)		231		232	100.0%	0.33 [0.03, 3.22]	
Total events	0		2				
Heterogeneity: Chi² = 0.00, df = 1 (P = 1.00); I² = 0%							
Test for overall effect: Z = 0.95 (P = 0.34)							
2.4.2 Combine VS IA							
Lin SY 2015	0	40	0	40		Not estimable	
Song EK 2016	0	50	0	50		Not estimable	
Subtotal (95% CI)		90		90		**Not estimable**	
Total events	0		0				
Heterogeneity: Not applicable							
Test for overall effect: Not applicable							

Fig. 6 Forest plot of thromboembolic complications when comparing the combined group with the IV group or the IA group

TXA in patients undergoing TKA can reduce blood loss with negligible side effects. Other studies [15, 16] that compared combined TXA with IV or IA TXA also reported that combined TXA was more effective than IV or IA TXA alone for patients undergoing TKA. In this meta-analysis, when compared with the IV group, we found that the combined group had reduced total blood loss by a mean of −148.64 mL (CI −194.28 to −103.01), and when compared with the IA group, it reduced total blood loss by a mean of −82.29 mL (CI −150.91 to −13.68). These results confirmed that combined TXA was more efficient for patients undergoing TKA in terms of reducing total blood loss.

Previous studies and several meta-analysis of IV TXA showed that administration of TXA intravenously reduced blood volume of drainage by up to 50% [12, 24]. Since IA administration of TXA can inhibit local activation of fibrinolysis and reduce time to vascular occlusion [25], it also has the advantage of limiting local blood loss [26]. Then, combined use of TXA has the advantages of both IV TXA and IA TXA in terms of reducing blood volume of drainage. Our meta-analysis also suggested that TXA administration that used the combination method resulted in a lower blood volume of drainage than TXA administration that used IV or IA alone (−38.19 and −42.34 mL, respectively, P < 0.05). Interestingly, there was a slightly higher transfusion rate in the combined group when compared with the IV or the IA group (0.46, 0.33, respectively), even though there was no significant difference (P > 0.05). These results may be attributed to the fact that the transfusion criteria were inconsistent among these studies. In addition, a limited number of RCTs and patients may also lead to these results.

It is well known that patients undergoing TKA will take risks of DVT or PE [27, 28]. TXA has been widely used in TKA, while the risk of thromboembolic events are increasingly concerned [29]. Our meta-analysis had shown that there was no significant difference in thromboembolic complications when comparing the combined group with the IV or the IA group. This result was consistent with those studies that recommend the use of combined TXA on TXA [15, 19]. One highly observable time of DVT or PE was the postoperative of TKA within 30 days [30], and chemoprophylaxis [31, 32] has been recommended to those patients. All of our studies observed the DVT or PE at least 30 days, and chemical prophylaxis was given to all patients or to those high-risk patients. Only one case of DVT was detected in the IV group 3 days after operation [15]. It should be noted that pneumatic tourniquet application could increase the risk of DVT or PE [33]. All patients reported by Huang et al. [15] used pneumatic tourniquet, and one case of DVT was detected in the IV group. In addition, Song [20] reported that three patients from the IV group, two from the combined group, and one patient from the IA group had clinical suspicion of DVT based on calf swelling and tenderness. Then, which one was the main reason for increased DVT or PE, TXA, or pneumatic tourniquet? The reason should be further confirmed. In addition, some included studies [19, 20] had evaluated symptomatic patients only, which may have caused a lower incidence of thromboembolic complications and missed the real patients who have DVT or PE. Considering the above factors, the results need to be further confirmed.

There was significant heterogeneity in the administration of IV TXA on total blood loss. The leave-one-out analysis showed that the key contributor to this high heterogeneity was one study conducted by Jain et al. [19]. After excluding this study, heterogeneity was reduced to $I^2 = 73\%$ for total blood loss. By comparing these four studies that compared the combined group with the IV group, we found that the total blood loss in this study was calculated by hemoglobin balance method, whereas the total blood loss in other studies was calculated by gross formula [34]. Therefore, we infer that the calculation formula of total blood loss might be partly responsible for the heterogeneity.

There are several limitations in this meta-analysis. Firstly, the present meta-analysis focused only on papers published in English; the ones that were reported in other languages may increase heterogeneity and change the present results. Secondly, because four studies included subjects coming from Asia and one from Europe, the results cannot be extended to populations elsewhere. Besides, the dose and the timing of administrate IV TXA or IA TXA in the combined group were inconsistent among those studies. Further rigorously designed RCTs with larger sample sizes are needed to confirm the efficacy of combined TXA in primary TKA.

Conclusions

Present meta-analysis results demonstrated that combined use of TXA in TKA significantly reduce the total blood loss and blood volume of drainage without increasing the adverse effect of DVT or PE. Further studies are needed to investigate an appropriate dose and times of administering IV TXA combined with IA TXA in patients undergoing TKA.

Abbreviations

IA: Intraarticular; IV: Intravenous; OA: Osteoarthritis; TKA: Total knee arthroplasty; TXA: Tranexamic acid

Acknowledgements

Thanks are due to Wu Zhou for assistance with the analysis of the data and Xi Chen for valuable discussion.

Funding

No external funding was received for the initiation or completion of this study.

Authors' contributions

BM and HL conceptualized the study. YL and QW helped in the data curation. KZ and HL carried out the formal analysis. JL and QW performed the investigation. BM and YL provided the methodology. BM and JL helped in the project administration. YL and KZ are responsible for the software. KZ supervised the study. HL and QW participated in the validation. GL wrote the original draft. BM and GL wrote, reviewed, and edited the paper. All authors read and approved the final manuscript.

Competing interests

The authors declare that they have no competing interests.

Author details

^{1}Department of Orthopedics, Union Hospital, Tongji Medical College, Huazhong University of Science and Technology, 1277, Jiefang Avenue, Wuhan, China. ^{2}Department of Rheumatology, Tangdu Hospital, The Fourth Military Medical University, 1, Xinsi Avenue, Xi'an, China.

References

1. Visuri T, Makela K, Pulkkinen P, Artama M, Pukkala E. Long-term mortality and causes of death among patients with a total knee prosthesis in primary osteoarthritis. Knee. 2016;23:162–6. doi:10.1016/j.knee.2015.09.002.
2. Kim DH, Lee GC, Lee SH, Pak CH, Park SH, Jung S. Comparison of blood loss between neutral drainage with tranexamic acid and negative pressure drainage without tranexamic acid following primary total knee arthroplasty. Knee Surg Relat Res. 2016;28:194–200. doi:10.5792/ksrr.2016.28.3.194.
3. Seol YJ, Seon JK, Lee SH, et al. Effect of tranexamic acid on blood loss and blood transfusion reduction after total knee arthroplasty. Knee Surg Relat Res. 2016;28:188–93. doi:10.5792/ksrr.2016.28.3.188.
4. Liu JJ, Mullane P, Kates M, et al. Infectious complications in transfused patients after radical cystectomy. Can J Urol. 2016;23:8342–7.
5. Wang Q, Du T, Lu C. Perioperative blood transfusion and the clinical outcomes of patients undergoing cholangiocarcinoma surgery: a systematic review and meta-analysis. Eur J Gastroenterol Hepatol. 2016. doi:10.1097/MEG.0000000000000706.
6. Liu D, Dan M, Martinez MS, Beller E. Blood management strategies in total knee arthroplasty. Knee Surg Relat Res. 2016;28:179–87. doi:10.5792/ksrr.2016.28.3.179.
7. Samujh C, Falls TD, Wessel R, et al. Decreased blood transfusion following revision total knee arthroplasty using tranexamic acid. J Arthroplasty. 2014; 29:182–5. doi:10.1016/j.arth.2014.03.047.
8. Shimizu M, Kubota R, Nasu M, et al. [The influence of tourniquet during total knee arthroplasty on perioperative blood loss and postoperative complications]. Masui. 2016;65:131–5.
9. Oremus K. Tranexamic acid for the reduction of blood loss in total knee arthroplasty. Ann Transl Med. 2015;3:S40. doi:10.3978/j.issn.2305-5839.2015.03.35.
10. Rozen L, Faraoni D, Sanchez TC, et al. Effective tranexamic acid concentration for 95% inhibition of tissue-type plasminogen activator induced hyperfibrinolysis in children with congenital heart disease: a prospective, controlled, in-vitro study. Eur J Anaesthesiol. 2015;32:844–50. doi:10.1097/EJA.0000000000000316.
11. Charoencholvanich K, Siriwattanasakul P. Tranexamic acid reduces blood loss and blood transfusion after TKA: a prospective randomized controlled trial. Clin Orthop Relat Res. 2011;469:2874–80. doi:10.1007/s11999-011-1874-2.
12. Tan J, Chen H, Liu Q, Chen C, Huang W. A meta-analysis of the effectiveness and safety of using tranexamic acid in primary unilateral total knee arthroplasty. J Surg Res. 2013;184:880–7. doi:10.1016/j.jss.2013.03.099.
13. Wong J, Abrishami A, El BH, et al. Topical application of tranexamic acid reduces postoperative blood loss in total knee arthroplasty: a randomized, controlled trial. J Bone Joint Surg Am. 2010;92:2503–13. doi:10.2106/JBJS.I.01518.
14. Buntting C, Sorial R, Coffey S, et al. Combination intravenous and intra-articular tranexamic acid compared with intravenous only administration and no therapy in total knee arthroplasty: a case series study. Reconstructive Review. 2016;6:13–20. doi:10.15438/rr.6.2.138.
15. Huang Z, Ma J, Shen B, Pei F. Combination of intravenous and topical application of tranexamic acid in primary total knee arthroplasty: a prospective randomized controlled trial. J Arthroplasty. 2014;29:2342–6. doi:10.1016/j.arth.2014.05.026.
16. Lin SY, Chen CH, Fu YC, Huang PJ, Chang JK, Huang HT. The efficacy of combined use of intraarticular and intravenous tranexamic acid on reducing blood loss and transfusion rate in total knee arthroplasty. J Arthroplasty. 2015;30:776–80. doi:10.1016/j.arth.2014.12.001.
17. Nielsen CS, Jans O, Orsnes T, Foss NB, Troelsen A, Husted H. Combined intra-articular and intravenous tranexamic acid reduces blood loss in total knee arthroplasty: a randomized, double-blind, placebo-controlled trial. J Bone Joint Surg Am. 2016;98:835–41. doi:10.2106/JBJS.15.00810.
18. Higgins JP, Thompson SG, Deeks JJ, Altman DG. Measuring inconsistency in meta-analyses. BMJ. 2003;327:557–60. doi:10.1136/bmj.327.7414.557.
19. Jain NP, Nisthane PP, Shah NA. Combined administration of systemic and topical tranexamic acid for total knee arthroplasty: can it be a better regimen and yet safe? A randomized controlled trial. J Arthroplasty. 2016;31: 542–7. doi:10.1016/j.arth.2015.09.029.

20. Song EK, Seon JK, Prakash J, et al. Combined administration of iv and topical tranexamic acid is not superior to either individually in primary navigated TKA. J Arthoplasty. 2016. doi:10.1016/j.arth.2016.06.052.

21. Akgul T, Buget M, Salduz A, et al. Efficacy of preoperative administration of single high dose intravenous tranexamic acid in reducing blood loss in total knee arthroplasty: a prospective clinical study. Acta Orthop Traumatol Turc. 2016. doi:10.1016/j.aott.2016.06.007.

22. Goyal N, Chen DB, Harris IA, Rowden NJ, Kirsh G, MacDessi SJ. Intravenous vs intra-articular tranexamic acid in total knee arthroplasty: a randomized, double-blind trial. J Arthroplasty. 2016. doi:10.1016/j.arth.2016.07.004.

23. Karaaslan F, Karaoglu S, Mermerkaya MU, Baktir A. Reducing blood loss in simultaneous bilateral total knee arthroplasty: combined intravenous-intra-articular tranexamic acid administration. A prospective randomized controlled trial. Knee. 2015;22:131–5. doi:10.1016/j.knee.2014.12.002.

24. Good L, Peterson E, Lisander B. Tranexamic acid decreases external blood loss but not hidden blood loss in total knee replacement. Br J Anaesth. 2003;90:596–9.

25. Sperzel M, Huetter J. Evaluation of aprotinin and tranexamic acid in different in vitro and in vivo models of fibrinolysis, coagulation and thrombus formation. J Thromb Haemost. 2007;5:2113–8. doi:10.1111/j.1538-7836.2007.02717.x.

26. Gomez-Barrena E, Ortega-Andreu M, Padilla-Eguiluz NG, Perez-Chrzanowska H, Figueredo-Zalve R. Topical intra-articular compared with intravenous tranexamic acid to reduce blood loss in primary total knee replacement: a double-blind, randomized, controlled, noninferiority clinical trial. J Bone Joint Surg Am. 2014;96:1937–44. doi:10.2106/JBJS.N.00060.

27. Chotanaphuti T, Ongnamthip P, Silpipat S, Foojareonyos T, Roschan S, Reumthantong A. The prevalence of thrombophilia and venous thromboembolism in total knee arthroplasty. J Med Assoc Thai. 2007;90:1342–7.

28. Levy YD, Hardwick ME, Copp SN, Rosen AS, Colwell CJ. Thrombosis incidence in unilateral vs. simultaneous bilateral total knee arthroplasty with compression device prophylaxis. J Arthroplasty. 2013;28:474–8. doi:10.1016/j.arth.2012.08.002.

29. Izumi M, Migita K, Nakamura M, et al. Risk of venous thromboembolism after total knee arthroplasty in patients with rheumatoid arthritis. J Rheumatol. 2015;42:928–34. doi:10.3899/jrheum.140768.

30. Mantilla CB, Horlocker TT, Schroeder DR, Berry DJ, Brown DL. Risk factors for clinically relevant pulmonary embolism and deep venous thrombosis in patients undergoing primary hip or knee arthroplasty. Anesthesiology. 2003;99:552–60. 5A.

31. Odeh K, Doran J, Yu S, Bolz N, Bosco J, Iorio R. Risk-stratified venous thromboembolism prophylaxis after total joint arthroplasty: aspirin and sequential pneumatic compression devices vs aggressive chemoprophylaxis. J Arthroplasty. 2016;31:78–82. doi:10.1016/j.arth.2016.01.065.

32. Mostafavi TR, Rasouli MR, Maltenfort MG, Parvizi J. Cost-effective prophylaxis against venous thromboembolism after total joint arthroplasty: warfarin versus aspirin. J Arthroplasty. 2015;30:159–64. doi:10.1016/j.arth.2014.08.018.

33. Mori N, Kimura S, Onodera T, Iwasaki N, Nakagawa I, Masuda T. Use of a pneumatic tourniquet in total knee arthroplasty increases the risk of distal deep vein thrombosis: a prospective, randomized study. Knee. 2016;23:887–9. doi:10.1016/j.knee.2016.02.007.

34. Kvederas G, Porvaneckas N, Andrijauskas A, et al. A randomized double-blind clinical trial of tourniquet application strategies for total knee arthroplasty. Knee Surg Sports Traumatol Arthrosc. 2013;21:2790–9. doi:10.1007/s00167-012-2221-1.

2

Metal-on-metal hip resurfacing in patients younger than 50 years: a retrospective analysis

1285 cases, 12-year survivorship

Melissa D. Gaillard* and Thomas P. Gross

Abstract

Background: The Nordic registry reports patients under 50 years old with total hip replacements realize only 83% 10-year implant survivorship. These results do not meet the 95% 10-year survivorship guideline posed by the UK's National Institute for Health and Care Excellence (NICE) in 2014.

Methods: The purpose of this study is threefold: First, we evaluate if metal-on-metal hip resurfacing arthroplasty meets these high standards in younger patients. Next, we compare outcomes between age groups to determine if younger patients are at higher risk for revision or complication. Lastly, we assess how outcomes between sexes changed over time. From January 2001 to August 2013, a single surgeon performed 1285 metal-on-metal hip resurfacings in patients younger than 50 years old. We compared these to an older cohort matched by sex and BMI.

Results: Kaplan-Meier implant survivorship was 96.5% at 10 years and 96.3% at 12 years; this did not differ from implant survivorship for older patients. Implant survivorship at 12 years was 98 and 93% for younger men and women, respectively; survivorship for women improved from 93 to 97% by using exclusively Biomet implants. There were four (0.3%) adverse wear-related failures, with no instances of wear or problematic ion levels since 2009. Activity scores improved from 5.4 ± 2.3 preoperatively to 7.6 ± 1.9 postoperatively ($p < 0.0001$), with 43% of patients reporting a UCLA activity score of 9 or 10.

Conclusions: Hip resurfacing exceeds the stricter 2014 NICE survivorship criteria independently in men and women even when performed on patients under 50 years old.

Keywords: Hip resurfacing, Metal-on-metal, Younger patients, Hip arthroplasty

Background

Total hip arthroplasty (THA) is durable in elderly populations [1] but does not meet functional demands or durability requirements for younger patients [2–5]. In 2014, the UK's National Institute for Health and Care Excellence (NICE) raised their benchmark criteria for hip implants from 90 to 95% 10-year survivorship. The Orthopaedic Data Evaluation Panel listed only 32 THA femoral stems which met this new, stricter benchmark [6], with potentially far fewer meeting NICE criteria in younger patients.

Sir John Charnley warned against performing THA in younger patients, citing that the procedure was not robust enough [7]; as an increasing number of younger patients demanded better, longer-lasting solutions [8], hip resurfacing arthroplasty (HRA) emerged as an alternative, bone-preserving option. It is well known THA implants display markedly lower survivorship in patients younger than 50 years old [2–4]. In the Scandinavian registry, 10-year implant survivorship for these patients was only 83% [5]. Considering underestimation of failure in the registry, 10-year survivorship could be lower. In a literature review by De Kam on THA in patients under 50 [9], only 15 of 37 papers met the outdated NICE

* Correspondence: dani.gaillard@midlandsortho.com
Midlands Orthopaedics & Neurosurgery, 1910 Blanding Street, Columbia, SC 29201, USA

criteria, and of these, only two studies met the new standard.

Experts attribute reduced implant survivorship in younger patients to more complex procedures and naturally higher activity levels [3, 10, 11]. The most common diseases of the younger hip include osteonecrosis, dysplasia, Legg-Perthes disease, and post-traumatic arthritis, all of which carry a worse prognosis [12]. Aside from having higher expectations, younger patients often require eventual revision; in an analysis of over 109 studies on patients under 50, only 37 had a mean survivorship greater than 10 years [9]. These combined risks make THA challenging in patients under 50.

McMinn et al. [13] and Amstutz [14] introduced metal-on-metal (MOM) HRA as a bone-preserving, temporizing measure to delay disease progression in younger patients, but HRA far surpassed these modest, early goals. Recent advancements in MOM bearing design have improved durability and lowered wear rate, with many studies reporting 93% implant survivorship for patients in their 40s [15–17]. Furthermore, several studies suggest that gait characteristics are more nearly normal in those receiving HRA versus THA [18, 19], appealing especially to younger patients.

HRA, compared to THA, allows for a more natural reconstruction of the hip and endows biomechanics more closely resembling a normal, healthy joint. The naturally stable bearing size and femoral offsets are preserved, leading to superior hip stability [20, 21]. The lack of a large stem has resolved issues with thigh pain [10, 22]. Gait lab studies demonstrate THA patients do not fully load the operative leg and take smaller strides than HRA patients [18]. These combined advantages of HRA allow more nearly normal function in younger patients who often still desire to participate in high range-of-motion (ROM) activities and impact sports. The available scientific studies amply confirm that HRA is a more functional arthroplasty than THA [23–25].

Despite many HRA studies with excellent outcomes, registry results have been mixed. While the Australian registry [26] confirms 10-year HRA implant survivorship surpasses that of THA in men under 60, the reverse is true for women and older men. In the UK's National Joint Registry, Smith et al. demonstrated HRA only outlives THA in men with larger implant sizes [27], but the study included inexperienced surgeons performing an average of only 2.6 HRA cases a year. Publications from inexperienced surgeons with weak results, high failure rates from poorly designed implants, and excessive publicity on adverse wear-related failures (AWRF) from a small number of outlier centers [28] have called into question the value of HRA. However, experienced surgeons, including the present senior author (TPG), have routinely surpassed HRA and THA outcomes in

arthroplasty registers [5, 27, 29]. Due to the mixed available results, the scarcity of published outcomes on younger patients, and the poor viability of THA in younger patients, we aim to establish a successful example for HRA implant survivorship in patients under 50 years old.

In 2001, the senior author began performing HRA on the basis that bone preservation in younger patients is paramount. We present the results of 1285 HRA procedures performed on patients under 50 years old and compare these data with a demographically similar, older cohort to evaluate several hypotheses:

1. MOM HRA meets the 2014 NICE criteria in our patients under 50 years old.
2. There is no difference in HRA implant survivorship due to age.
3. Outcome disparity between sexes of our younger cohort has improved.

Methods
Patients and follow-up
We used OrthoVault (Midlands Orthopaedics & Neurosurgery, Columbia, SC), our database of over 4200 HRA procedures, to retrospectively identify 1285 consecutive cases from January 2001 to August 2013 in 1062 patients under 50 years old at the time of surgery as our group 1 study cohort. Ages for group 1 ranged from 11 to 49 years. From the same date range, we identified 1984 HRA devices in 1614 patients as the older control group (group 2); ages among the group 2 cohort ranged from 50 to 78 years. These patients received surgery at the age of 50 years or older. All patients had a minimum of 2 years' follow-up. Between January 2001 and January 2005, the primary surgeon performed 372 HRA procedures in 329 patients using the hybrid Corin Cormet 2000 resurfacing system. Subsequently, from January 2005 to March 2007, the primary surgeon performed 739 HRA procedures in 652 patients using the hybrid Biomet ReCap™-Magnum™ implant system. Lastly, we shifted to our current uncemented method, and from March 2007 to August 2013, 1803 patients received 2158 fully porous-coated Biomet ReCap™-Magnum™ resurfacings.

Table 1 presents demographic information for both cohorts. The average age at the time of surgery for group 1 was 44 ± 6 years and for group 2 was 57 ± 4 years. Bone density was greater for younger patients (see "Statistical methods"). Sex distribution and BMI were not statistically different between the two groups. Group 1 presented a higher percentage of patients with more complex diagnoses, which are those that typically result in worse outcomes.

This study is a level II, retrospective review of prospectively collected data. Approval for this study and manuscript was granted by the Institutional Review Board of Providence Health in Columbia, SC.

Table 1 Group demographics for patients under and over 50 years old

	Group 1, <50 (N = 1285)	Group 2, ≥50 (N = 1984)	p value
Sex (no. of hips)			
Male	951 (74%)	1426 (72%)	0.1802
Female	334 (26%)	558 (28%)	
Deceased#	10 (0.8%)	29 (1.5%)	0.0784
F/U mean years	3.4 ± 2.98	2.8 ± 2.59	*<0.0001**
Lost to F/U	17 (1.3%)	23 (1.2%)	0.6745
Case date range	1/2001–8/2013		–
Age (years)	44 ± 6.02	57 ± 4.23	*<0.0001**
BMI	28 ± 4.92	28 ± 4.56	0.0750
T-score	0.26 ± 1.36	−0.14 ± 1.18	*<0.0001**
Uncemented fixation (no. of hips)	776 (60%)	1380 (70%)	*<0.0001**
10-year survivorship (no. of hips)	1234 (96%)	1924 (97%)	0.1443
Diagnosis (no. of hips)			
Dysplasia	149 (12%)	214 (11%)	0.4715
Osteoarthritis (OA)	866 (67%)	1589 (80%)	*<0.0001**
Osteonecrosis (ON)	107 (8.3%)	63 (3.2%)	*<0.0001**
Rheumatoid arthritis (RA)	9 (0.7%)	2 (0.1%)	*0.0039**
Post-trauma	40 (3.1%)	20 (1.0%)	*<0.0001**
Legg-Calve-Perthes disease (LCP)	32 (2.5%)	7 (0.4%)	*<0.0001**
Slipped capital femoral epiphysis (SCFE)	12 (0.9%)	9 (0.5%)	0.0930
Other	22 (1.7%)	21 (1.1%)	0.1096
Implants (no. of hips)			
Corin Cormet 2000	187 (14%)	185 (9.3%)	*<0.0001**
Biomet ReCap™-Magnum™ hybrid	330 (26%)	409 (21%)	*0.0007**
Biomet ReCap™-Magnum™ uncemented	768 (60%)	1390 (70%)	*<0.0001**
ASA score	1.6 ± 0.57	1.7 ± 0.58	*<0.0001**
Femoral component <48 mm (no. of hips)	199/973 (20%)	334/1641 (20%)	0.9522
Femoral component size	50.0 ± 3.92	50.2 ± 3.53	0.1793

Statistically significant p values are italicized and denoted by an asterisk (*)
#indicates deaths unrelated to the patients' hip arthroplasties

Implant systems

The primary surgeon (TPG) performed HRAs using three unique implant systems in a consecutive fashion. We began using the hybrid Corin Cormet 2000 (Corin, Cirencester, UK) implant system in March 2001 as part of a multicenter US Food and Drug Administration clinical trial. This device was fully approved in 2007 but is no longer sold. We partnered with Biomet (now Zimmer Biomet) to develop the hybrid ReCap™-Magnum™ (Biomet, Warsaw, IN), which we began using in 2005. We further collaborated with Biomet to develop the fully porous-coated ReCap™-Magnum™, which became available in March 2007; we have used this exclusively for all resurfacing cases after January 2008. In the USA, employing the ReCap™-Magnum™ system for HRA is considered off-label use. We published

comprehensive metallurgy and design details for all implant systems previously [30, 31].

Procedure

The primary surgeon (TPG) performed all HRA operations through the posterior approach as described previously [32]. We have taken normalized to standing intraoperative radiographs since 2009 to confirm the acetabular component position meets our relative acetabular inclination limit (RAIL) guideline [33]. Table 2 presents a summary of surgical information.

Postoperative protocol

Patients progress to weight-bearing as tolerated unless they present notably low preoperative bone density. Most patients use crutches for 2 weeks and a cane for

Table 2 Surgical summary for two groups

Variable	Group 1	Group 2	p value
Length of incision (in.)	4.4 ± 1.44	4.3 ± 0.77	0.0100*
Operation time (min)	106 ± 19.4	102 ± 28.8	<0.0001*
Estimated blood loss (mL)	208 ± 171	183 ± 137	<0.0001*
Hospital stay (day)	2.1 ± 1.11	2.1 ± 5.17	1.0000
Transfusion received (no. of cases)	0 (0.0%)	2 (0.1%)	0.2543
Transfusion volume (cm³)	–	375 ± 0	–
Outpatient (no. of cases)	10 (0.8%)	21 (1.1%)	0.4179

Statistically significant p values are italicized and denoted by an asterisk (*)

2 weeks thereafter. We require no formal physical therapy following hospital discharge. Patients may progress to moderate aerobic exercise at 6 weeks and unlimited activity at 6 months after surgery. The establishment of a multimodal pain management protocol and comprehensive blood management protocol has accelerated patient recovery and eliminated the need for transfusion, allowing many patients to receive HRA as an outpatient procedure since 2012.

Metal ion testing

The OrthoVault database facilitates collection of metal ion test results, which we routinely requested from all patients at 2 years postoperatively since 2007; we also requested metal ion results from all patients operated on prior to this time at least once. Metal ion levels are useful indicators of potential failure from excessive implant wear [34] even before the onset of symptoms. We converted serum and plasma test results for cobalt (Co) and chromium (Cr) to whole blood ion level values using Smolders' method [35, 36] and subsequently used whole blood values for all comparisons. Based on previous research [33–35], we define five ion level categories (Table 3): normal, optimal, acceptable, problematic, and potentially toxic.

Clinical and radiographic analysis

We request patients return for an office visit or to complete a remote follow-up package at 6 weeks, 1 and 2 years, and every other year thereafter. Each follow-up comprises a clinical questionnaire, radiographic analysis, and a physical examination testing ROM and strength. Physical examinations are no longer necessary after the 1-year postoperative visit for patients completing remote follow-up. OrthoVault supported the collection of demographic, clinical, and radiographic data for all patients.

We use clinical questionnaires to collect information for calculating the following scores: Harris hip score (HHS) [37], University of California, Los Angeles (UCLA) activity score [38], and visual analog scale (VAS) pain scores [39]. We use the HHS for quantitative measurement of overall clinical outcome, based on function and ROM. UCLA activity scores measure patient activity level on a scale of 1 to 10, for which 10 represents regular participation in impact sports. VAS pain scores provide a simple indication of overall pain on normal and worst days based on a scale of 0, or no pain, to 10, or maximum, debilitating pain.

Radiographs are obtained at every follow-up; these x-rays are analyzed for component position, shifting, and radiolucencies. We determine the acetabular inclination angle (AIA) by measuring the angle formed between a horizontal reference line running across the face of the inferior pubic rami and a measurement line running across the face of the acetabular component on the patient's standing anterior-posterior x-ray (Fig. 1). All measurements were performed using OrthoVault and InteleViewer® (InteleRAD, Chicago, IL, USA).

Statistical methods

Statistical analyses were performed using Microsoft® Excel (Microsoft, Redmond, WA, USA) and SAS® (SAS Institute Incorporated, Cary, NC, USA). All tests used a significance level of $\alpha = 0.05$. Paired, two-tailed Student's t tests were used to find significant differences between numeric results. Two-sample proportion Z-tests were performed to compare percentages. Kaplan-Meier (KM) implant survivorship curves were plotted using XLSTAT® (Addinsoft, New York, NY, USA), and log-rank and Wilcoxon tests were performed to determine significant difference in implant survivorship between groups.

Table 3 Whole blood metal ion reference table

	Normal[a]	Optimal[b]	Acceptable[c]	Problematic[c]	Potentially toxic[b]
Unilateral					
Co (µg/L)	<1.5	<4.0	4–10	10–20	>20
Cr (µg/L)	<1.5	<4.6	4.6–10	10–20	>20
Bilateral					
Co (µg/L)	<1.5	<5.0	5–10	10–20	>20
Cr (µg/L)	<1.5	<7.4	7.4–10	10–20	>20

[a]Laboratory normal for patients without metal bearings
[b]According to DeSmet/Van der Straeten [34, 35]
[c]According to our previous analysis

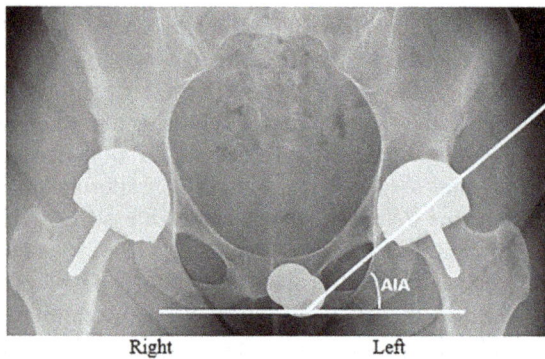

Fig. 1 Pelvic radiograph acetabular inclination angle measurement lines. Anterior-posterior pelvis radiograph taken 5 years after a hybrid metal-on-metal Corin hip resurfacing on the right hip and 2 years after a hybrid metal-on-metal Biomet ReCap™ hip resurfacing on the left hip. Better AIA is noted in the most recent HRA on the patient's left side

Results

Survivorship

KM implant survivorship (Fig. 2) at 10 years was 96.5% and at 12 years was 96.3% for patients under 50. Overall survivorship also improved with each successive implant type (Fig. 3); for both age groups, the uncemented ReCap™-Magnum™ system exhibited significantly better survivorship than all other implants at 8 years (group 1 $p < 0.0001$, group 2 $p = 0.001$). Survivorship did not vary by age for any implant (log-rank $p = 0.199$ and Wilcoxon $p = 0.206$).

Survival rates varied by sex (Fig. 4), with males displaying significantly greater implant survivorship at 12 years than females in both group 1 (98 vs. 93%, respectively, log-rank and Wilcoxon $p < 0.0001$) and group 2 (99 vs. 95%, respectively, log-rank and Wilcoxon $p < 0.0001$). Sex

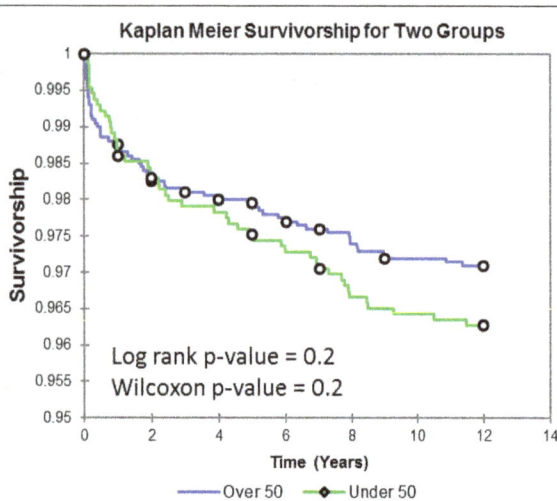

Fig. 2 Kaplan-Meier implant survivorship curves for two study cohorts. *Open circles* represent deaths unrelated to the patients' hip arthroplasties

disparity decreased with each successive implant type. Disparity in male-female results was minimal in cases with the uncemented Biomet ReCap™-Magnum™, with an 8-year failure rate of 99.5 and 97.0% for group 1 males and females, respectively (log-rank and Wilcoxon $p = 0.01$) (Fig. 5).

Failures

Table 4 details modes of failure and indicates for each failure type whether there is or is not significant difference. The only statistically significant difference in occurrence of any failure mode was that of recurrent instability, with which was greater in group 1 (0.2% in group 1 and 0.0% in group 2, $p = 0.03$). AWRF was rare (0.3% in group 1 and 0.4% in group 2, $p = 0.84$) with no instances of wear in cases performed after July 2009; there was no significant difference in AWRF between age groups ($p = 0.84$). One of four total cases of unexplained pain occurred in group 1 ($p = 0.55$). This female patient received revision surgery 1 year after her original operation. Preceding revision, whole blood Co and Cr ion levels were 10.8 and 4.5 µg/L, respectively. Her CT scan prior to revision revealed a small, 3-cm fluid collection anteriorly. While this evidence suggests mild AWRF, implants were found well fixed at the time of surgery, with minimal osteolysis of the acetabulum and femur. All symptoms resolved by 3 months post-revision, and the patient scored a 100 HHS on their most recent 2-year follow-up.

Complications and reoperations

Table 5 lists complications, and Table 6 details reoperations. Group 2 patients were more likely to experience acetabular component shift not resulting in reoperation or revision than group 1 (0.9 vs. 0.2%, respectively, $p = 0.007$). All 21 recognized cases of acetabular shift occurred before 6 weeks and stabilized. All shifted components, with a single exception, became more horizontal than their initial position, and all patients presented optimal metal ion levels.

The overall rate of instability not resulting in revision surgery was 0.3% in group 1 and 0.6% in group 2 ($p = 0.24$). These were treated nonoperatively, and all patients scored a HHS ≥ 92 by 1-year post-revision and presented acceptable blood metal ion levels after surgery.

Ion data and adverse wear-related failure

Approximately 65% of patients from both groups complied with our request for metal ion levels (Table 7). Group 2 unilateral patients expressed slightly higher mean Cr levels ($p = 0.05$), although the difference in mean Cr levels was nonsignificant between the two bilateral cohorts ($p = 0.28$). Average Co ion levels were not statistically different between age groups for either unilateral ($p = 1.0$) or bilateral ($p = 0.26$) patients. Cobalt

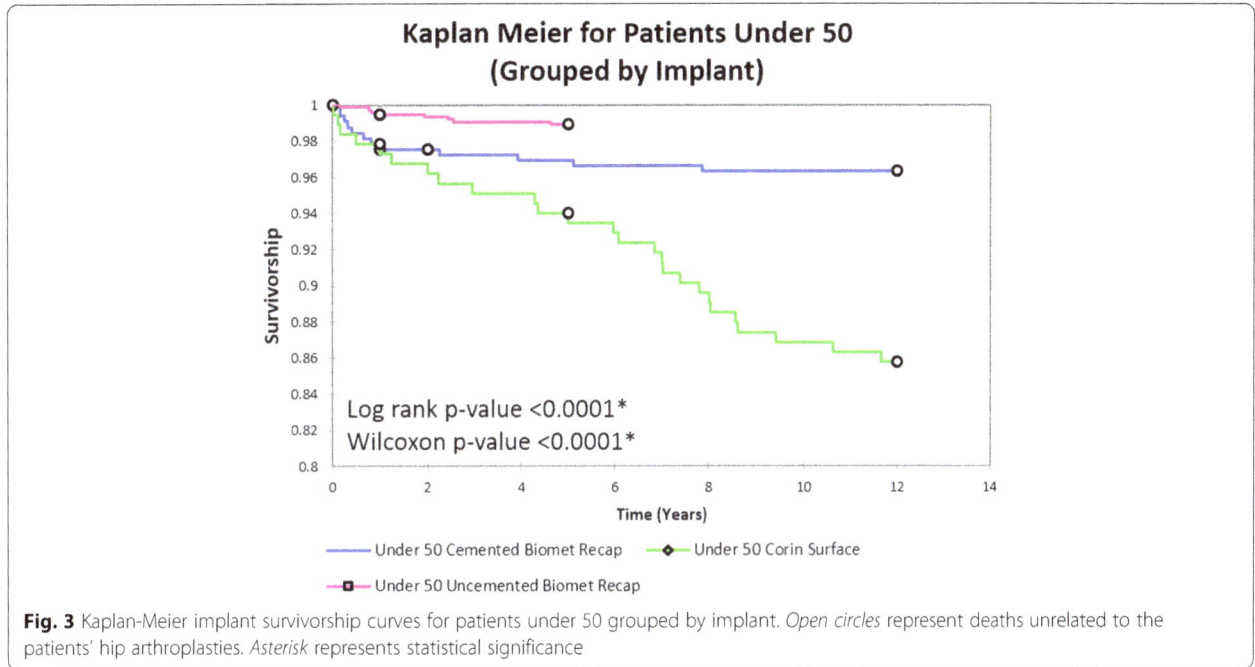

Fig. 3 Kaplan-Meier implant survivorship curves for patients under 50 grouped by implant. *Open circles* represent deaths unrelated to the patients' hip arthroplasties. *Asterisk* represents statistical significance

levels in 825 group 1 patients were optimal in 99% of unilateral cases and 97% of bilateral cases, with no levels greater than 10 µg/L, excluding revised cases. All patients presenting with AWRF in group 1 had ion levels ≥14 µg/L and were revised successfully. Four patients from group 1, and seven from group 2, have developed AWRF to date ($p = 0.84$) (Table 2). The most recent case that resulted in ion levels greater than 10 µg/L was a

case from June 2009; this was the last case to require revision for AWRF. Seven years have elapsed, and in this study, 1530 cases have been performed since that time.

Clinical data

Clinical outcomes for unrevised cases are presented in Table 8. Postoperative average HHS (97 ± 7) was similar for the two groups ($p = 1.0$). Postoperative UCLA activity

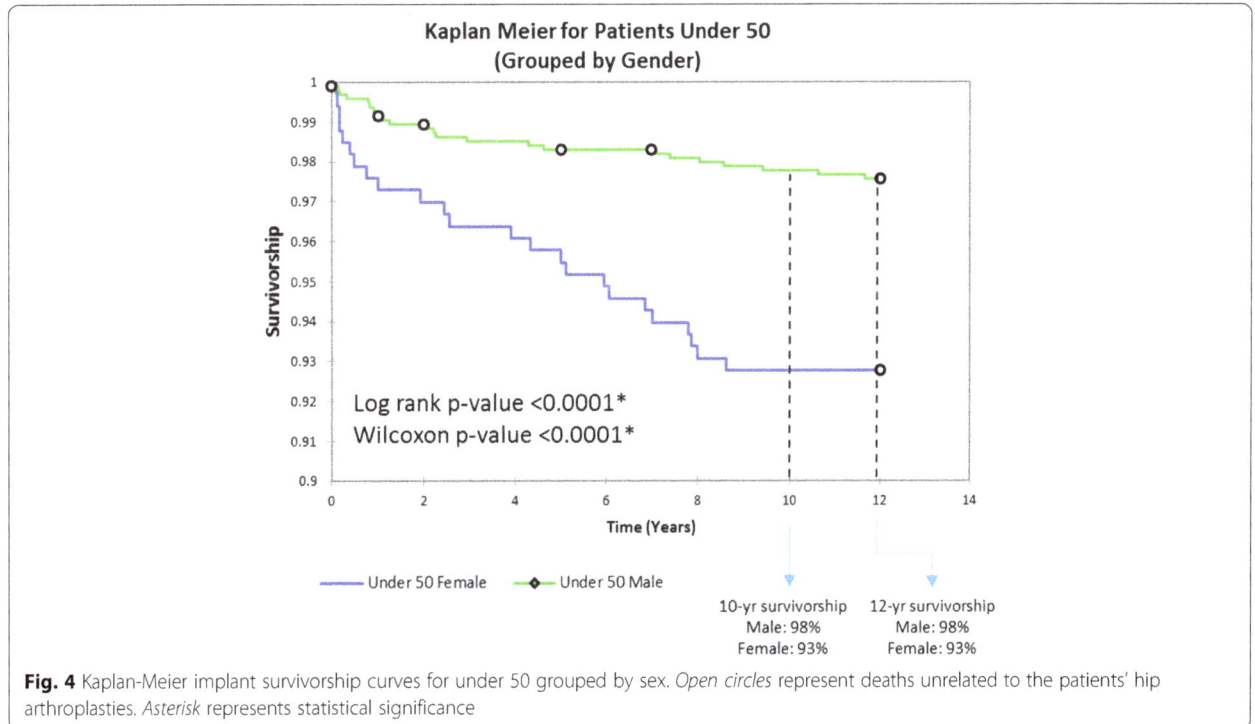

Fig. 4 Kaplan-Meier implant survivorship curves for under 50 grouped by sex. *Open circles* represent deaths unrelated to the patients' hip arthroplasties. *Asterisk* represents statistical significance

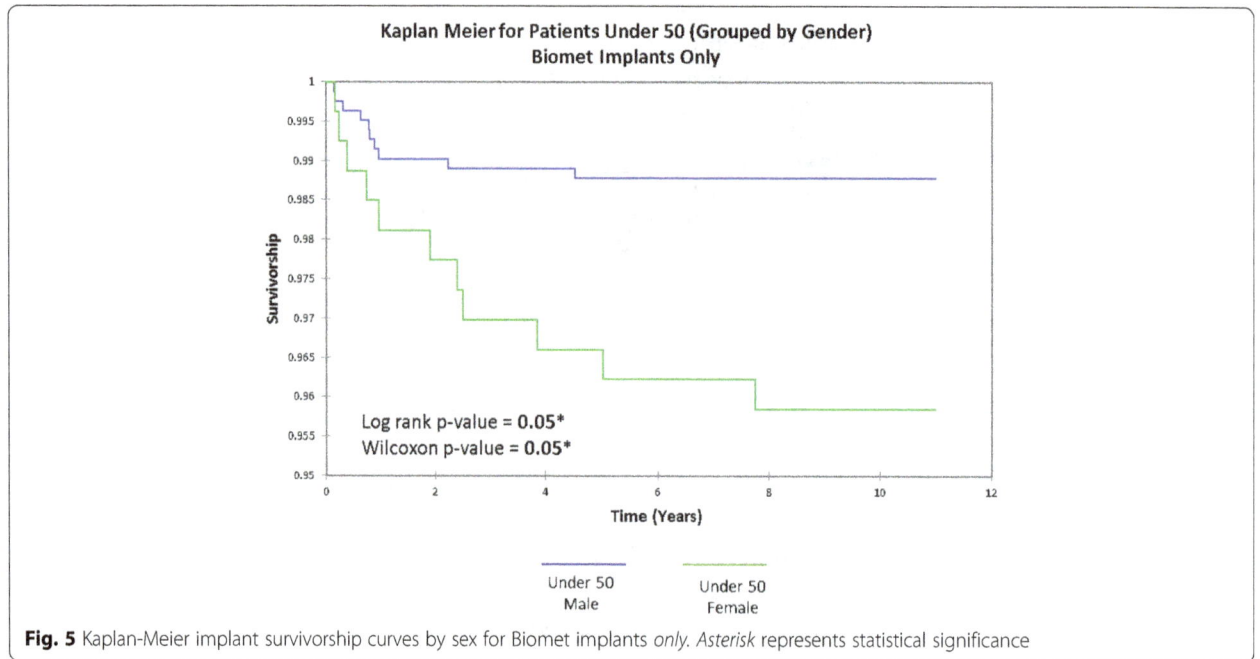

Fig. 5 Kaplan-Meier implant survivorship curves by sex for Biomet implants *only*. *Asterisk* represents statistical significance

Table 4 Failures for two study groups

Type	Group 1	Group 2	p value
No. of cases	1285	1984	–
1) Acetabular failures			
Adverse wear	4 (0.3%)	7 (0.4%)	0.8415
Loose acetabular component	6 (0.5%)	4 (0.2%)	0.1802
Failure of acetabular ingrowth	10 (0.8%)	9 (0.5%)	0.2340
Acetabular component shift	0 (0%)	1 (0.1%)	0.4237
2) Femoral failures			
Early femoral neck fracture	5 (0.4%)	15 (0.8%)	0.1902
Loose femoral component	12 (1.0%)	9 (0.5%)	0.0930
Femoral head collapse	2 (0.2%)	4 (0.2%)	0.7642
3) Other failures			
Unexplained pain	1 (0.1%)	3 (0.2%)	0.5552
Late infection	2 (0.2%)	0 (0%)	0.0784
Early infection	1 (0.1%)	1 (0.1%)	0.7566
Late fracture	2 (0.2%)	1 (0.1%)	0.3320
Recurrent instability	3 (0.2%)	0 (0%)	*0.0316**
Psoas tendonitis	1 (0.1%)	0 (0%)	0.2150
Other failures[a]	0 (0%)	4 (0.2%)	0.1074
Total failures	48 (3.7%)	58 (2.9%)	0.2005

Statistically significant p values are italicized and denoted by an asterisk (*)
[a]Other causes include diarrhea, UTI, urinary retention, squeaking implant, frostbite, and other uncommon causes not built into the database

Table 5 Complications for two study groups

Type	Group 1	Group 2	p value
No. of cases	1285	1984	–
Complications			
1) Acetabular complications			
Loose acetabular component	1 (0.1%)	0 (0%)	0.2150
Acetabular component shift	2 (0.2%)	18 (0.9%)	*0.0071**
2) Femoral complications			
Loose femoral component	1 (0.1%)	1 (0.1%)	0.7566
Femoral component shift	0 (0%)	1 (0.1%)	0.4237
3) Other complications			
Psoas tendonitis	1 (0.1%)	0 (0%)	0.2150
Sciatic nerve palsy	3 (0.2%)	2 (0.1%)	0.3421
Hip dislocation	4 (0.3%)	12 (0.6%)	0.2420
Late fracture	2 (0.2%)	2 (0.1%)	0.6599
Pulmonary embolus	3 (0.2%)	2 (0.1%)	0.3421
Spinal headache	2 (0.2%)	1 (0.1%)	0.3320
Embolic stroke	1 (0.1%)	2 (0.1%)	0.8337
Unexplained pain	0 (0%)	3 (0.2%)	0.1645
Psoas hematoma	1 (0.1%)	0 (0%)	0.2150
Abductor tear	0 (0%)	3 (0.2%)	0.1645
Deep vein thrombosis	2 (0.2%)	5 (0.3%)	0.5619
Other complications[a]	1 (0.1%)	9 (0.5%)	0.0574

Statistically significant p values are italicized and denoted by an asterisk (*)
[a]Other complications include diarrhea, spinal headache, urinary retention, squeaking implant, and other uncommon causes not built into the database

Table 6 Reoperations for two study groups

Type	Group 1	Group 2	p value
No. of cases	1285	1984	–
Reoperations			
Femoral neck fracture	0 (0%)	1 (0.1%)	0.4237
Early fracture	0 (0%)	1 (0.1%)	0.4237
Late fracture	2 (0.2%)	2 (0.1%)	0.6599
Fascial healing defect	1 (0.1%)	0 (0%)	0.2150
Psoas tendonitis	1 (0.1%)	1 (0.1%)	0.7566
Late infection	0 (0%)	2 (0.1%)	0.2543
Early infection	2 (0.2%)	4 (0.2%)	0.7642
Wound dehiscence	2 (0.2%)	2 (0.1%)	0.6599
Other causes[a]	2 (0.2%)	0 (0%)	0.0784

[a]Other causes include suture reaction, frostbite, and other uncommon causes not built into the database

scores were significantly higher for group 1 ($p = 0.003$). VAS pain scores on regular days were statistically equivalent between the two groups ($p = 1.0$). VAS pain scores on worst days were lower for group 2 ($p < 0.0001$).

Radiographic data

Radiographic data for unrevised cases are presented in Table 8. The mean AIA was 40° for both groups ($p = 1.0$). Fewer group 1 cases met our RAIL criteria for proper component position (92 vs. 94%, $p = 0.04$). There were no cases exhibiting lysis ($p = 1.0$), while three cases in the older cohort displayed limited partial radiolucency ($p = 0.16$).

Surgical data

Length of incision, operation time, and estimated blood loss were greater in group 1 ($p = 0.01$, $p < 0.0001$, and $p < 0.0001$, respectively). However, no transfusions were required, and hospital stay did not differ between the two age groups ($p = 1.0$).

Discussion

These data evince the validity of all of our original hypotheses. In the largest single-center report of hip arthroplasty yet published for patients under 50 years old, we demonstrated that MOM hip resurfacing exceeds the stricter 2014 NICE benchmark of 95% 10-year implant survivorship. We achieved 96.5% at 10 years and 96.3% at 12 years in this unselected, consecutive group of 1285 patients under 50 years of age.

Similar to other studies [40–43], we confirmed that hip resurfacing has better implant survivorship in men ($p < 0.0001$) (Fig. 4). However, disparity in results by sex was reduced when we considered only the latest uncemented Biomet cohort, with 8-year survivorship at 99.5% in males and 97.0% in females; per the Orthopaedic Data Evaluation Panel [6], both groups are independently on track to exceed the 2014 NICE criteria. These data show that HRA in women now achieves similar outcomes as in men and that the sex disparity has nearly been resolved.

From the current data, it becomes evident that as hip resurfacing matures, as the scientific body of evidence in resurfacing grows, as failure modes are studied and solutions are found, as implant designs improve, and as

Table 7 Whole blood metal ion results

Under 50 case study Variables	Group 1 (under 50)			Group 2 (over 50)			p values between group 1 and group 2	
	Unilateral (N = 494)	Bilateral (N = 331)	p value	Unilateral (N = 836)	Bilateral (N = 559)	p value	Unilateral 1 vs. 2	Bilateral 1 vs. 2
Co (μg/L)	1.1 ± 0.83	1.8 ± 1.25	<0.0001*	1.1 ± 0.93	1.9 ± 1.31	<0.0001*	1.000	0.2633
Cr (μg/L)	0.9 ± 0.84	1.6 ± 1.32	<0.0001*	1.0 ± 0.93	1.5 ± 1.32	<0.0001*	0.0498*	0.2750
Follow-up date (years)	4.4 ± 2.58	4.9 ± 2.75	0.0080*	3.9 ± 2.38	4.4 ± 2.55	0.0002*	0.0003*	0.0062*
No. (%) of patients tested	825 (64%)		–	1359 (70%)		–	0.0108*	
No. (%) of levels converted	117 (24%)	72 (22%)	0.5157	191 (23%)	138 (25%)	0.4295	0.7279	0.3173
Normal, no. (%)	393 (80%)	169 (51%)	<0.0001*	657 (79%)	234 (42%)	<0.0001*	0.6745	0.0078*
Optimal, no. (%)	488 (99%)	320 (97%)	0.0366*	815 (97%)	533 (95%)	0.0300*	0.1052	0.3371
Acceptable, no. (%)	6 (1.2%)	11 (3.3%)	0.0366*	21 (2.5%)	26 (4.7%)	0.0300*	0.1052	0.3371
Problematic, no. (%)	0 (0%)	0 (0%)	1.000	0 (0%)	0 (0%)	1.000	1.000	1.000
Potentially toxic, no. (%)	0 (0%)	0 (0%)	1.000	0 (0%)	0 (0%)	1.000	1.000	1.000

Statistically significant p values are italicized and denoted by an asterisk (*)

Table 8 Clinical follow-up information for two study groups

Variable	Group 1—under 50	Group 2—over 50	p value
Preoperative			
HHS	58 ± 6.47	49 ± 7.56	<0.0001*
Postoperative			
HHS	97 ± 6.80	97 ± 6.60	1.000
UCLA activity score	7.6 ± 1.91	7.4 ± 1.90	0.0033*
High-impact UCLA, no. of cases (%)	230/539 (43%)	377/1031 (37%)	0.0183*
VAS pain: regular	0.2 ± 0.80	0.2 ± 0.74	1.000
VAS pain: worse	1.5 ± 2.07	1.1 ± 1.78	<0.0001*
Combined ROM	258 ± 46.1	264 ± 41.9	<0.0001*
Radiographic data			
AIA	39.6 ± 8.14	39.6 ± 8.15	1.000
Under RAIL, no. of hips (%)	1138/1238 (92%)	1807/1918 (94%)	0.0366*
Radiolucency, no. of hips (%)	0 (0.0%)	3 (0.2%)	0.1645
Osteolysis, no. of hips (%)	0 (0.0%)	0 (0.0%)	1.000

Statistically significant p values are italicized and denoted by an asterisk (*)

surgeon experience grows, clinical outcomes and implant survivorship improve. It is impossible to determine the exact interplay of these complex factors without further studies, but Fig. 2 undeniably shows dramatic improvement in overall implant survivorship over the 12-year period that encompasses this study. In this short time, 8-year implant survivorship increased from 88 to 99% (log-rank $p < 0.0001$, Wilcoxon $p < 0.0001$). While implant survivorship in THA is generally much lower in younger patients, this does not hold true for hip resurfacing at our center. KM implant survivorship curves comparing our younger and older patient cohorts (Fig. 2) show no statistical difference in failure rates. These KM data show hip resurfacing implants in younger, active patients are at no higher risk of failure.

It is noteworthy that we have achieved 2014 NICE survivorship in our younger, high-risk population, as this group typically presents poor outcomes in THA [2, 9]. Our study produced better outcomes than most THA reports and compare favorably to other smaller, youth-centered resurfacing studies, such as those by Sayeed et al., Haddad et al., and Krantz et al. (Table 9) [11, 23, 44]. Similar survivorship in patients under 50 has been achieved with the Birmingham hip resurfacing, with one report of 100% 10-year survivorship in 20 hips [23] and another report of 96% 10-year survivorship in 447 hips [45]. We are aware of two recent series of uncemented THAs that have achieved similar success, including a report by Facek et al. [46] of 120 consecutive, ceramic THAs in patients under 55 with 96.5% 10-year implant survivorship and another report by Murphy and Murphy

Table 9 Literature comparison of survivorship between treatment options for younger patients

Study	Procedure	Prosthesis	Date range	Diagnosis (years)	Patient cohort Hips	Female (%)	Avg FU (years)	Survivorship FU	Rate (%)
Jameson et al. [51]	HRA	Birmingham	2004–2007	<55	254	39	2.3	3.8	97
Matharu et al. [45]	HRA	Birmingham	1997–2006	<50	447	28	10.1	10	96
Woon et al. [52]	HRA	Conserve Plus	1996–2010	<30	53	39	8.2	8	95
Amstutz et al. [53]	HRA	Conserve Plus	1998–2007	<50	350	25	5.5	5	97.8
Krantz et al. [44]	HRA	Conserve Plus and Durom	2007–2008	<30	24	32	4.2	4.9	100
Haddad et al. [23]	HRA	Birmingham	1999–2002	<55	40	25	12	10	100
Matharu et al. [54]	HRA	Conserve Plus and Corin Cormet 2000	2001–2007	<25 + osteonecrosis	20	50	5.2	8.6	100
Matharu et al. [54]	THA	Stryker Accolade II stem and Trident cup	2001–2007	<25 + osteonecrosis	20	38	5.2	7.3	93
Wroblewski et al. [55]	THA	Charnley	1962–1990	<51	1434	61	15	17	83
Current study	HRA	Corin Surface and Biomet ReCap™	2008–2013	<50	1285	26	3.4	12	96

[47] of 220 alumina ceramic THAs in patients under 50 with 94.9% 15-year survivorship.

Outcomes for resurfacing are mixed, with registries typically showing lower implant survivorship than published series from dedicated resurfacing surgeons. Hip resurfacing requires a significant learning curve compared to THA [48] and is seldom taught in residency programs.

The most common failure mode for either group was loosening of the femoral component (1.0% in group 1 and 0.5% in group 2). Converting to exclusively uncemented implants eliminated this failure mode. The second most common cause for revision was failure of acetabular ingrowth (0.8% in group 1 and 0.5% in group 2). After introduction of the acetabular component with Magnum™ Tri-Spike supplemental fixation in high-risk cases in 2007, this failure mode reduced from 1.1 to 0.5%. Since 2010, there have been no instances of failure of acetabular ingrowth in patients under 50 years old.

AWRF is a well-publicized and widely feared complication of MOM HRA. Particle-driven tissue inflammation has long been associated with polyethylene, polymethyl methacrylate, and metallic debris between modular junctions [28]. Tissue inflammation due to metallic particles from excessive MOM bearing wear came to widespread attention around 2007 [34]. At first, many speculated that these represented allergic reactions to metal [22]. Later, studies revealed the cause of the problem as edge-loading on the malpositioned acetabular component [35]. When this occurs, the fluid film lubrication of the hip joint breaks down, and a high wear rate ensues. Metal particles settle in surrounding tissue, activating an inflammatory response. Poor implant design and improper acetabular component positioning cause this abnormal edge-loading wear; thus, smaller bearing sizes, used primarily in women, are more prone to edge-loading because of their lower coverage arc. In response to these findings, we published the RAIL guideline [33], which indicates safe positions for all implant sizes. Patients under 50 presented significantly reduced ion levels when their implant was placed under the RAIL limit, with a mean Co level of 1.4 compared to 2.1 in patients over RAIL ($p < 0.0001$). No instances of AWRF, problematic ion levels, or potentially toxic ion levels occurred in cases under RAIL, which has been achieved in all cases since 2009. These results justify that AWRF is completely preventable in MOM implants, even in cases previously considered high-risk.

This study contains a few notable limitations. First, all HRAs reported herein were performed by a single, experienced HRA surgeon. Registry results are inferior, but numerous publications from experienced HRA surgeons show similar survivorship. Although studies have shown proper HRA surgical technique requires an extended learning curve [27, 48, 49], this curve is expected to shorten with increased availability of HRA research. The next limitation derives from excellent patient outcomes, which recently have been so good that our current clinical measurement, the HHS, suffers from a ceiling effect [50]; a younger patient who outperforms an older patient with a clinical HHS of 100 would still score the same, limiting comparison. Finally, a larger proportion of group 2 received the superior uncemented Biomet ReCap™ device ($p < 0.0001$), potentially skewing results in favor of the older patient cohort. Despite this, postoperative results for the younger study group were similar to, and in many instances better than, those for group 2.

Conclusions

We make the following conclusions:

- In the largest ($n = 1285$) single series of hip arthroplasty ever published for patients under 50, MOM HRA exceeds the 2014 NICE implant survivorship criteria, with 96.5% at 10 years and 96.4% at 12 years.
- Results in women have improved rapidly, reducing the disparity in outcomes between sexes; furthermore, after eliminating the initial Corin cohort, 10-year implant survivorship for men and women Biomet implants both exceed the 2014 NICE criteria independently at 99 and 97%, respectively.
- There is no difference in survivorship by age among our patients (96.5 vs. 96.3% at 12 years for under and over 50, respectively).
- AWRF is a rare complication (0.3%). Blood ion testing is an effective screening tool. When the acetabular component position meets RAIL guidelines, this failure mode is completely avoidable. None have occurred in 1530 consecutive cases since July 2009.

Abbreviations
AWRF: Adverse wear-related failure; Co: Cobalt; Cr: Chromium; HHS: Harris hip score; HRA: Hip resurfacing arthroplasty; KM: Kaplan-Meier; MOM: Metal-on-metal; NICE: National Institute for Health and Care Excellence; RAIL: Relative acetabular inclination limit; ROM: Range of motion; THA: Total hip arthroplasty; UCLA: University of California, Los Angeles; VAS: Visual analog scale

Acknowledgements
Not applicable.

Funding
Funding for this entirety of this project was provided by the primary surgeon (TPG).

Authors' contributions

TPG performed all surgeries and follow-ups, took radiographic measurements, designed questionnaires, developed the present study design, and made multiple rounds of edits on this manuscript. MDG is responsible for data collection, for statistical analyses, for writing most of the content herein, and for manuscript development and submission. Both authors were involved in data acquisition, data analysis and interpretation, drafting, and final revisions. Both authors have read and approved the final submitted manuscript.

Competing interests

The authors declare that they have previously received royalties and research support (<$50,000) from Zimmer Biomet and Corin during preceding studies.

References

1. Amstutz HC, Beaule PE, Dorey FJ, Le Duff MJ, Campbell PA, Gruen TA. Metal-on-metal hybrid surface arthroplasty: two to six-year follow-up study. J Bone Jt Surg Am. 2004;86–A:28–39. doi:10.2106/JBJS.F.00273.
2. Innmann MM, Weiss S, Andreas F, Merle C, Streit MR. Sports and physical activity after cementless total hip arthroplasty with a minimum follow-up of 10 years. Scand J Med Sci Sports. 2016;26:550–6. doi:10.1111/sms.12482.
3. Ollivier M, Frey S. Does impact sport activity influence total hip arthroplasty durability? Clin Orthop Relat Res. 2012;470:3060–6. doi:10.1007/s11999-012-2362-z.
4. Havelin LI, Robertsson O, Fenstad AM, Overgaard S, Garellick G, Furnes O. A Scandinavian experience of register collaboration: the Nordic Arthroplasty Register Association (NARA). J Bone Jt Surg. 2011;93:13–9. doi:10.2106/JBJS.K.00951.
5. Mäkelä KT, Matilainen M, Pulkkinen P, Fenstad AM, Havelin LI, Engesaeter L, et al. Countrywise results of total hip replacement. An analysis of 438,733 hips based on the Nordic Arthroplasty Register Association database. Acta Orthop. 2014;85:107–16. doi:10.3109/17453674.2014.893498.
6. Orthopaedic Data Evaluation Panel. http://www.odep.org.uk. Accessed 22 May 2017.
7. Charnley J. Arthroplasty of the hip—a new operation. Lancet. 1961;1:1129.
8. Aldinger PR, Jung AW, Pritsch M, Breusch S, Thomsen M, Ewerbeck V, et al. Uncemented grit-blasted straight tapered titanium stems in patients younger than fifty-five years of age. Fifteen to twenty-year results. J Bone Jt Surg Am. 2009;91:1432–9. doi:10.2106/JBJS.H.00297.
9. De Kam D. Total hip arthroplasties in young patients under 50 years: limited evidence for current trends. A descriptive literature review. Hip Int. 2011;21:518–25.
10. Baker RP, Pollard TCB, Eastaugh-Waring SJ, Bannister GC. A medium-term comparison of hybrid hip replacement and Birmingham hip resurfacing in active young patients. J Bone Jt Surg [Br]. 2011;93:158–63. doi:10.1302/0301-620X.93B2.
11. Sayeed SA, Johnson AJ, Bs DAS, Gross TP, Mont MA. Hip resurfacing in patients who have osteonecrosis and are 25 years or under. Clin Orthop Relat Res 2011:1582–8. doi:10.1007/s11999-010-1629-5
12. Torchia ME, Klassen RA, Bianco AJ. Total hip arthroplasty with cement in patients less than twenty years old. J Bone Jt Surg. 1996;78:995–1003.
13. McMinn DJW, Treacy RBC, Lin K, Pynsent PB. Metal on metal surface replacement of the hip: experience of the McMinn prothesis. Clin Orthop Relat Res. 1996;329S:S89–98.
14. Amstutz HC. Treatment of primary osteoarthritis of the hip: a comparison of total joint and surface replacement arthroplasty. J Bone Jt Surg. 1984.
15. Amstutz HC, Le Duff MJ. Hip resurfacing results for osteonecrosis are as good as for other etiologies at 2 to 12 years. Clin Orthop Relat Res. 2010;468:375–81. doi:10.1007/s11999-009-1077-2.
16. Beaulé PE. Surface arthroplasty of the hip: a review and current indications. Semin Arthroplasty. 2005;16:70–6. doi:10.1053/j.sart.2004.12.008.
17. Mont M a, Seyler TM, Marker DR, Marulanda G a, Delanois RE. Use of metal-on-metal total hip resurfacing for the treatment of osteonecrosis of the femoral head. J Bone Joint Surg Am 2006;88 Suppl 3:90–7. doi:10.2106/JBJS.F.00543.
18. Aqil A, Drabu R, Bergmann JH, Masjedi M, Manning V, Andrews B, et al. The gait of patients with one resurfacing and one replacement hip: a single blinded controlled study. n.d. doi:10.1007/s00264-013-1819-3
19. Mont MA, Seyler TM, Ragland PS, Starr R, Erhart J, Bhave A. Gait analysis of patients with resurfacing hip arthroplasty compared with hip osteoarthritis and standard total hip arthroplasty. n.d. doi:10.1016/j.arth.2006.03.010

20. Gross TP, Liu F, Webb LA. Clinical outcome of the metal-on-metal hybrid Corin Cormet 2000 hip resurfacing system. An up to 11-year follow-up study. J Arthroplasty 2012;27:533–538.e1. doi:10.1016/j.arth.2011.06.019.
21. Gross TP, Liu F. Current status of modern fully porous coated metal-on-metal hip resurfacing arthroplasty. J Arthroplast. 2014;29:181–5. doi:10.1016/j.arth.2013.04.010.
22. Howie DW. Metal-on-metal resurfacing versus total hip replacement-the value of a randomized clinical trial. Orthop Clin North Am. 2005;36:195. doi:10.1016/j.ocl.2004.12.001.
23. Haddad FS, Konan S, Tahmassebi J. A prospective comparative study of cementless total hip arthroplasty and hip resurfacing in patients under the age of 55 years. Bone Jt J 2015;97–B:617–22. doi:10.1302/0301-620X.97B5.
24. Mont MA, Schmalzried T. Modern metal-on-metal hip resurfacing: important observations from the first ten years. J Bone Jt Surg. 2008;90:3–11. doi:10.2106/JBJS.H.00750.
25. Barrack RL. Metal-on-metal hip resurfacing offers advantages over traditional arthroplasty in selected patients. Orthopedics. 2007;30.
26. Prosser GH, Yates PJ, Wood DJ, Graves SE, De Steiger RN, Miller LN. Outcome of primary resurfacing hip replacement: evaluation of risk factors for early revision 12,093 replacements from the Australian Joint Registry. Acta Orthop. 2010;81:66–71. doi:10.3109/17453671003685434.
27. Smith AJ, Dieppe P, Howard PW, Blom AW. Failure rates of metal-on-metal hip resurfacings: analysis of data from the National Joint Registry for England and Wales. Lancet. 2012;380:1759–66. doi:10.1016/S0140-6736(12)60989-1.
28. Williams S, Leslie I, Isaac G, Jin Z, Ingham E, Fisher J. Tribology and wear of metal-on-metal hip prostheses: influence of cup angle and head position. JBJSAm. 2008;90:111–7. doi:10.2106/JBJS.H.00485.
29. Malchau H, Herberts P, Eisler T, Gerllick G, Soderman P. The Swedish Total Hip Replacement Register. J Bone Jt Surg. 2004;86.
30. Gaillard MD, Gross TP. Reducing the failure rate of hip resurfacing in dysplasia patients: a retrospective analysis of 363 cases. BMC Musculoskelet Disord. 2016;17:251. doi:10.1186/s12891-016-1095-7.
31. O'Leary R, Gaillard MD, Gross TP. Comparison of cemented and bone ingrowth fixation methods in hip resurfacing for osteonecrosis. J Arthroplasty. 2016. doi:10.1016/j.arth.2016.07.028.
32. Gross TP, Liu F. Minimally invasive posterior approach for hip resurfacing. Tech Orthop. 2010;25:39–49.
33. Liu F, Gross TP. A safe zone for acetabular component position in metal-on-metal hip resurfacing arthroplasty: winner of the 2012 HAP PAUL award. J Arthroplast. 2013;28:1224–30. doi:10.1016/j.arth.2013.02.033.
34. Langton DJ, Joyce TJ, Mangat N, Lord J, Van Orsouw M, De Smet K, et al. Reducing metal ion release following hip resurfacing arthroplasty. Orthop Clin North Am. 2011;42:169–80. doi:10.1016/j.ocl.2011.01.006. viii.
35. Smolders JMH, Bisseling P, Hol A, Van Der Straeten C, Schreurs BW, van Susante JLC. Metal ion interpretation in resurfacing versus conventional hip arthroplasty and in whole blood versus serum. How should we interpret metal ion data? Hip Int. 2011;21:587–95. doi:10.5301/HIP.2011.8643.
36. Van Der Straeten C. Systemic symptoms of metal toxicity in metal-on-metal hip arthroplasty. Palm Beach ISTA Meet. 2013.
37. Harris W. Endosteal errosion in association with stable uncemented femoral components. J Bone Jt Surg. 1990.
38. Zahiri CA, Schmalzried TP, Szuszczewicz ES, Amstutz HC. Assessing activity in joint replacement patients. J Arthroplast. 1998;13:890–5. doi:10.1016/S0883-5403(98)90195-4.
39. Scott J. Graphic representation of pain. Pain 1976;2. doi:10.1016/0304-3959(76)90113-5
40. Gross TP, Liu F. Prevalence of dysplasia as the source of worse outcome in young female patients after hip resurfacing arthroplasty. Int Orthop. 2012;36:27–34. doi:10.1007/s00264-011-1290-y.
41. Jameson SS, Langton DJ, Natu S, Nargol TVF. The influence of age and sex on early clinical results after hip resurfacing. An independent center analysis. J Arthroplasty. 2008. doi:10.1016/j.arth.2008.03.019.
42. Carrothers a D, Gilbert RE, Jaiswal a, Richardson JB. Birmingham hip resurfacing: the prevalence of failure. J Bone Joint Surg Br 2010. doi:10.1302/0301-620X.92B10.23504.
43. Witzleb WC, Hanisch U, Ziegler J, Guenther K-P. In vivo wear rate of the Birmingham Hip Resurfacing arthroplasty: a review of 10 retrieved components. J Arthroplasty. 2009;24:951–6. doi:10.1016/j.arth.2008.06.022.
44. Krantz N, Miletic B, Migaud H, Girard J. Hip resurfacing in patients under thirty years old: an attractive option for young and active patients. Int

Orthop. 2012;36:1789–94. doi:10.1007/s00264-012-1555-0.

45. Matharu, Uppal HS, Peterson BE, Misfeldt ML, Della Rocca GJ, Volgas DA, et al. The outcome of the Birmingham Hip Resurfacing in patients aged < 50 years up to 14 years post-operatively. Bone Jt J 2013. doi:10.1302/0301-620X.95B9.

46. Facek M, Tilley S, Walter WK, Zicat B, Walter WL. Ceramic-on-ceramic bearings in young patients. Bone Jt J. 2013;95:1603–9. doi:10.1302/0301-620X.95B12.30917.

47. Murphy S, Murphy W. Alumina ceramic ceramic THA at 15 years in patients less than 50. New Engl. Baptist Hosp. 2014;98-B(Suppl 3):69.

48. Nunley RM, Zhu J, Brooks PJ, Engh CAJ, Raterman SJ, Rogerson JS, et al. The learning curve for adopting hip resurfacing among hip specialists. Clin Orthop Relat Res. 2010;468:382–91. doi:10.1007/s11999-009-1106-1.

49. Amstutz HC, Le Duff MJ. Eleven years of experience with metal-on-metal hybrid hip resurfacing: a review of 1000 conserve plus. J Arthroplasty. 2008;23(6 Suppl 1):36–43.

50. Wamper KE, Sierevelt IN, Poolman RW, Bhandari M, Haverkamp D. The Harris hip score: do ceiling effects limit its usefulness in orthopedics? Acta Orthop. 2010;81:703–7. doi:10.3109/17453674.2010.537808.

51. Jameson SS, Langton DJ, Natu S, Nargol TVF. The influence of age and sex on early clinical results after hip resurfacing. An independent center analysis. J Arthroplasty. 2008;23:50–5. doi:10.1016/j.arth.2008.03.019.

52. Woon RP, Johnson AJ, Amstutz HC. The results of metal-on-metal hip resurfacing in patients under 30 years of age. J Arthroplasty. 2013;28:1010–4. doi:10.1016/j.arth.2012.07.043.

53. Amstutz HC, Ball ST, Le Duff MJ, Dorey FJ. Resurfacing THA for patients younger than 50 year: results of 2- to 9-year followup. Clin Orthop Relat Res. 2007;460:159–64.

54. Matharu GS, Mcbryde CW, Pynsent WB, Pynsent PB, Treacy RBC, Matharu GS. The outcome of the Birmingham Hip Resurfacing in patients aged < 50 years up to 14 years post-operatively. Bone Jt J. 2013;95:1172–7. doi:10.1302/0301-620X.95B9.

55. Wroblewski BM, Siney PD, Fleming PA. Charnley low-frictional torque arthroplasty in patients under the age of 51 years. J Bone Jt Surg. 2002;84-B:540–3.

3

Extramedullary versus intramedullary femoral alignment technique in total knee arthroplasty

Qian Tang[1†], Ping Shang[2†], Gang Zheng[1], Hua-Zi Xu[1] and Hai-Xiao Liu[1*] (iD)

Abstract

Background: There is no consensus whether the use of the extramedullary femoral cutting guide takes advantage over the intramedullary one in total knee arthroplasty. The aim of this study was to compare the extramedullary femoral alignment guide system with the conventional intramedullary alignment guide system for lower limb alignment, blood loss, and operative time during total knee arthroplasty.

Methods: The Medline, Embase, Cochrane Library, China National Knowledge Infrastructure (CNKI), Wan Fang Chinese Periodical, Google, and reference lists of all the included studies were searched for randomized controlled trials. The following parameters were compared between the extramedullary technique and the intramedullary technique: (1) lower limb coronal alignment, (2) coronal alignment of femoral component, (3) sagittal alignment of femoral component, (4) blood loss, (5) and operation time.

Results: Four randomized controlled trials consisting of 358 knees were included in our study. There was no significant difference between the extramedullary and intramedullary groups for the lower limb coronal alignment (RR = 1.20, 95%CI 0.28~5.21, n.s.), coronal alignment of femoral component (RR = 0.65, 95%CI 0.19~2.22, n.s.), and sagittal alignment of femoral component (RR = 0.73, 95%CI 0.38~1.41, n.s.). A reduced blood loss was associated with the use of the extramedullary guide (MD = −120.34, 95%CI −210.08~−30.59, P = 0.009). No significant difference in operation time was noted between the two groups (MD = 1.41, 95%CI −1.82~4.64, n.s.).

Conclusions: Neither extramedullary nor intramedullary femoral alignment is more accurate than the other in facilitating the femoral cut in total knee arthroplasty. Use of the extramedullary guide results in less blood loss and exhibits a similar operation time as compared with the intramedullary guide.

Keywords: Total knee arthroplasty, Meta-analysis, Blood loss

Background

In total knee arthroplasty (TKA), the prosthetic placement and overall limb alignment has been demonstrated to be most influential in determining implant survival [1–4]. The ideal position for the components recreates a neutral mechanical axis. Most surgeons currently favor intramedullary (IM) alignment for its ease of use and accuracy as compared with extramedullary (EM) alignment. Previous comparisons of IM and EM femoral alignment systems have shown the former to be more accurate in performing the distal femoral cut [5–7]. In these studies, the IM alignment technique has ranged from 85 to 96% in the normal range as compared with 69 to 86% for the EM alignment technique.

However, the IM femoral alignment system does not always guarantee the accuracy of the component position in TKA. Previous studies used only the anterosuperior iliac spine as an intraoperative landmark for the EM referencing instruments [5–7]. Intraoperative visual

* Correspondence: spineliu@163.com
†Equal contributors
[1]Department of Orthopaedic Surgery, The Second Affiliated Hospital and Yuying Children's Hospital of Wenzhou Medical University, 109, Xueyuanxi road, 325027 Wenzhou, China
Full list of author information is available at the end of the article

assessment of the longitudinal femur axis and the ante-rosuperior iliac spine by EM rods is difficult owing to the large soft tissue cover and tourniquets. TKAs using extramedullary femoral alignment guides have been extensively studied in recent years. Extramedullary instruments using newly designed mechanical axis marker systems have provided as accuracy in reproducing a neutral distal femoral resection on the coronal and sagittal planes during TKA as standard IM instruments [8–10].

Recent advances in TKA have focused on the reduction of damage during the procedure [11–13]. One of the most invasive parts of TKA is the violation of the intramedullary femoral canal and the subsequent use of IM instruments. The use of an intramedullary guide for the femur can result in various complications such as blood loss, postoperative hypoxia, intraoperative fractures, and fat embolism [11, 14, 15], while the EM method has less morbidity in terms of blood loss because it does not invade bone marrow. In addition, the IM instrument may not be applicable when a long-stemmed femoral component implanted during a previous surgery remains or a rod cannot be inserted due to severe deformity of the femur [9].

In this study, we conducted a meta-analysis of pooled the data from relevant RCTs to evaluate whether an IM or EM femoral guide is more accurate in assuring correct femoral positioning. Moreover, the blood loss and operation time were also compared between these two techniques. Our hypothesis was that the EM femoral guide provided similar accuracy for femoral positioning and less blood loss compared with the IM femoral guide during TKAs. If the hypothesis is confirmed, the EM femoral guide may provide an alternative approach for femoral cuts and display clinical benefit for particular cases, such as a previous surgery remains and severe deformity of the femur.

Methods

Database retrieval

The present study was conducted using the Preferred Reporting Items for Systematic Reviews and Meta Analyses (PRISMA) statement. We conducted this meta-analysis of all English and non-English articles identified from electronic databases including Medline, Embase, Cochrane Library, China National Knowledge Infrastructure, Wan Fang Chinese Periodical, and Google. In addition, we also manually searched for other relevant studies including those from the reference lists of all included studies. The last search was conducted on December 6, 2015. We used the following key words: arthroplasty, replacement, femoral, total knee arthroplasty, randomized, randomised, intramedullary, extra-medullary, in combination with the Boolean operators AND or OR. The search strategy is presented in Fig. 1.

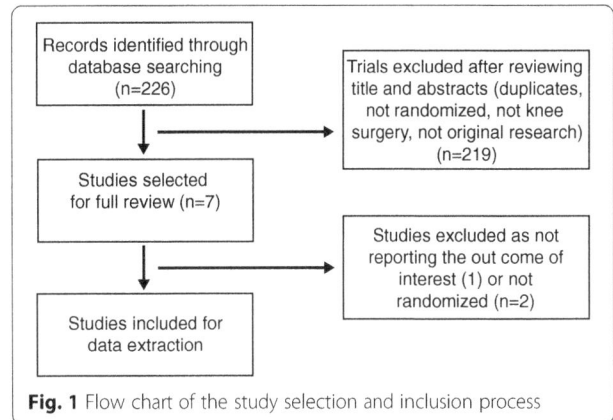

Fig. 1 Flow chart of the study selection and inclusion process

Quality criteria of trials and data extraction

We included all published RCTs comparing EM guide with IM guide in patients undergoing primary TKA. Exclusion criteria comprised the following: trials with a retrospective design and trials that did not randomize patients into two relevant groups. Quality criteria included the randomization method, concealment of allocation, blinding, and intention-to-treat analysis.

For each eligible study, two of the authors of this meta-analysis independently extracted all relevant data. Disagreement was resolved by discussion with a third investigator. The following data were extracted: (1) the participants' demographic data; (2) the lower limb coronal alignment; (3) the coronal alignment of femoral component; (4) the sagittal alignment of femoral component; (5) the blood loss; (6) and the operation time. When data were incomplete or unclear, attempts were made to contact the investigators for clarification. The lower limb coronal alignment was defined as a line bisecting the center of the femoral head, the center of the knee, and the center of the ankle. The coronal alignment of femoral component (which represents varus-valgus angulation) was measured in the coronal plane on the full-limb anteroposterior film. The sagittal alignment of femoral component (which represents flexion-extension angulation) was measured in the sagittal plane on the lateral film [9].

Statistical methods

This meta-analysis was conducted using RevMan 5.0 (Cochrane Collaboration, Oxford, UK). We assessed the statistical heterogeneity using a standard chi-square test (statistical heterogeneity was considered to be present at $P < 0.1$ and I^2 values >50%). When comparing trials exhibiting heterogeneity, pooled data were meta-analyzed using a random effects model; otherwise, a fixed effects model was used. Mean differences and 95% confidence intervals (CIs) were calculated for continuous outcomes and risk ratio (RR) and 95% CIs for dichotomous outcomes. Ethical approval was obtained.

Results

The included studies

A total of 226 potentially relevant papers were identified. By screening titles and reading the abstracts and entire articles, four studies with 358 knees (178 in the EM group and 180 in the IM group) were included in the final meta-analysis. All of the included studies were RCTs which were level I evidence studies and all published in English. The sample sizes ranged from 50 to 100 knees. The key characteristics of the included RCTs are summarized in Table 1. And the detailed data of the comparison of blood loss between femoral EM and IM technique was showed in Additional file 1.

Quality of studies

The methodologic quality of the four included studies was variable. The reported methods of generating allocation sequences were adequate in two studies and one trial reported allocation concealment. Blinding of surgeon and patients were reported in one study and one of the studies blinded their assessors to the outcome. The methodologic quality of the studies is presented in Fig. 2. Judgment with respect to each risk of bias item is presented as a percentage for all of the included studies, as shown in Fig. 3.

The pooled results of meta-analysis

The pooled results indicated that there was no significant difference between the two groups in terms of the lower limb coronal alignment (RR = 1.20, 95%CI 0.28~5.21, n.s. Fig. 4a). For coronal alignment of femoral component, no significant difference was noted between the two groups (RR = 0.65, 95%CI 0.19~2.22, n.s. Fig. 4b). No significant difference was noted between the two groups in the sagittal alignment of femoral component (RR = 0.73, 95%CI 0.38~1.41, n.s. Fig. 4c). The blood loss was less in the EM group compared with the IM group (MD = −120.34, 95%CI −210.08~−30.59, P =0.009, Fig. 5a). There was no significant difference between the two groups in terms of the operation time (MD = 1.41, 95%CI -1.82~4.64, n.s. Fig. 5b).

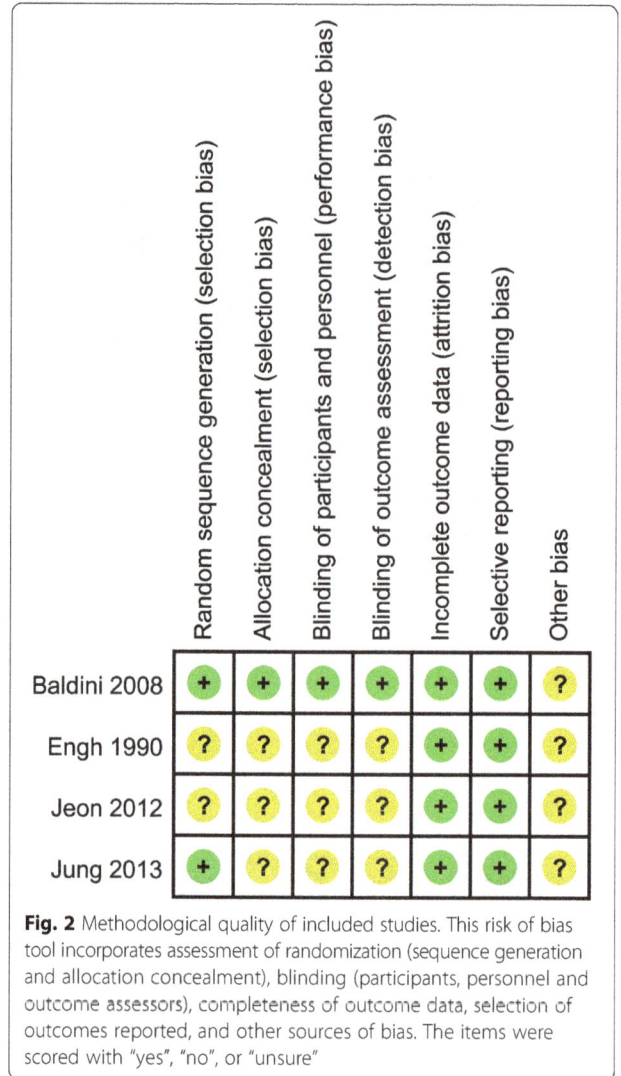

Fig. 2 Methodological quality of included studies. This risk of bias tool incorporates assessment of randomization (sequence generation and allocation concealment), blinding (participants, personnel and outcome assessors), completeness of outcome data, selection of outcomes reported, and other sources of bias. The items were scored with "yes", "no", or "unsure"

Discussion

Our meta-analysis compared the radiographic outcomes between the EM and the IM femoral guiding technique in patients undergoing TKA. No significant differences were found between the two groups in terms of the lower limb coronal alignment, the coronal alignment of

Table 1 Characteristics of the included studies

Author	Country	Patients (EM)/(IM)	Age (EM)/(IM)	Gender (EM)/(IM)	Total knee system	EM system
Jung 2013 [9]	South Korea	56/50	70.4/68.5	Female:male 6:1/5.3:1	PS prosthesis (Stryker)	Mechanical axis marker with IFD measurement
Jeon 2012 [28]	South Korea	40/40	70.1/69.2	Female	PS prosthesis (Stryker)	Markers attached to skin
Baldini 2008 [8]	Italy	50/50	71/70	Female:male 2:1/1.7:1	Posterior stabilized flex fixed-bearing prosthesis (Zimmer)	An extramedullary device with preoperative templated data
Engh 1990 [7]	USA	32/40	69.11(38-88)	Female: 53 Male: 19	Depuy	HDisc–peg taped to skin for intraoperative location

EM extramedullary group, *IM* intramedullary group, *IFD* inter-femoral head distance, *ASIS* anterosuperior iliac spine

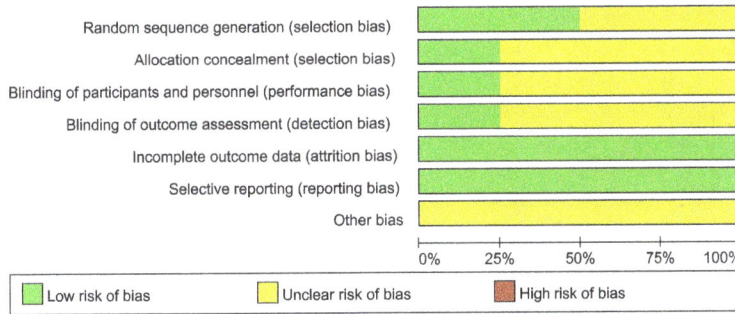

Fig. 3 Risk of bias. Each risk of bias item presented as percentages across all included studies which indicated the proportion of different level risk of bias for each item

femoral component, and the sagittal alignment of femoral component. The EM guide was associated with a less blood loss and exhibited a similar operation time as the IM guide.

Long-term success after TKA is dependent especially on proper intraoperative component positioning [1–4]. Most authors have reported favorable femoral cuts made with the IM guide and it is considered to be the most accurate with a statistically significant increase in the percentage of distal femoral cuts [6, 7]. Several studies found 85–96% of IM femoral cuts to be acceptable compared with 69–86% of EM cuts. The EM femoral alignment technique had inferior accuracy with approximately 10% more outliers on the coronal plane compared with the IM technique [9]. Historically, all the authors were using the EM instruments referring only to the anterosuperior iliac spine (ASIS) intraoperatively

[7, 16]. However, the use of the ASIS to locate the femoral head center (FHC) might not be an accurate method since the FHC was indirectly determined by and dependent on anatomical structures adjacent to the femoral head. Identification of the FHC using the two finger-breadths medial to the ASIS method was unreliable and a wide variation of inter-ASIS distances was found among patients [17].

Recently, some studies have introduced new techniques to improve the accuracy of the extramedullary alignment guide system. Baldini and Adravanti [8] developed a set of EM instruments calibrated with preoperative templating radiograph measurements of inter-femoral head center distance (IFD), which allowed one to perform distal femoral resection without violating the femoral canal. They reported that the femoral component coronal alignment was within $0° \pm 2°$ of the

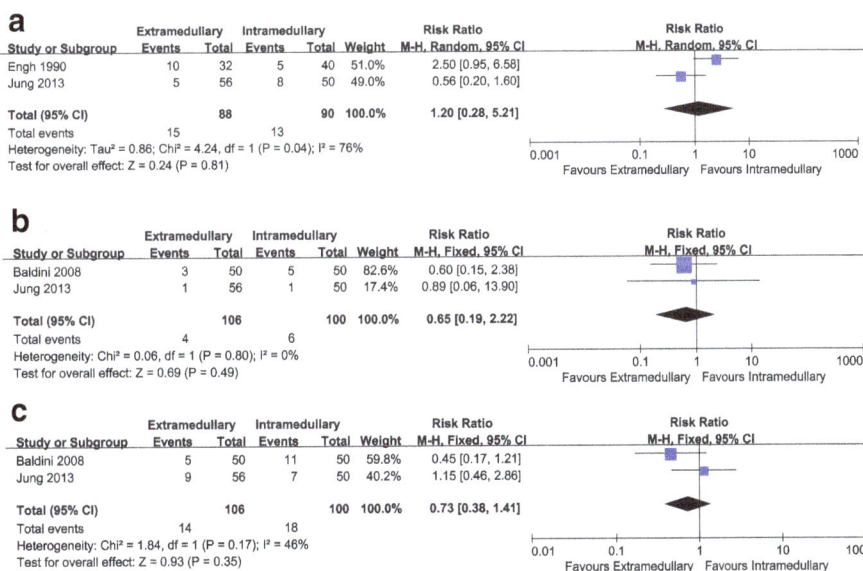

Fig. 4 a Comparison of the lower limb coronal alignment between femoral EM and IM techniques. **b** Comparison of coronal alignment of femoral component between femoral EM and IM techniques. **c** Comparison of sagittal alignment of femoral component between femoral EM and IM techniques

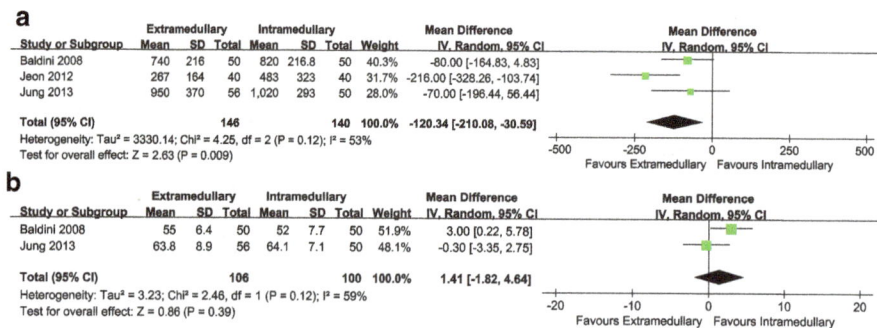

Fig. 5 a Comparison of blood loss between femoral EM and IM techniques. **b** Comparison of operative time between femoral EM and IM techniques

mechanical axis in 84% of the IM group and 86% of the EM group. Matsumoto et al. [18] reported that the femoral component coronal alignment was within $0° ± 3°$ of the mechanical axis in 98% of patients by using a similar EM instrument. Seo et al. [19] using preoperative templating radiograph measurements of IFD showed that outliers ($±3°$) of the femoral component coronal alignment were observed in 9.4% of all cases. However, the proximal reference point in the coronal plane was considered to be incorrect when the lower limb was abducted or adducted during surgery. Therefore, Seo et al. [20] reported the extramedullary technique assisted by a mechanical axis marker, which could easily identify the center of femoral head and result in 98.2% of patients achieving acceptable alignment in the range of $0° ± 3°$ in the coronal plane. Jung et al. [9] reported that the femoral component coronal alignment was within $90° ± 5°$ in 98.4% of patients using the mechanical axis marker system. This new EM alignment guide system was accurate since it included proximal and distal coronal axis markers to indicate the IFD, which was independent of leg posture. The use of an intramedullary guide for the femur was associated with increased risks of fat embolism, blood loss, postoperative hypoxia, and intraoperative fractures [11, 14, 15]. In addition, the IM femoral alignment system did not always guarantee accuracy of the component position in the TKA. The femoral bowing was a common phenomenon and could affect axial alignment of TKA when IM alignment systems were used, especially in East Asian populations [21, 22]. In these cases, the EM femoral alignment system was a useful alternative surgical option to adjust femoral component alignment [9]. In patients with a more bowed femur, malalignment of lower limb may occur in IM technique, while Computer-assisted techniques could improve the accuracy in both sagittal and coronal planes and EM technique could improve the accuracy in coronal planes. Although the computer-assisted TKA enabled more accurate component alignment [23, 24], the

10-year outcomes of computer-assisted TKA are not superior to that of the conventional technique in function, patient satisfaction and implant survivorship [25, 26].

The opening of the medullary canal using intramedullary jigs was postulated to cause significant blood loss during TKA, although most surgeons have closed the femoral canal opening with bone plug. The application of EM technique was associated with minimal invasiveness since the femoral canal was not breached and the blood loss could be reduced by 145–396 mL [8, 14, 27–29]. Computer-assisted TKA and patient-specific instrumentation (PSI) were recently introduced with the aim of improving alignment without violating the femoral canal [30–32]. TKA using PSI did not result in significantly better femoral component alignment in the sagittal and axial planes than TKA using conventional instrumentation [32]. However, the blood loss was significantly reduced by using the PSI system compared with the IM system for femoral cut. While, the computer-assisted TKA enabled more accurate component alignment. However, it did not reduce the hidden blood loss since the blood loss avoided by not opening the canal might be compensated by greater post tourniquet bleeding due to greater tourniquet time [31].

This present meta-analysis has several limitations. First, only four studies were included and the sample size of the included studies was small, which might have affected our results. Second, we could not perform a valid statistical comparison of the functional outcomes between the two groups. Therefore, further high-quality RCTs with long-term follow-up should be designed to assess radiographic outcomes, knee function, and implant survival rate.

Conclusions

A satisfactory alignment can be obtained with the use of either intramedullary or extramedullary alignment guide system in TKAs. The use of the extramedullary guide results in less blood loss and exhibits a similar operation time as the intramedullary guide.

Abbreviations
CI: Confidence interval; CNKI: China National Knowledge Infrastructure; EM: Extramedullary; IM: Intramedullary; MD: Mean differences; RCTs: Randomized controlled trials; RR: Risk ratio; TKA: Total knee arthroplasty

Acknowledgements
We thank all authors of the included studies and the authors listed have made substantial contributions to the study HXL conceived the study design.

Funding
This work was supported by National Natural Science Foundation of China (81501869).

Authors' contributions
HXL conceived the study design. QT, GZ, and HXL performed the study, collected the data, and contributed to the study design. QT and HXL prepared the manuscript. PS and HZX edited the manuscript. All authors read and approved the final manuscript.

Competing interests
The authors declare that they have no competing interests.

Author details
[1]Department of Orthopaedic Surgery, The Second Affiliated Hospital and Yuying Children's Hospital of Wenzhou Medical University, 109, Xueyuanxi road, 325027 Wenzhou, China. [2]Department of Rehabilitation, The Second Affiliated Hospital and Yuying Children's Hospital of Wenzhou Medical University, 109 Xueyuanxi road, Wenzhou 325027, China.

References
1. Fang DM, Ritter MA, Davis KE. Coronal alignment in total knee arthroplasty: just how important is it? J Arthroplasty. 2009;24:39–43.
2. Fujimoto E, Sasahige Y, Tomita T, Kashiwagi K, Inoue A, Sawa M, et al. Different femorotibial contact on the weight-bearing: midflexion between normal and various aligned knees after total knee arthroplasty. Knee Surg Sports Traumatol Arthrosc. 2015;23:1720–8.
3. Kim YH, Park JW, Kim JS, Park SD. The relationship between the survival of total knee arthroplasty and postoperative coronal, sagittal and rotational alignment of knee prosthesis. Int Orthop. 2014;38:379–85.
4. Ritter MA, Davis KE, Meding JB, Pierson JL, Berend ME, Malinzak RA. The effect of alignment and BMI on failure of total knee replacement. J Bone Joint Surg Am. 2011;93:1588–96.
5. Brys DA, Lombardi Jr AV, Mallory TH, Vaughn BK. A comparison of intramedullary and extramedullary alignment systems for tibial component placement in total knee arthroplasty. Clin Orthop Relat Res. 1991;263:175–9.
6. Dennis DA, Channer M, Susman MH, Stringer EA. Intramedullary versus extramedullary tibial alignment systems in total knee arthroplasty. J Arthroplasty. 1993;8:43–7.
7. Engh GA, Petersen TL. Comparative experience with intramedullary and extramedullary alignment in total knee arthroplasty. J Arthroplasty. 1990;5:1–8.
8. Baldini A, Adravanti P. Less invasive TKA extramedullary femoral reference without avigation. Clin Orthop Relat Res. 2008;466:2694–700.
9. Jung WH, Chun CW, Lee JH, Ha JH, Jeong JH. The accuracy of the extramedullary and intramedullary femoral alignment system in total knee arthroplasty for varus osteoarthritic knee. Knee Surg Sports Traumatol Arthrosc. 2013;21:629–35.
10. Seo JG, Moon YW, Kim YS. A comparison of extramedullary and intramedullary femoral component alignment guide systems in TKA. J Korean Knee Soc. 2006;18:47–54.
11. Laskin RS. Minimally invasive total knee arthroplasty: the results justify its use. Clin Orthop Relat Res. 2005;440:54–9.
12. Liu HC, Kuo FC, Huang CC, Wang JW. Mini-midvastus total knee arthroplasty in patients with severe varus deformity. Orthopedics. 2015;38:112–7.
13. Xu SZ, Lin XJ, Tong X, Wang XW. Minimally invasive midvastus versus standard parapatellar approach in total knee arthroplasty: a meta-analysis of randomized controlled trials. PLoS One. 2014;9:e95311.
14. Kandel L, Vasili C, Kirsh G. Extramedullary femoral alignment instrumentation reduces blood loss after uncemented total knee arthroplasty. J Knee Surg. 2006;19:256–8.
15. Kumar N, Saleh J, Gardiner E, Devadoss VG, Howell FR. Plugging the intramedullary canal of the femur in total knee arthroplasty: reduction in postoperative blood loss. J Arthroplasty. 2000;15:947–9.
16. Ishii Y, Ohmori G, Bechtold JE, Gustilo RB. Extramedullary versus intramedullary alignment guides in total knee arthroplasty. Clin Orthop Relat Res. 1995;318:167–75.
17. Mullaji A, Shetty GM, Kanna R, Sharma A. Variability in the range of inter-anterior superior iliac spine distance and its correlation with femoral head centre. A prospective computed tomography study of 200 adults. Skeletal Radiol. 2010;39:363–8.
18. Matsumoto K, Mori N, Ogawa H, Akiyama H. Accuracy of novel extramedullary femoral alignment guide system in primary total kneearthroplasty. Arch Orthop Trauma Surg. 2015;135:1743–8.
19. Seo JG, Lim JS, Lee HI, Woo KJ. An extramedullary femoral alignment system in total knee arthroplasty using the inter-femoral head center distance. J Korean Orthop Assoc. 2010;45:24293–300.
20. Seo JG, Moon YW, Park SH, Shim JW, Kim SM. An alternative method to create extramedullary references in total knee arthroplasty. Knee Surg Sports Traumatol Arthrosc. 2012;20:1339–48.
21. Kim JM, Hong SH, Kim JM, Lee BS, Kim DE, Kim KA, et al. Femoral shaft bowing in the coronal plane has more significant effect on the coronal alignment of TKA than proximal or distal variations of femoral shape. Knee Surg Sports Traumatol Arthrosc. 2015;23:1936–42.
22. Lasam MP, Lee KJ, Chang CB, Kang YG, Kim TK. Femoral lateral bowing and varus condylar orientation are prevalent and affect axial alignment of TKA in Koreans. Clin Orthop Relat Res. 2013;471:1472–83.
23. Blakeney WG, Khan RJ, Wall SJ. Computer-assisted techniques versus conventional guides for component alignment in total knee arthroplasty: a randomized controlled trial. J Bone Joint Surg Am. 2011;93(15):1377–84.
24. Todesca A, Garro L, Penna M, Bejui-Hugues J.Conventional versus computer-navigated TKA: a prospective randomized study. Knee Surg Sports Traumatol Arthrosc. 2016. [Epub ahead of print].
25. Khuangsirikul S, Lekkreusuwan K, Chotanaphuti T. 10-Year patient satisfaction compared between computer-assisted navigation and conventional techniques in minimally invasive surgery total knee arthroplasty. Comput Assist Surg (Abingdon). 2016;21(1):172–5.
26. Ouanezar H, Franck F, Jacquel A, Pibarot V, Wegrzyn J. Does computer-assisted surgery influence survivorship of cementless total knee arthroplasty in patients with primary osteoarthritis? A 10-year follow-up study. Knee Surg Sports Traumatol Arthrosc. 2016;24(11):3448–56.
27. Dutton AQ, Yeo SJ, Yang KY, Lo NN, Chia KU, Chong HC. Computer-assisted minimally invasive total knee arthroplasty compared with standard total knee arthroplasty. A prospective, randomized study. J Bone Joint Surg Am. 2008;90:2–9.
28. Jeon SH, Kim JH, Lee JM, Seo ES. Efficacy of extramedullary femoral component alignment guide system for blood saving after total knee arthroplasty. Knee Surg Relat Res. 2012;24:99–103.
29. Kalairajah Y, Simpson D, Cossey AJ, Verrall GM, Spriggins AJ. Blood loss after total knee replacement: effects of computer-assisted surgery. J Bone Joint Surg (Br). 2005;87:1480–2.
30. Conteduca F, Iorio R, Mazza D, Ferretti A. Patient-specific instruments in total knee arthroplasty. Int Orthop. 2014;38:259–65.
31. Singla A, Malhotra R, Kumar V, Lekha C, Karthikeyan G, Malik V. A Randomized controlled study to compare the total and hidden blood loss in computer-assisted surgery and conventional surgical technique of total knee replacement. Clin Orthop Surg. 2015;7:211–6.
32. Yan CH, Chiu KY, Ng FY, Chan PK, Fang CX. Comparison between patient-specific instruments and conventional instruments and computer navigation in total knee arthroplasty: a randomized controlled trial. Knee Surg Sports Traumatol Arthrosc. 2015;23:3637–45.

4

Comparison of local infiltration analgesia and sciatic nerve block for pain control after total knee arthroplasty

Li-ping Ma[1], Ying-mei Qi[1] and Dong-xu Zhao[2*]

Abstract

Background: This meta-analysis aimed to perform a meta-analysis to evaluate the efficiency and safety between local infiltration analgesia (LIA) and sciatic nerve block (SNB) when combined with femoral nerve block (FNB) after total knee arthroplasty (TKA).

Methods: A systematic search was performed in MEDLINE (1966-2017.04), PubMed (1966-2017.04), Embase (1980-2017.04), ScienceDirect (1985-2017.04), and the Cochrane Library. Only high-quality studies were selected. Meta-analysis was performed using Stata 11.0 software.

Results: Four randomized controlled trials (RCTs) and two non-randomized controlled trials (non-RCTs), including 273 patients met the inclusion criteria. The present meta-analysis indicated that there were significant differences between groups in terms of visual analogue scale (VAS) score at 12 h (SMD = −0.303, 95% CI −0.543 to −0.064, P = 0.013), VAS score at 24 h (SMD = −0.395, 95% CI −0.636 to −0.154, P = 0.001), morphine equivalent consumption at 24 h (SMD = −0.395, 95% CI −0.636 to −0.154, P = 0.001), and incidence of nausea (RD = 0.233, 95% CI 0.107 to 0.360, P = 0.000) and vomiting (RD = 0.131, 95% CI 0.025 to 0.237, P = 0.015).

Conclusion: FNB-combined SNB provides superior pain relief and less morphine consumption within the first 24 h compared FNB-combined LIA in total knee arthroplasty. In addition, there were fewer side effects associated with SNB. Because the sample size and the number of included studies were limited, a multicenter RCT is needed to identify the effects of the two kinds of methods and further work must include range of motion analyses and functional test.

Keywords: Sciatic nerve block, Local infiltration analgesia, Total knee arthroplasty, Pain control, Meta-analysis

Background

Total knee arthroplasty (TKA) is a common procedure for improving mobility and quality of life in patients with osteoarthritis or rheumatoid arthritis. However, it is reported that 30–60% of patients suffer moderate to severe postoperative pain [1]. Adequate and effective pain relief is requested, mainly to improve patient satisfaction, to expedite mobilization and rehabilitation, to decrease the duration of hospital stay, and consequently

to lower the risk of deep vein thrombosis or nosocomial infections [2–4]. Femoral nerve block (FNB) could provide effective analgesia and is a well-accepted method for regional anesthesia following TKA [5, 6]; however, some patients still experienced significant postoperative pain. Compared with FNB, local infiltration anesthesia (LIA) is an alternative and cost-effective anesthetic technique which has been promoted for a few decades and shows excellent outcome for pain relief after TKA [7, 8]. Previous studies have reported that LIA was comparable to epidural anesthesia and FNB for analgesic effect in total joint arthroplasty. LIA is considered as a promising method with few side effects and prospective of early

* Correspondence: 2556574588@qq.com
[2]Department of Orthopedics, China-Japan Union Hospital of Jilin University, 126 Xiantai Street, Changchun, Jilin, People's Republic of China
Full list of author information is available at the end of the article

mobilization without weakness of quadriceps muscle strength [9, 10]. Therefore, LIA is a major choice for supplementing FNB after TKA. However, fundamental research has shown that knee joint is also innervated by sciatic nerves; thus, FNB combined sciatic nerves block (SNB) has become growing practice to provide improved pain relief.

However, there is no consensus regarding which anesthesia method is preferable to relieve pain as an adjunct to FNB. Thus, a meta-analysis of randomized controlled trials (RCTs) was conducted to compare the efficacy and safety of pain control with SNB versus LIA when combined with FNB after TKA.

Methods

Search strategy

Potentially relevant studies were identified from electronic databases including MEDLINE (1966-2017.4), PubMed (1966-2017.4), Embase (1980-2017.4), ScienceDirect (1985-2017.4), and the Cochrane Library. The following keywords were used in combination with the Boolean operators AND or OR: "total knee replacement OR arthroplasty," "femoral nerve block," "sciatic nerves block," "local infiltration anesthesia," and "pain control." The bibliographies of the retrieved trials and other relevant publications were cross-referenced to identify additional articles. We placed no restrictions on the publication language. The search process was performed as presented in Fig. 1.

Inclusion and exclusion criteria

Studies were considered eligible if they met the following criteria: (1) Published clinical randomized control trails (RCTs) and non-RCTs; (2) Patients undergoing TKA, experiment group received SNB-combined FNB for pain control and control group received LIA-combined FNB; (3) Reported surgical outcomes, including visual analogue scale (VAS) scores, morphine consumption, length of stay, and postoperative adverse effects including the risk of nausea and vomiting. Studies would be excluded from present meta-analysis for incomplete data, case reports, conference abstract, or review articles.

Selection criteria

Two reviewers independently review the abstract of the potential studies. After an initial decision, full text of the studies that potentially met the inclusion

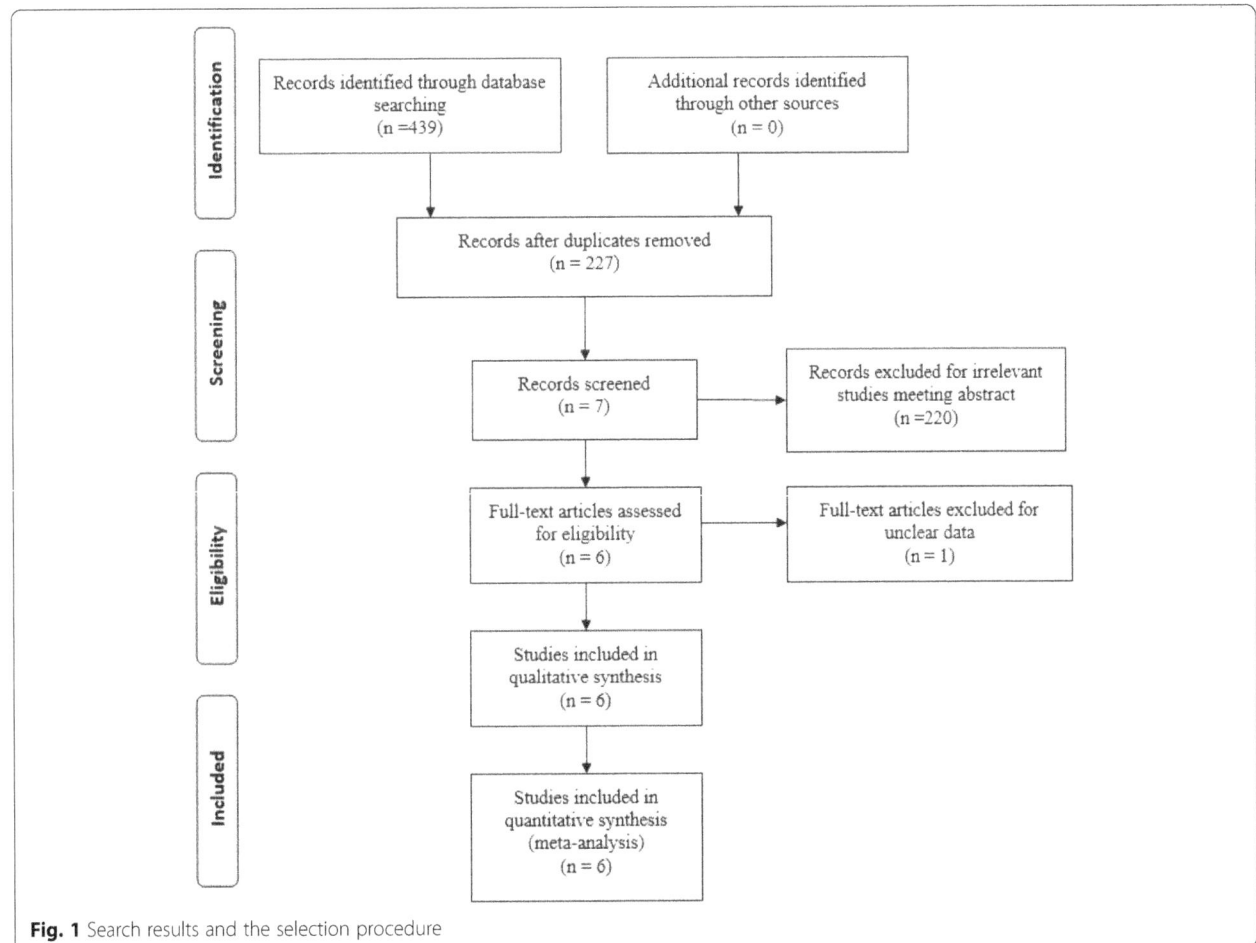

Fig. 1 Search results and the selection procedure

Table 1 Trials characteristics

Studies	Reference type	Cases (SNB/LIA)	Mean age (SNB/LIA)	Female patient (SNB/LIA)	Anesthesia	Drug dose of FNB	Drug dose of SNB	Drug dose of LIA	Concomitant Pain	Follow-up
Tanikawa 2014 [11]	RCT	23/23	72/71	19/20	General anesthesia	20 ml of 0.375% ropivacaine	20 ml of 0.375% ropivacaine	200 mg of ropivacaine and 0.5 ml of adrenaline	IV ketorolac 30 mg, ketoprofen 100 mg, or diclofenac 75 mg	3 months
Gi 2014 [13]	RCT	24/25	78/77	21/24	General anesthesia	20 ml 0.375% ropivacaine	20 ml 0.375% ropivacaine	60 ml 0.5% ropivacaine with 0.3 mg epinephrine	400 mg celecoxib, 20 mg oxycontin, and a 6 mg scopolamine patch topically	1 month
Safa 2014 [12]	RCT	33/32	61/61	18/15	Spinal anesthesia	20 mL of 0.5% ropivacaine	20 mL of 0.5% ropivacaine	50 mL of 0.2% ropivacaine	Celecoxib 200 mg, gabapentin 200 mg and acetaminophen 1 g	1.5–3 months
Nagafuchi 2015 [14]	RCT	17/16	72/73	15/13	General anesthesia	20 mL of 0.375% ropivacaine	20 ml of 0.375% ropivacaine	100 mL of 0.2% ropivacaine	Celecoxib 200 mg, gabapentin 200 mg and acetaminophen 1 g	1 months
Cip 2016 [15]	Non-RCT	16/18	73.4/71.8	12/11	Spinal or general anesthesia	0.2% ropivacaine (4 ml/h)	20 ml ropivacaine 0.2%	0.33% ropivacaine (5 mL/h)	Celecoxib and Oxycodone	NS
Aikawa 2016 [16]	Non-RCT	23/23	72/71	19/20	general anesthesia	20 ml 0.375% ropivacaine	20 ml 0.375% ropivacaine	20 mL of 0.375% levobupivacaine	NS	6 months

SNB sciatic nerve block, *LIA* local infiltration of analgesia, *IV* intravenous, *NS* not stated

corresponding author. Following data was extracted: first author names, published year, study design, comparable baseline, anesthesia methods, and dosage and type of anesthetic drug. Outcome parameters included VAS scores at different periods, the cumulative morphine consumption, length of stay, and postoperative adverse effects. Other relevant data was also extracted from individual studies.

Quality assessment

Quality assessment of included studies was performed by two reviewers independently. Modified Jadad score (7-point scale) which was based on Cochrane Handbook for Systematic Reviews of Interventions is used for assessment of RCTs. Studies which scores greater than four points was considered high quality. We conducted "risk of bias" table including the following key points: random sequence generation, allocation concealment, blinding, incomplete outcome data, free of selective reporting, and other bias. The Methodological Index for Non-Randomized Studies (MINORS) scale was used to assess non-RCTs with scores ranging from 0 to 24. A consensus is reached through a discussion.

Data analysis and statistical methods

All calculation was carried out by Stata 11.0 (The Cochrane Collaboration, Oxford, UK). Statistical heterogeneity was assessed based on the value of P and I^2 using standard chi-square test. When $I^2 > 50\%$, $P < 0.1$ was considered to be significant heterogeneity; random-effect model was performed for meta-analysis. Otherwise, fixed-effect model was used. If possible, sensibility analysis is conducted to explore the origins of heterogeneity. The results of dichotomous outcomes were expressed as risk difference (RD) with a 95% confidence intervals (CIs). For continuous various outcomes, mean difference (MD) and

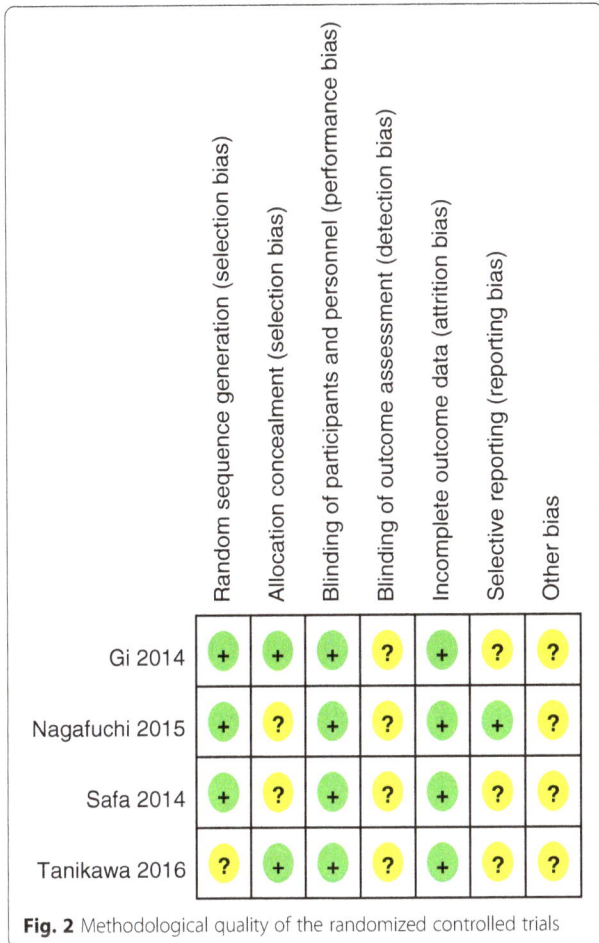

Fig. 2 Methodological quality of the randomized controlled trials

criteria were reviewed and final decision was made. A senior reviewer is consulted in case of disagreement.

Date extraction

Two reviewers independently extracted the relevant data from the included studies. Details of incomplete data of included articles are received by consulting the

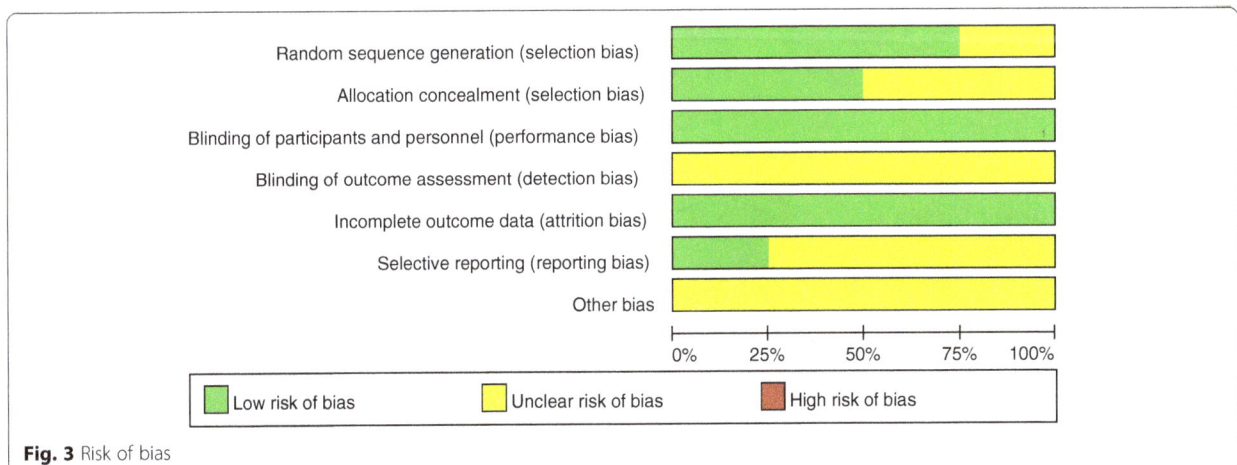

Fig. 3 Risk of bias

Table 2 Methodological quality of the non-randomized controlled trials

Quality assessment for non-randomized trials	Cip 2016 [15]	Aikawa 2016 [16]
A clearly stated aim	2	2
Inclusion of consecutive patients	2	2
Prospective data collection	2	2
Endpoints appropriate to the aim of the study	2	2
Unbiased assessment of the study endpoint	0	0
A follow-up period appropriate to the aims of study	2	2
Less than 5% loss to follow-up	2	2
Prospective calculation of the sample size	0	2
An adequate control group	2	2
Contemporary groups	0	1
Baseline equivalence of groups	2	2
Adequate statistical analyses	2	2
Total score	18	21

standard mean difference (SMD) with a 95% confidence intervals (CIs) were applied for assessment.

Results

Search result

A total of 439 studies were preliminarily reviewed. By reading the title and abstracts, 433 reports were excluded from current meta-analysis followed inclusion criteria. No gray reference was obtained. Finally, four RCTs [11–14] and two non-RCTs [15, 16] which had been published between 2014 and 2016 were enrolled in present meta-analysis and includes 136 participates in the SNB groups and 137 patients in the LIA groups.

Risk of bias assessment

Demographic characteristics, the details about the included studies are summarized in Table 1. Modified Jadad score which was based on Cochrane Handbook for Systematic Reviews of Interventions is used for assessment of RCTs (Fig. 2). All RCTs [11–14] provide clear inclusion and exclusion criteria and suggest a methodology of randomization, two [12–14] of which described that randomization algorithm was generated

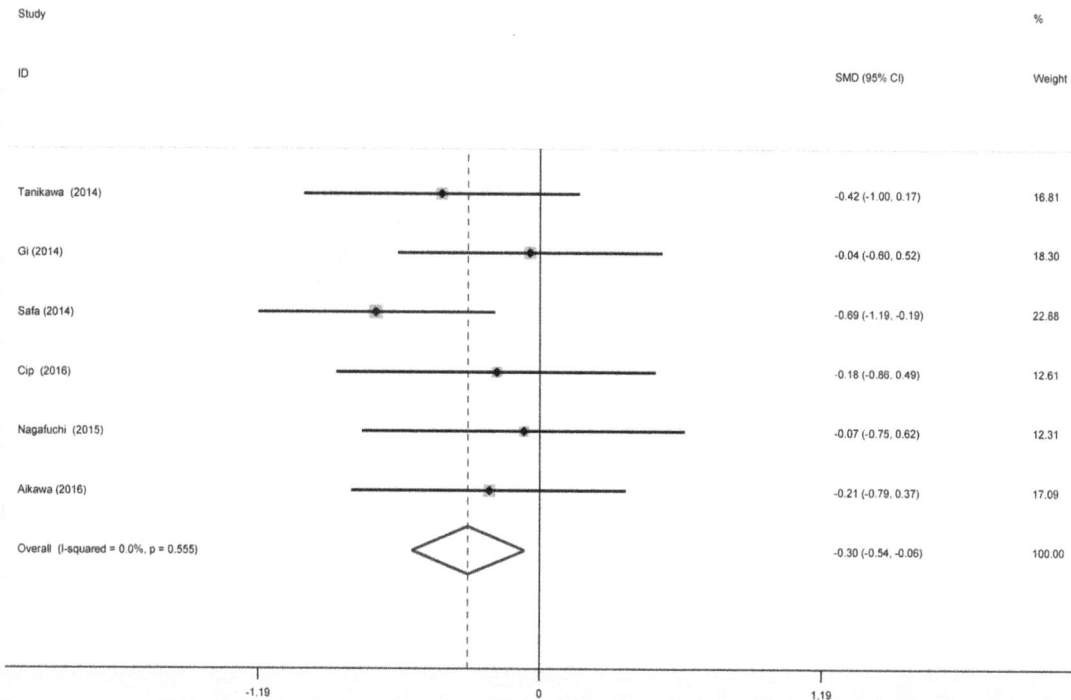

Fig. 4 Forest plot diagram showing VAS scores at 12 h following TKA

from computer. Two of them [11, 13] stated alloca-tion concealment was achieved by sealed envelope. Double blinding was provided in all RCTs. None of them had stated assessors were blinded. Each risk of bias item is presented as the percentage across all included studies, which indicates the proportion of different levels of risk of bias for each item (Fig. 3). All RCTs demonstrated complete outcome data. The MINORS scale was used to assess non-RCTs by assigning scores ranging from 0 to 24 (Table 2).

Study characteristics

The sample size of the included studies ranged from 33 to 65. All of them compared efficiency and safety be-tween SNB and LIA as a supplement for pain control in TKA. Experimental groups received SNB-combined FNB, while control groups received LIA-combined FNB. There is variation dosage and type of anesthetic drugs in included studies. Four studies [11, 13–15] applied gen-eral anesthesia and one [12] applied spinal anesthesia. Five [11–15] studies reported that surgical procedure was performed by same surgeons. All studies reported that postoperative medication was used for concomitant pain management. All of them suggest the outcomes for at least 95% of the patients. The follow-up period ranged from 1 to 3 months.

Outcomes for meta-analysis

VAS scores at 12 h

Six studies [11–16] reported VAS scores at 12 h fol-lowing TKA. There was no significant heterogeneity ($\chi2 = 3.96$, df = 5, $I^2 = 0\%$, $P = 0.555$); therefore, a fixed-effects model was used. The result of meta-analysis showed that there was significant difference between the SNB and LIA groups regarding the VAS scores at 12 h (SMD = –0.303, 95% CI –0.543 to –0.064, $P = 0.013$; Fig. 4).

VAS scores at 24 h

Six studies [11–16] reported VAS scores at 24 h following TKA. No statistical heterogeneity was observed in present meta-analysis ($\chi2 = 5.53$, df = 5, $I^2 = 9.6\%$, $P = 0.355$); therefore, a fixed-effects model was applied. We found that there was significant dif-ference between the SNB and LIA groups regarding the VAS scores at 24 h (SMD = –0.395, 95% CI –0.636 to –0.154, $P = 0.001$; Fig. 5).

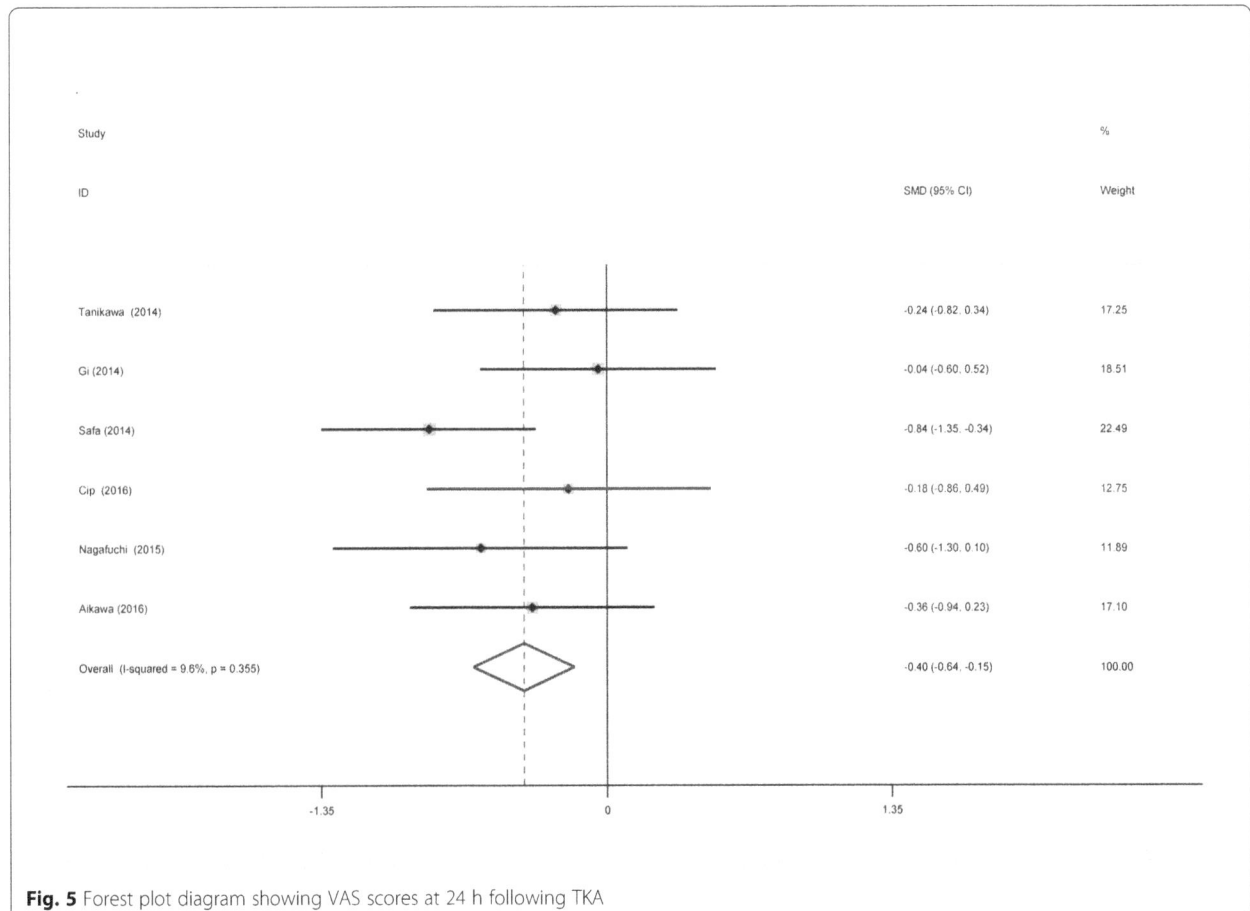

Fig. 5 Forest plot diagram showing VAS scores at 24 h following TKA

VAS scores at 48 h

Six reports [11–16] showed VAS scores at 48 h following TKA. There was no significant heterogeneity and a fixed-effects model was performed ($\chi2 = 5.06$, df = 5, $I^2 = 1.2\%$, $P = 0.408$). Current meta-analysis indicated that no significant difference was found in terms of VAS scores at 48 h (SMD = –0.137, 95% CI –0.375 to 0.102, $P = 0.262$; Fig. 6).

Morphine consumption at 24 h

Morphine consumption at postoperative 24 h was presented in four studies [11–13, 16] following TKA. There was no significant heterogeneity ($\chi2 = 0.78$, df = 3, $I^2 = 0\%$, $P = 0.854$) and a fixed-effects model was used. The present meta-analysis showed that there was significant difference between the SNB and LIA groups in terms of morphine consumption at postoperative 24 h (SMD = –0.330, 95% CI –0.606 to –0.055, $P = 0.019$; Fig. 7).

Morphine consumption at 48 h

Four studies [11–13, 16] provided morphine consumption at postoperative 48 h following TKA. No significant heterogeneity was found ($\chi2 = 1.25$, df = 3, $I^2 = 0\%$, $P = 0.742$); therefore, a fixed-effects model was used. Meta-

analysis revealed that there was no significant difference between the SNB and LIA groups in terms of morphine consumption at postoperative 48 h (SMD = –0.063, 95% CI –0.337 to 0.210, $P = 0.649$; Fig. 8).

Length of hospital stay (LOS)

Six studies [11–16] reported the length of hospital stay between groups. No significant heterogeneity was identified in the pooled results; therefore, a fixed-effects model was used ($\chi2 = 0.24$, df = 5, $I^2 = 0\%$, $P = 0.999$). There was no significant difference between the two groups in LOS (SMD = –0.118, 95% CI –0.356 to 0.120, $P = 0.330$; Fig. 9).

The occurrence of nausea

The occurrence of nausea was reported in five studies [11, 13–16]. No significant heterogeneity among these studies was found; therefore, a fixed-effects model was used ($\chi2 = 2.99$, df = 4, $I^2 = 0\%$, $P = 0.560$). There was significant difference between the two groups in the incidence of nausea (RD = 0.233, 95% CI 0.107 to 0.360, $P = 0.000$; Fig. 10).

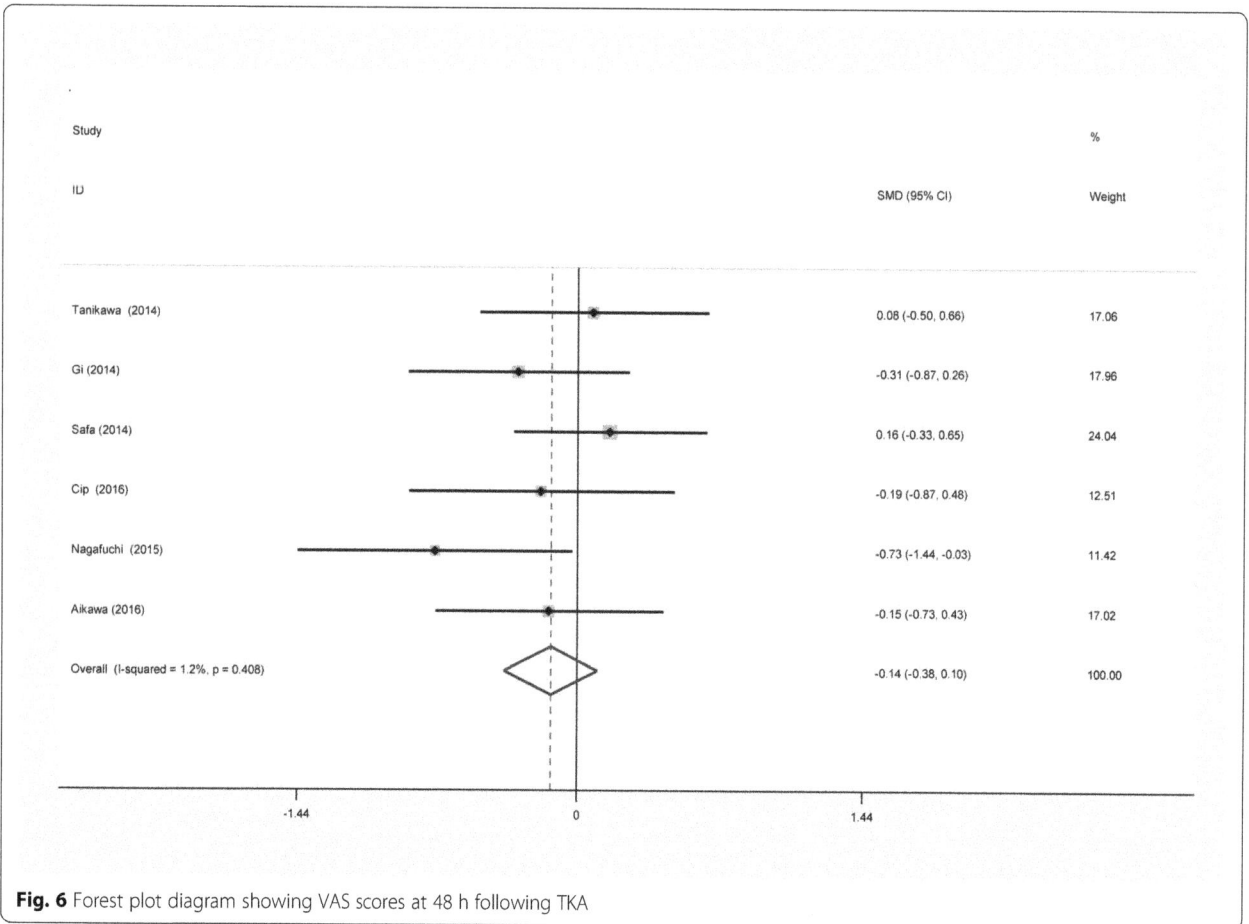

Fig. 6 Forest plot diagram showing VAS scores at 48 h following TKA

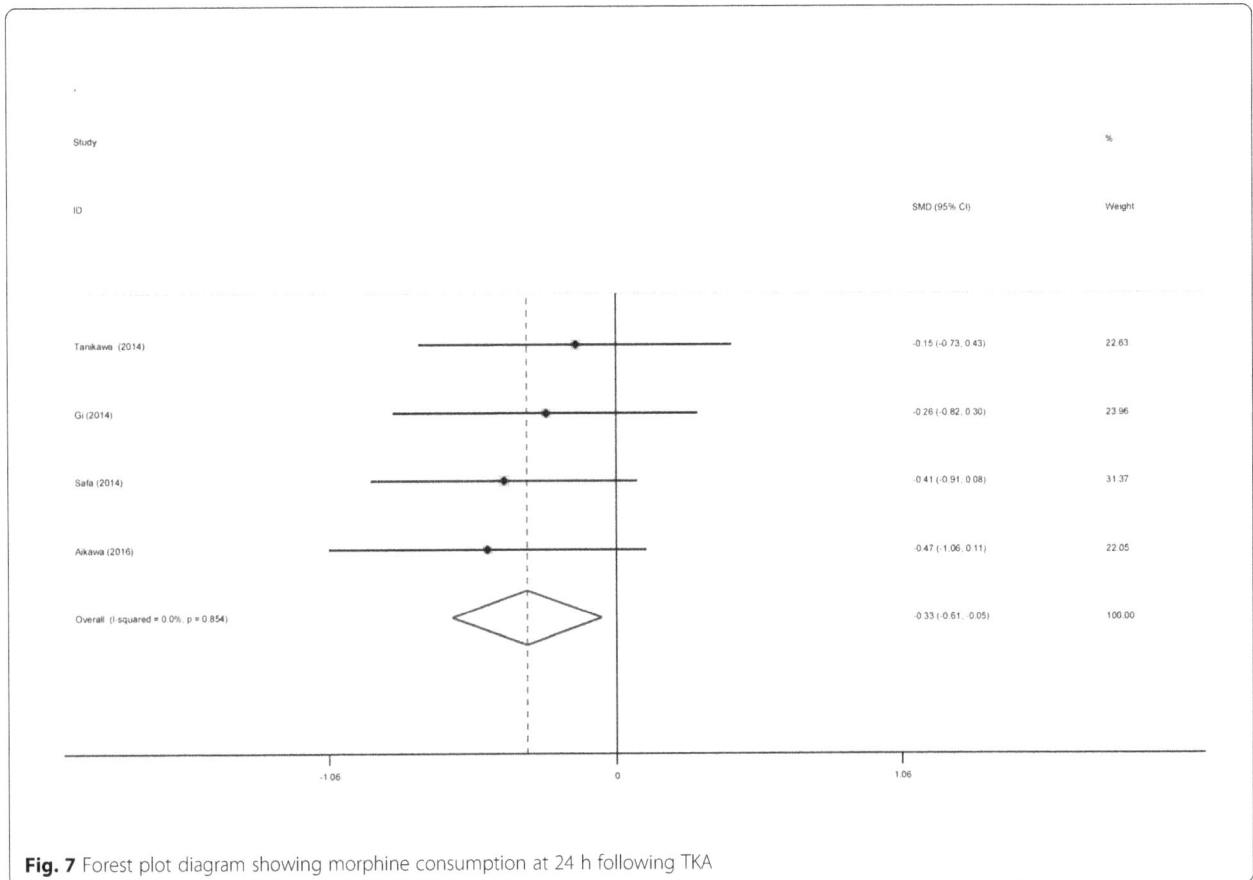

Fig. 7 Forest plot diagram showing morphine consumption at 24 h following TKA

The occurrence of vomiting

Five studies [11, 13–16] reported the incidence of vomiting. We found no statistical heterogeneity and a fixed-effects model was applied ($\chi2 = 2.89$, df = 4, $I^2 = 0\%$, $P = 0.577$). Present meta-analysis showed significant difference regarding the frequency of vomiting between groups (RD = 0.131, 95% CI 0.025 to 0.237, $P = 0.015$; Fig. 11).

Discussion

This is the first systematic review and meta-analysis to compare the efficiency and safety of combined femoral and SNB versus combined femoral with LIA for pain control in TKA. The most important finding of the present meta-analysis was that SNB-combined FNB was associated with significantly decreased pain scores at 12- to 48-h point and reduced opioids consumption at 24-h point following TKA. In addition, there was a decreased risk of complications in the SNB groups.

With the aging population, the occurrence of knee osteoarthritis is increasing, and TKA is a popular treatment. However, pain control following TKA can be very challenging. Optimal analgesia may shorten hospital stays and result in decreased risks of deep vein thrombosis (DVT) and pulmonary embolism (PE).

Furthermore, early rehabilitation exercise contributes to a satisfied sufficient functional recovery. Postoperative pain control is an interesting topic in orthopedic surgery. Multiple perioperative pain management strategies have been implemented following TKA, including femoral nerve block, spinal analgesia, and periarticular or intra-articular injection of anesthetics.

Sciatic nerve block is performed as an adjunct to femoral nerve block in TKA. Several articles have reported its efficiency for pain control compared FNB alone in TKA. Cook et al. [17] suggest that the combined femoral and sciatic provides superior pain management in the early postoperative period after TKA. Pham et al. [18] showed that the combination of continuous femoral and SNB improves analgesia and decreasing opioids consumption and risk of complications.

Quadriceps strength is a major concern following TKA, as quadriceps function is closely associated with postoperative walking and stair climbing ability. The possible etiologies may be muscle strength reduction before operation, patient positioning during operation, long tourniquet times, and inadequate postoperative pain control. Peripheral nerve injury is iatrogenic factor which may cause an increased risk

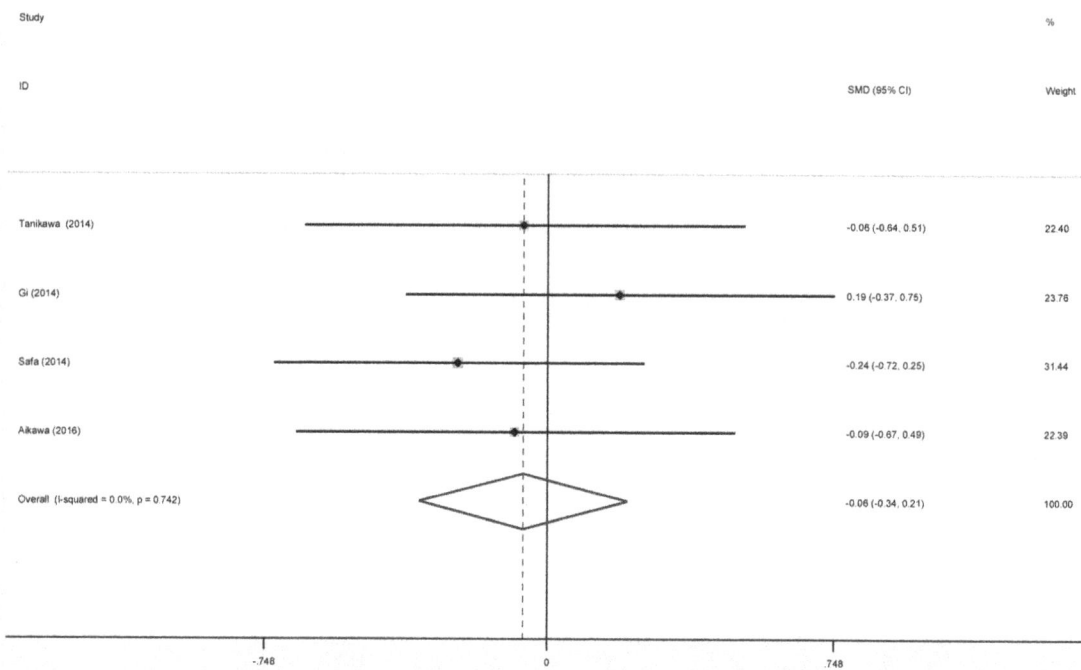

Fig. 8 Forest plot diagram showing morphine consumption at 48 h following TKA

of falls. It has been reported that the rate of peripheral nerve injury is 2.9/10,000 for FNB and 2.4/10,000 for SNB, and the incidence of permanent nerve damage is 1.5/10,000 [19]. Sciatic nerve injury is also a generally known complication after TKA, with an incidence of 1.3 to 2.2% [20, 21]. However, some degree of quadriceps weakness was also observed in LIA group. The data were not sufficient for a meta-analysis; larger sample size of RCTs was needed to reach a conclusion.

LIA was alternative choice to achieve comparable pain control. It was more and more popular for the ease of preform and less motor block. Many kinds of local anesthetics have been applied in TKA. Long-acting local anesthetics including ropivacaine and levobupivacaine are commonly used. In present meta-analysis, all included articles used local ropivacaine for peripheral nerve block whose concentration ranged from 0.2 to 0.5%. Five used ropivacaine for local infiltration anesthesia and one applied levobupivacaine. The present meta-analysis indicated that SNB-combined FNB had an analgesic effect that was superior to that of LIA-combined FNB at 24 and 48 h following TKA. Considering that only six studies were

included in present meta-analysis, we did not perform a subgroup analysis for types of anesthetics. Further investigation was necessary.

TKA is usually associated with severe pain in 60% and moderate pain in 30% of patients, especially in the first 48 h, and after postoperative mobilization, pain remains intense [22]. Additional opioids, including oral and patient-controlled analgesia (PCA) administration, were applied as concomitant pain control. Opioid consumption is considered an objective method to measure pain. Opioid-related adverse effects, such as nausea, vomiting, respiratory depression, and pruritus, were reported in previous studies [23, 24]. Besides the side effects described above, drug dependence is also an important issue that should be considered. Minimizing opioid consumption would improve patient satisfaction and expedite mobilization and rehabilitation. The present meta-analysis showed that there was a decreased morphine consumption in the SNB groups compared to LIA groups at postoperative 24 h; however, no significant difference was found between groups regarding the morphine consumption at postoperative 48 h.

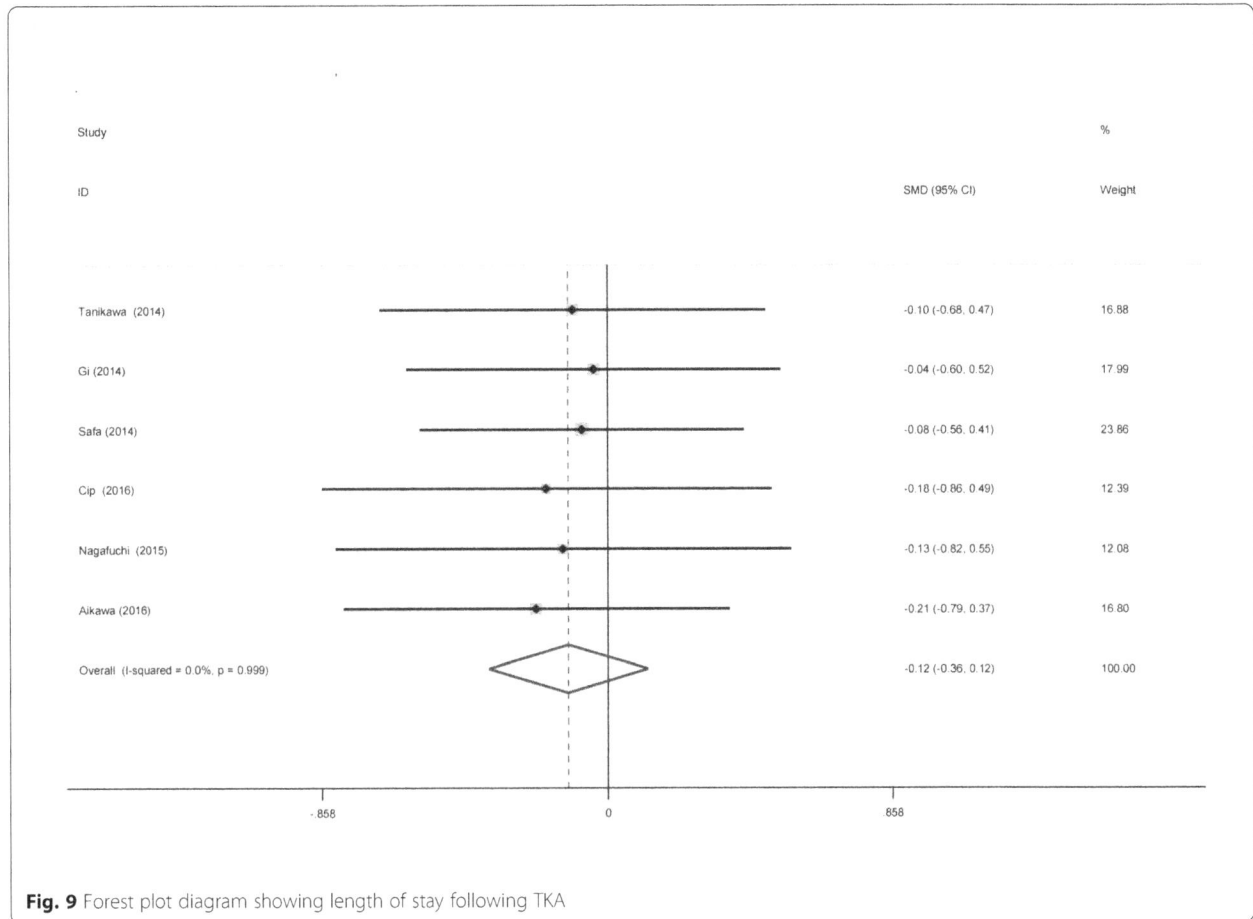

Fig. 9 Forest plot diagram showing length of stay following TKA

Nausea and vomiting are common side effects that are frequently associated with PCA of morphine. Sufficient anesthetic techniques can reduce morphine consumption and subsequently decrease the risk of complications. The present meta-analysis showed that there was a decreased risk of nausea and vomiting in SNB groups compared controls. Considering that only six studies were included in our meta-analysis, we did not perform investigation on dose dependence. Large sample sizes from high-quality RCTs are needed.

There were several potential limitations that should be noted. (1) Only six studied were included in present meta-analysis; although all of them are recently published studies, the sample size is relatively small. We also included non-RCTs; thus, the evidence level would be decreased. (2) Some methodological weakness existed in some included studies which generated potential bias. (3) Functional outcome is an important parameter; due to the insufficiency of relevant data, we fail to perform a meta-analysis; (4) Dose of anesthetics is varied, and concomitant pain management regime differs from each other, which may influence the results of the meta-analysis. (5)

Subgroup analysis was not performed due to the small included studies. (6) The duration of follow-up is relatively short which leads to underestimating complications. (7) Publication bias in present meta-analysis may influence the results.

Despite the limitations above, this is the first meta-analysis from recently published studies to assess the efficiency and safety between LIA and SNB when combined with FNB following TKA. Long term of high-quality RCTs were needed to explore the functional outcome of the knees and other adverse effects.

Conclusion

FNB-combined SNB provides superior pain relief and less morphine consumption within the first 24 h compared FNB-combined LIA in total knee arthroplasty. In addition, there were fewer side effects associated with SNB. Because the sample size and the number of included studies were limited, a multicenter RCT is needed to identify the effects of the two kinds of methods and further work must include range of motion analyses and functional test.

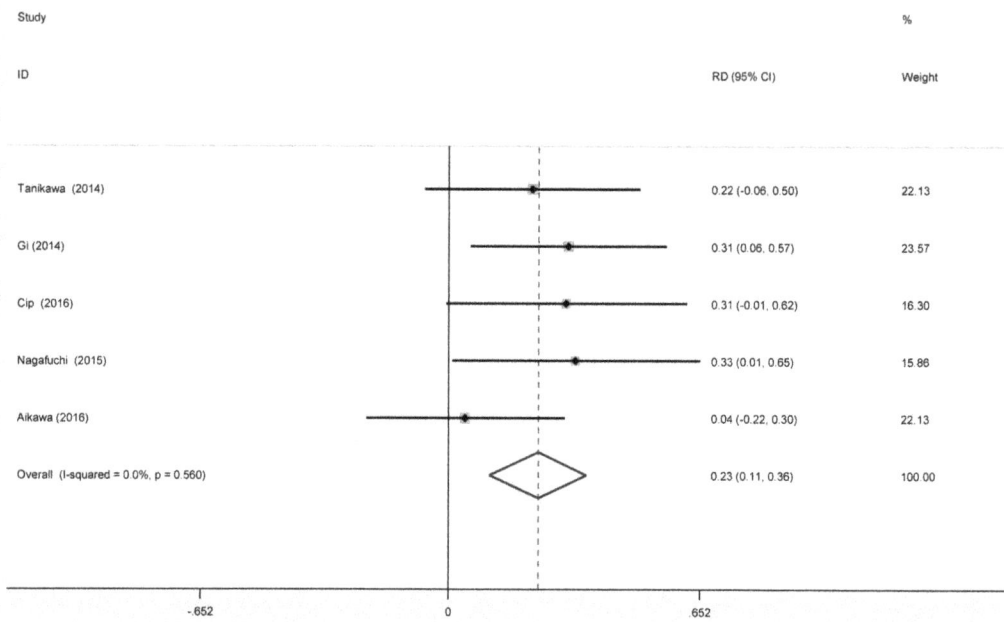

Fig. 10 Forest plot diagram showing incidence of nausea following TKA

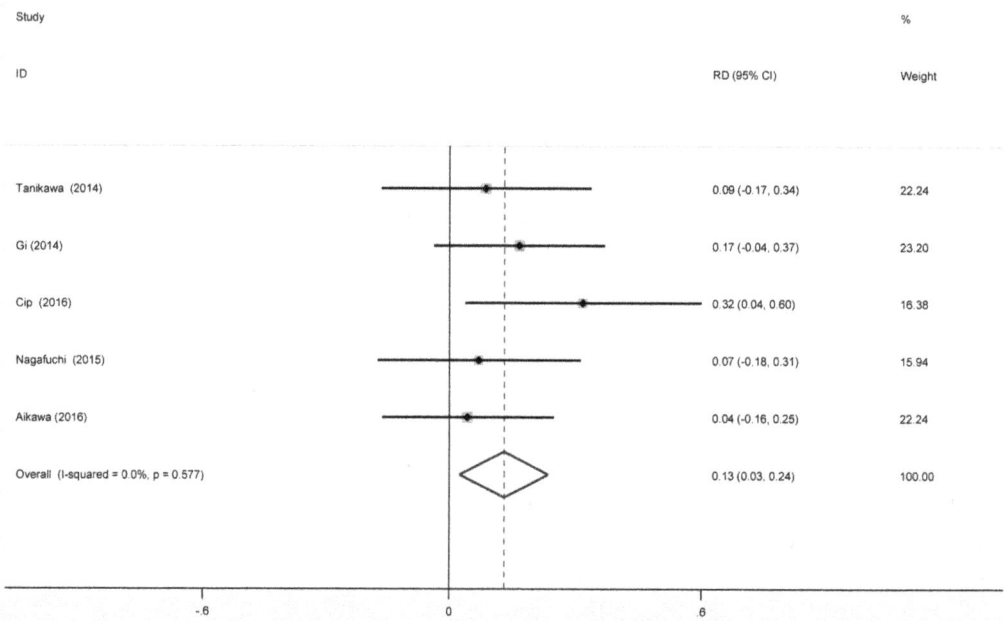

Fig. 11 Forest plot diagram showing incidence of vomiting following TKA

Abbreviations
LIA: Local infiltration analgesia; RCT: Randomized controlled trials; SNB: Sciatic nerve block; TKA: Total knee arthroplasty; VAS: Visual analogue scale

Acknowledgements
Thank you Dong-xu Zhao for the document printing.

Funding
None.

Authors' contributions
LM and YQ contributed to the data collections and revised the manuscript and writing. DZ contributed to the study design. All authors read and approved the final manuscript.

Authors' information
None.

Competing interests
The authors declare that they have no competing interests.

Author details
[1]China-Japan Union Hospital of Jilin University, Changchun, People's Republic of China. [2]Department of Orthopedics, China-Japan Union Hospital of Jilin University, 126 Xiantai Street, Changchun, Jilin, People's Republic of China.

References
1. Albrecht E, Guyen O, Jacot-Guillarmod A, Kirkham KR. The analgesic efficacy of local infiltration analgesia vs femoral nerve block after total knee arthroplasty: a systematic review and meta-analysis. Br J Anaesth. 2016;116(5):597–609.
2. Tripuraneni KR, Woolson ST, Giori NJ. Local infiltration analgesia in TKA patients reduces length of stay and postoperative pain scores. Orthopedics. 2011;34(3):173.
3. Mullaji A, Kanna R, Shetty GM, Chavda V, Singh DP. Efficacy of periarticular injection of bupivacaine, fentanyl, and methylprednisolone in total knee arthroplasty:a prospective, randomized trial. J Arthroplast. 2010;25(6):851–7.
4. Duellman TJ, Gaffigan C, Milbrandt JC, Allan DG. Multi-modal, pre-emptive analgesia decreases the length of hospital stay following total joint arthroplasty. Orthopedics. 2009;32(3):167.
5. Choy WS, Lee SK, Kim KJ, Kam BS, Yang DS, Bae KW. Two continuous femoral nerve block strategies after TKA. Knee Surg Sports Traumatol Arthrosc. 2011;19(11):1901–8.
6. Wang D, Yang Y, Li Q, Tang SL, Zeng WN, Xu J, Xie TH, Pei FX, Yang L, Li LL, et al. Adductor canal block versus femoral nerve block for total knee arthroplasty: a meta-analysis of randomized controlled trials. Sci Rep. 2017;7:40721.
7. Affas F, Nygards EB, Stiller CO, Wretenberg P, Olofsson C. Pain control after total knee arthroplasty: a randomized trial comparing local infiltration anesthesia and continuous femoral block. Acta Orthop. 2011;82(4):441–7.
8. Tran J, Schwarzkopf R. Local infiltration anesthesia with steroids in total knee arthroplasty: a systematic review of randomized control trials. J Orthop. 2015;12 Suppl 1:S44–50.
9. Hofstad JK, Winther SB, Rian T, Foss OA, Husby OS, Wik TS. Perioperative local infiltration anesthesia with ropivacaine has no effect on postoperative pain after total hip arthroplasty. Acta Orthop. 2015;86(6):654–8.
10. Thorsell M, Holst P, Hyldahl HC, Weidenhielm L. Pain control after total knee arthroplasty: a prospective study comparing local infiltration anesthesia and epidural anesthesia. Orthopedics. 2010;33(2):75–80.
11. Tanikawa H, Sato T, Nagafuchi M, Takeda K, Oshida J, Okuma K. Comparison of local infiltration of analgesia and sciatic nerve block in addition to femoral nerve block for total knee arthroplasty. J Arthroplast. 2014;29(12):2462–7.
12. Safa B, Gollish J, Haslam L, McCartney CJ. Comparing the effects of single shot sciatic nerve block versus posterior capsule local anesthetic infiltration on analgesia and functional outcome after total knee arthroplasty: a prospective, randomized, double-blinded, controlled trial. J Arthroplast. 2014;29(6):1149–53.
13. Gi E, Yamauchi M, Yamakage M, Kikuchi C, Shimizu H, Okada Y, Kawamura S, Suzuki T. Effects of local infiltration analgesia for posterior knee pain after total knee arthroplasty: comparison with sciatic nerve block. J Anesth. 2014; 28(5):696–701.
14. Nagafuchi M, Sato T, Sakuma T, Uematsu A, Hayashi H, Tanikawa H, Okuma K, Hashiuchi A, Oshida J, Morisaki H. Femoral nerve block-sciatic nerve block vs. femoral nerve block-local infiltration analgesia for total knee arthroplasty: a randomized controlled trial. BMC Anesthesiol. 2015;15:182.
15. Cip J, Erb-Linzmeier H, Stadlbauer P, Bach C, Martin A, Germann R. Continuous intra-articular local anesthetic drug instillation versus discontinuous sciatic nerve block after total knee arthroplasty. J Clin Anesth. 2016;35:543–50.
16. Aikawa K, Hashimoto T, Itosu Y, Fujii T, Horiguchi T, Amenomori H, Morimoto Y. Comparison of the effect of periarticular infiltration analgesia versus sciatic nerve block for total knee arthroplasty. Masui. 2016;65(1):50–5.
17. Cook P, Stevens J, Gaudron C. Comparing the effects of femoral nerve block versus femoral and sciatic nerve block on pain and opiate consumption after total knee arthroplasty. J Arthroplast. 2003;18(5):583–6.
18. Pham Dang C, Gautheron E, Guilley J, Fernandez M, Waast D, Volteau C, Nguyen JM, Pinaud M. The value of adding sciatic block to continuous femoral block for analgesia after total knee replacement. Reg Anesth Pain Med. 2005;30(2):128–33.
19. Auroy Y, Benhamou D, Bargues L, Ecoffey C, Falissard B, Mercier FJ, Bouaziz H, Samii K. Major complications of regional anesthesia in France: the SOS regional anesthesia hotline service. Anesthesiology. 2002;97(5):1274–80.
20. Schinsky MF, Macaulay W, Parks ML, Kiernan H, Nercessian OA. Nerve injury after primary total knee arthroplasty. J Arthroplast. 2001;16(8):1048–54.
21. Horlocker TT, Cabanela ME, Wedel DJ. Does postoperative epidural analgesia increase the risk of peroneal nerve palsy after total knee arthroplasty? Anesth Analg. 1994;79(3):495–500.
22. Strassels SA, Chen C, Carr DB. Postoperative analgesia: economics, resource use, and patient satisfaction in an urban teaching hospital. Anesth Analg. 2002;94(1):130–7. table of contents.
23. Khansari M, Sohrabi M, Zamani F. The usage of opioids and their adverse effects in gastrointestinal practice: a review. Middle East J Dig Dis. 2013;5(1):5–16.
24. Wanderer JP, Nathan N. Opioids and adverse effects: more than just opium dreams. Anesth Analg. 2016;123(4):805.

5

Analysis of factors that affect the precision of the radiographic lateral femoral bowing angle using a three-dimensional computed tomography-based modelling technique

Ye-Ran Li, Yu-Hang Gao, Xin Qi[*], Jian-Guo Liu, Lu Ding, Chen Yang, Zheng Zhang and Shu-Qiang Li

Abstract

Background: Precise measurement of lateral femoral bowing is important to achieve postoperative lower limb alignment. We aimed to investigate factors that affect the precision of the radiographic lateral femoral bowing (RLFB) angle using three-dimensional (3D) models and whether the angle affects surgery design.

Methods: Forty femurs in total were divided into two groups based on their preoperative RLFB angle. The flexion contracture angle, preoperative and postoperative RLFB angles, and intersection angle between the mechanical and anatomical axes were compared. The angle between the arc and sagittal planes, varus and valgus angles, and intersection angle between the mechanical and anatomical axes were measured on a 3D model.

Results: There was no significant between-group difference in 3D model measurements of the angle between the arc and sagittal planes ($p = 0.327$). There was no significant difference between the mechanical and anatomical axes measured by both imaging modalities ($p > 0.258$). When the RLFB was $>5°$, the flexion contracture angle and radiographic femoral bowing angle were positively correlated ($r = 0.535$, $p < 0.05$). Distal femur varus and valgus angles significantly differed between the two groups ($p = 0.01$). After total knee arthroplasty, the radiographic femoral bowing angle decreased significantly. When the cases' radiographic femoral bowing angle is larger and the angle between the arc and sagittal planes is smaller as measured in 3D models, the angle between the arc and coronal planes is larger.

Conclusion: The radiographic femoral bowing angle does not reflect the actual size of lateral femoral bowing, does not greatly affect surgery design, and is greatly affected by flexion contracture deformity. A RLFB angle larger than $15°$ indicates real lateral femoral bowing.

Keywords: Lateral femoral bowing, Radiograph, Imaging, Computed tomography, Three-dimensional model, Total knee arthroplasty

Background

Regaining lower limb alignment is crucial in total knee arthroplasty (TKA) [1, 2]. Preoperative planning based on long-leg weight-bearing anterior radiography aims to restore the alignment [3]. Precise femoral alignment relies on accurate femoral resection which depends on the angle between the mechanical and anatomical axes measured on a preoperative long-leg weight-bearing anterior

radiograph. This angle can be affected by lateral femoral bowing; thus, miscalculation of lateral femoral bowing can directly lead to distal femoral resection error and subsequently femoral misalignment [4, 5].

Some researchers concluded that the lateral femoral bowing angle measured on radiographs can affect preoperative planning [5–8]. Akamatsu et al. reported that computed tomography (CT)-based measurements of lateral femoral bowing are much smaller than radiography-based measurements [7]. Some studies based on the latest three-dimensional (3D) technology indicated that surgery

---

* Correspondence: qixindoc@163.com
Department of Orthopaedic Surgery, The First Hospital of Jilin University, Jilin University, Xinmin St 71, Chang Chun, China

design should rely on both radiographic measurement of lateral femoral bowing and 3D measurements [6, 9]. However, few studies have investigated the factors affecting the difference between the lateral femoral bowing angle measured on radiographs and 3D models and whether femoral lateral bowing measured on radiographs affects the angle between the mechanical and anatomical axes measured on 3D models.

The present study aimed to compare the difference between radiographic lateral femoral bowing (RLFB) and 3D model-based lateral femoral bowing, to analyse the factors that affect the precision of the RLFB angle, and to determine whether the RLFB angle affects surgery design.

Methods
Study subjects
We prospectively enrolled patients who underwent primary knee arthroplasty in our department from June 2016 to September 2016. Patients who had a history of knee trauma or surgery and those with preoperative knee infection were excluded. The medical history and radiographic findings were recorded. The ethics committee of our institution approved this study, and all patients gave their informed consent to participate in this study. All of the patients enrolled in this study were assessed by physical examination (e.g. the degree of flexion contracture preoperatively). Patients were also evaluated using long-leg weight-bearing anterior radiographs preoperatively and postoperatively [8, 10], and long-leg CT (GE Discovery CT750 HD scanner, GE Healthcare, Waukesha, WI, USA) of the bilateral limbs with 5-mm thickness preoperatively. The mean and median RLFB angle was measured before and after the surgery. The patients were divided into two groups: those with a preoperative RLFB angle <5° were assigned to group A, and those with marked preoperative RLFB angle ≥5° were assigned to group B. The dividing method is also used in previous studies [3, 7].

Imaging analysis
The RLFB angle [8, 10] and the angle between the mechanical axis and anatomical axis were measured on long-leg weight-bearing anterior radiographs preoperatively. All patients underwent full-length CT examination of the lower limbs before surgery, and the CT data were processed by Mimics 15 software (Materialise, Leuven, Belgium). The 3D data model of both lower limbs was obtained after modelling, and the model was anatomically measured by Mimics software. We defined a number of special anatomical landmarks by referring to previous literature [7, 11–15] (Figs. 1 and 2). With these landmarks in the 3D model, we could determine the coordinate system (Fig. 3). The measurement based on this coordinate system could effectively avoid the effect of flexion contracture, varus, valgus, or rotation. The following variables were measured in the 3D model coordinate system: the angle between the arc plane and sagittal plane and the angle between the mechanical axis and anatomical axis.

Regarding the angle between the arc plane and sagittal plane (3D lateral femoral bowing index), the femoral medullary cavity centre line was established through the Mimics software, and the centre line was fitted into a complete arc. The plane was determined by the two intersections of the arc and the femur, and the centre of the arch was defined as the arc plane. The angle between the arc plane and sagittal plane was measured in the coordinate system (Fig. 4) [9].

Regarding the angle between the mechanical axis and the anatomical axis, the central point of the planes in CT of the one third isthmus of the medullary cavity was fitted into a straight line. This line was defined as the anatomical axis of the femur in the 3D model. The angle between the two lines projected onto the femoral coronal plane was defined as the angle between the mechanical axis and the anatomical axis in the 3D model.

Regarding the degree of varus and valgus deformity, the lower extremity model obtained from patients' lower limb CT by using Mimics software was projected to the coronal plane, and then the "real" double lower extremity full-length "radiograph" was obtained without deviation caused by incorrect body position (e.g. internal and external rotation of the femur and knee flexion contracture). Then, the degree of varus and valgus deformity of the distal femur was measured by TRAUMA CAD 2.0 (Orthocrat, USA).

A high-volume senior orthopaedic surgeon performed all the surgeries in the present study. All the knee prostheses used in the present study were from the same company (PFC Sigma, Depuy, Warsaw, IN, USA).

The RLFB angle and radiographic angle between the mechanical axis and anatomical axis were also measured postoperatively. After the measurements were completed, the differences between the angles of the arc plane-sagittal plane and arc plane-coronal plane between the two groups; the difference in the degree of flexion contracture and the correlation between the RLFB angle and the degree of flexion contracture; the between-group difference in the angle of the distal end of the femur and its correlation with the RLFB angle; and the change in the RLFB angle before and after surgery were compared.

Statistical analysis
According to prior power analysis, this was the study size needed to meet the minimum requirement to achieve a power of 0.8 and an α value of 0.05. The Shapiro-Wilk test was used to evaluate the normality of the data

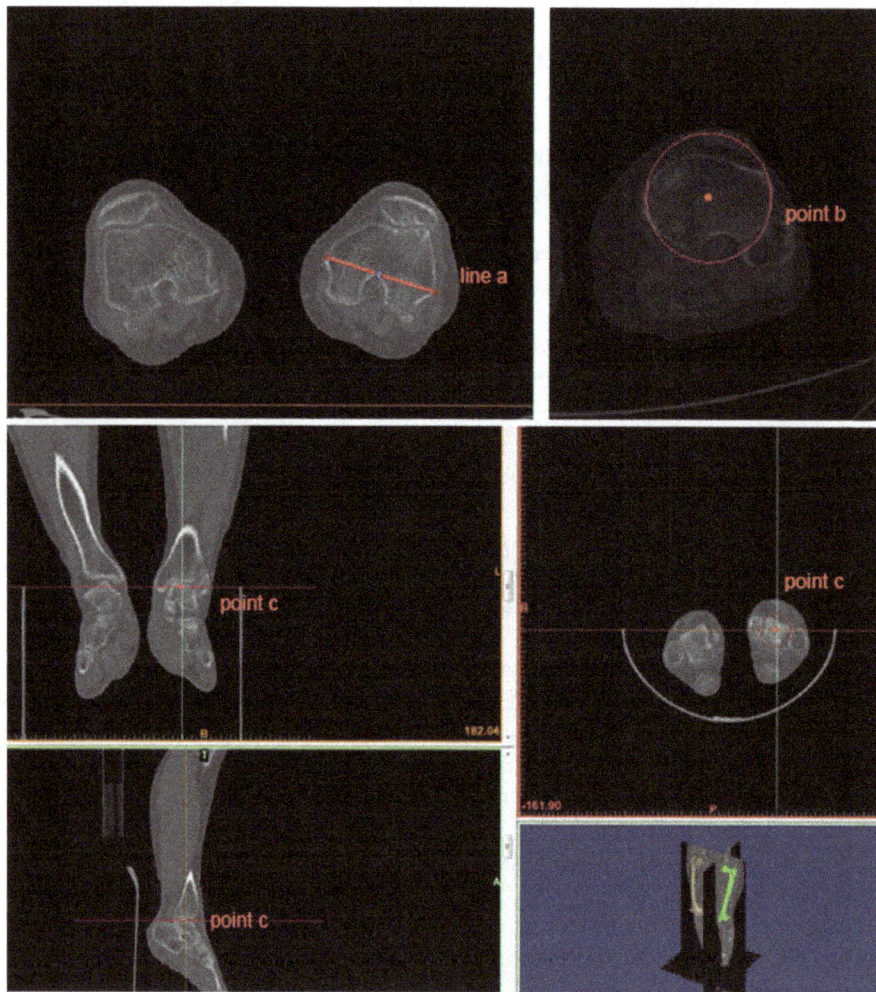

Fig. 1 Line **a**: transepicondylar axis; Point **b**: the midpoint of the proximal tibia; Point **c**: distal tibia center point

distributions. Data are expressed as median (range) and were compared using the Mann-Whitney U test. Correlations between two parameters were estimated by Pearson's test when the data had a Gaussian distribution. Data with non-Gaussian distributions were compared between groups using the Kruskal-Wallis test. A p value <0.05 was considered statistically significant. All statistical analyses were performed using SPSS Statistics 22 (IBM Corporation, Armonk, NY, USA).

Results

A total of 30 patients were enrolled in this study. Three of them were male and the remaining 27 were female. The mean age was 65.7 ± 7.16 (range, 51–83) years. Forty femurs were evaluated (left, 19; right, 21); 6 were from male patients and 34 were from female patients. The median of the RLFB angle was 4.95°. According to the preoperative RLFB angle, 20 femurs were included in the group with an RLFB angle <5° and 20 were included

in the group with an RLFB angle >5°. There were no significant differences in the baseline characteristics between the two groups (Table 1). When comparing the angle of the sagittal plane and arc plane, no significant between-group difference was found ($p = 0.327$) (Table 1).

The radiographic and 3D model-based angle between the mechanical axis and anatomical axis was $6.44° \pm 1.54°$ and $6.84° \pm 1.33°$, respectively. The absolute value of the difference between the two angles was not significantly correlated with the plain RLFB angle ($p = 0.258$). The difference between the angle of the two sets of mechanical axes and anatomical axes was not significantly different between the two groups ($p = 0.314$).

The relationship between the two groups according to the RLFB angle and the flexion contracture angle was compared. When the RLFB angle was >5°, the flexion contracture angle had a strong linear positive correlation with the RLFB angle ($r = 0.535$, $p < 0.05$), that is, the bigger the RLFB angle, the larger the flexion contracture

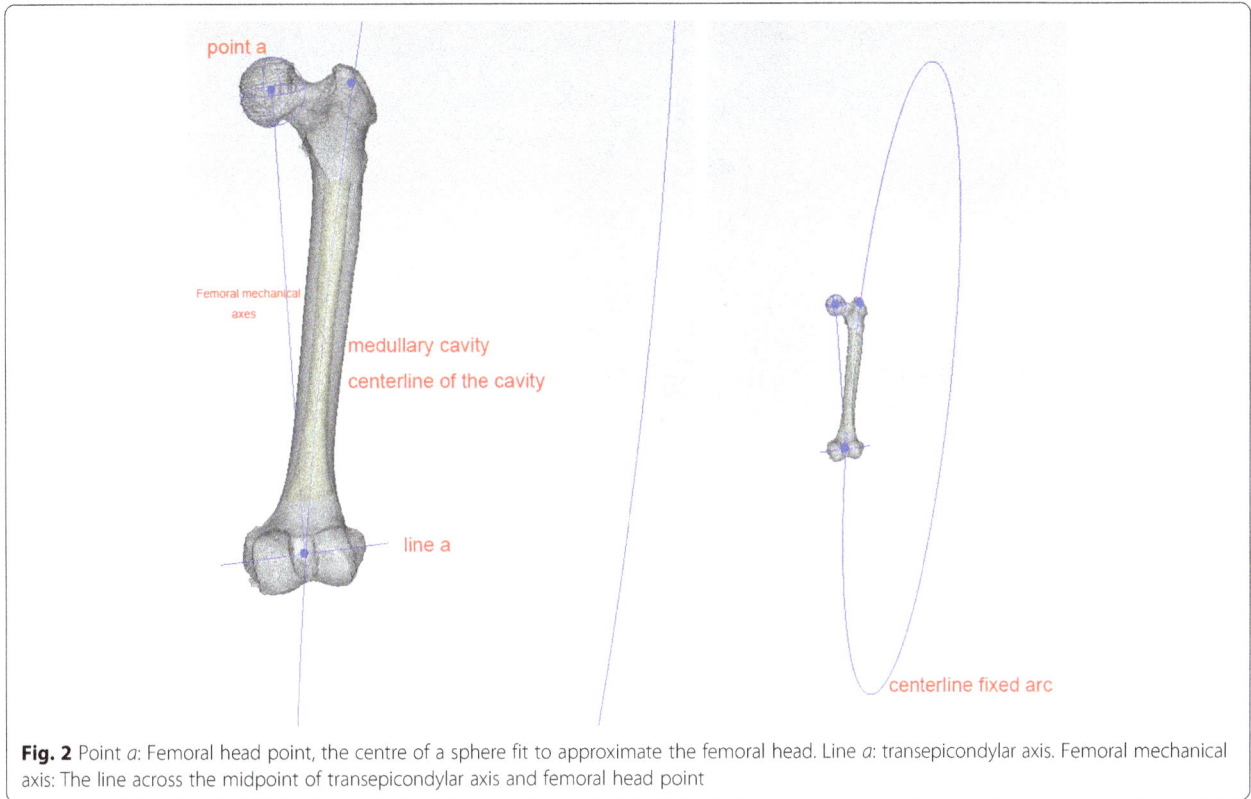

Fig. 2 Point *a*: Femoral head point, the centre of a sphere fit to approximate the femoral head. Line *a*: transepicondylar axis. Femoral mechanical axis: The line across the midpoint of transepicondylar axis and femoral head point

angle. When the RLFB angle was <5°, there was no strong correlation between the flexion contracture angle and the RLFB angle. The mean ± SD and median values of the flexion contracture angle of the group with an RLFB angle >5° were greater than those of the group with an RLFB angle <5° (11.20 ± 6.97 and 8.92 vs 9.59 ± 7.99 and 5.39, respectively).

When the RLFB angle was >5°, there was no linear correlation between the RLFB angle and varus and valgus deformity($r = 0.281$). However, a significant difference in varus and valgus deformity between the two groups was found ($p = 0.03$) (Table 2).

For patients whose RLFB angle was >5°, the mean ± SD and median angle between the arc and sagittal plane were 24.39 ± 14.07 and 20.40, respectively. This group of cases was divided into two groups using the arc-sagittal plane angle of 20° as an interface. When the RLFB angle was larger and the angle between the arc and sagittal plane smaller, the angle between the arc and coronal plane is larger (77.01 ± 5.91 vs 52.38 ± 11.95), and the two sets of data were statistically significant ($r = -0.954$, $p = 0.01$).

By measuring the preoperative and postoperative RLFB angle, the flexion contracture deformity and the varus and valgus deformity were corrected by surgery. The mean ± SD and median postoperative RLFB angle were 3.01 ± 1.99 and 2.60, respectively, which were significantly lower than the mean ± SD and median

preoperative RLFB angle (5.52 ± 4.56 and 4.57, respectively). The patients' RLFB angle disappeared after surgery (Fig. 5).

In the group with an RLFB angle >5°, a notable larger femoral bow angle >15° was found in six cases. In these six cases, the femoral bow angle remained greater than 5° after surgery.

Discussion

A total of 40 femurs from 30 patients were evaluated in the present study and were divided into two groups in accordance with the preoperative RLFB angle, where an RLFB angle of 5° was used as the cut-off value to divide both groups, *in accordance with previous publications* [3, 7]. A preoperative RLFB angle >5° could result in a wrong judgment regarding force alignment; therefore, special attention should be paid to the bone section intraoperatively [3, 7, 16].

According to the results of our research, the RLFB angle cannot reflect the real size of the lateral femoral bowing. Compared with previous research, the 3D method measurement for the difference between the mechanical axis and anatomical axis is more accurate. In the present study, there was no between-group difference in the angle between the mechanical axis and anatomical axis measured by 3D CT and radiography, indicating that the RLFB angle does not have a large effect on the surgery design.

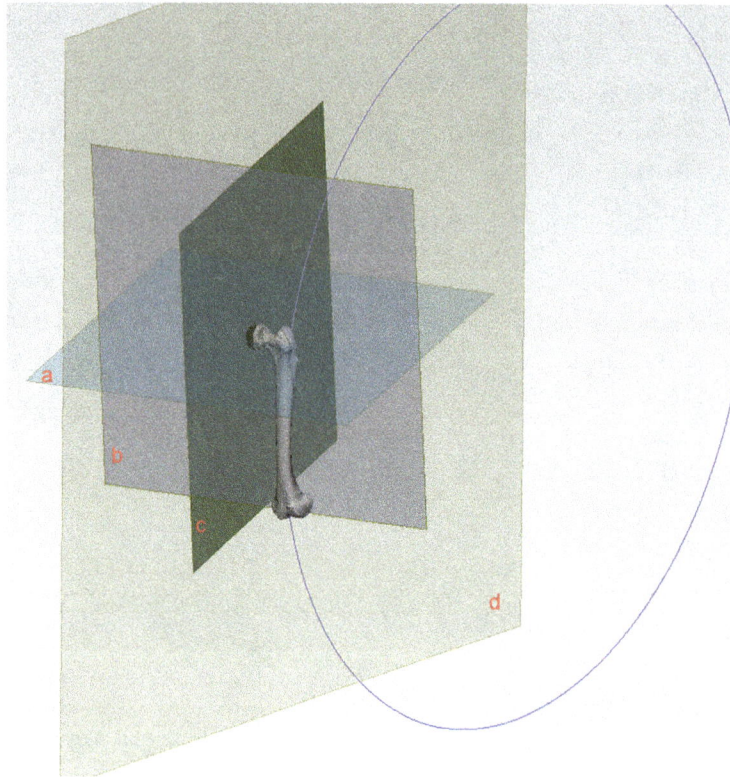

Fig. 3 Plane *a*: axial plane; Plane *b*: coronal plane; Plane *c*: sagittal plane; Plane *d*: arc plane. Lower limb coronal plane: The plane formed by femoral transepicondylar axis and femoral head point. Lower limb sagittal and axial plane: perpendicular to coronal plane, respectively, and mutually

The flexion contracture is a major factor that affects the RLFB angle. Patients with a larger preoperative flexion contracture deformity have a larger difference in the femoral bow angle. When the RLFB angle was >5°, a positive linear correlation was found between the flexion contracture angle and the RLFB angle, that is, the larger the flexion contracture angle, the larger the femoral bow angle.

The varus and valgus deformity at the distal femur can also affect the RLFB angle, but its effect is not greater than that of flexion contracture. There was no significant correlation between the varus and valgus angle and the RLFB angle, but the varus and valgus angle is significantly different between the two groups ($p = 0.03$). Therefore, the effect of the varus and valgus angle of the distal femur on the RLFB angle should still be acknowledged. In the present study, the varus and valgus angle of the distal femur was effectively measured on the femoral coronal plane. This measurement method avoids inaccurate measurements on a plain radiograph caused by incorrect position and flexion contracture.

Concerns about the effect of the RLFB angle on surgical design have been previously reported. Abdelaal et al. showed that after CT reconstruction, the larger lateral femoral bowing angle measured by CT had an effect on

the surgery design [16], but was not correlated to the radiographic examination. Their study showed that the femoral bowing is expressed through the axial plane measurement and in multiple sections. Compared with our research methods, their methods cannot show the lateral femoral bowing's overall situation very well. Shi et al. measured the femoral bowing based on preoperative radiographs and concluded that the RLFB angle can effectively guide surgery [17]. Although the measurement of femoral bowing on radiographs is a common practice, it cannot eliminate the effects caused by flexion and varus and valgus deformity.

Lee et al. suggested that the femoral bow affects the angle measurement of the mechanical and anatomical axes by misleading the positioning of the anatomical axis of the femur, which greatly affects the surgery design [5]. Their measurement, however, is based on radiographs and, in the preoperative period, often leads to shooting position inaccuracy because of the flexion contracture deformity and varus and valgus deformity of the distal femur. Our research is based on a 3D model, and the measurement of the angle between the mechanical axis and the anatomical axis rules out the influential factors on the quality of radiographs. No significant difference

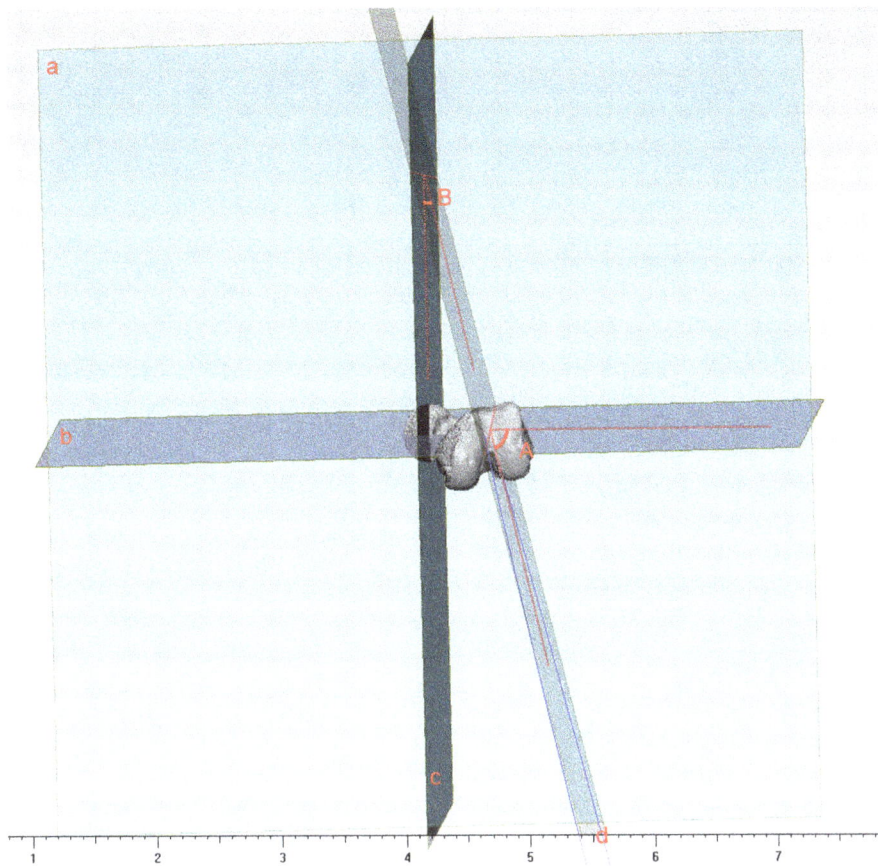

Fig. 4 Plane *a*: axial plane; Plane *b*: coronal plane ; Plane *c*: sagittal plane ; Plane *d*: arc plane. Angle *A*: angle between arc plane and coronal plane; Angle *B*: angle between arc plane and sagittal plane. The arc plane is the formed by the fitted arc of central point and the femoral medullary cavity; thus, the arc is commonly influenced by both the femoral anterior bowing and lateral bowing. For the femur, the lateral bowing is often accompanied by anterior bowing; therefore, it is not appropriate to analyse each one of them at a time. The angle between the femoral sagittal plane and the arc plane (defined as 3D lateral femoral bowing index) can clearly reflect the lateral bowing degree of the femur. That is, the larger the femoral anatomy of the lateral bowing, the greater the 3D lateral femoral bowing index. While the angle between the arc plane and the coronal plane of the femur reflects the anterior arch degree of the femur. That is, the larger the anterior arch of the femur, the greater the angle between the arc plane and the coronal plane

in the 3D measurement of the "real" angle between the mechanical axis and anatomical axis was found between large and small RLFB angle groups.

The present study also found that in the cases in which the RLFB angle was bigger and the 3D measurement of the angle between the sagittal and arc plane was smaller, the angle between the coronal and arc plane was larger and the difference was statistically significant. We believe that flexion contracture or deformity causes lateral femoral rotation, which can lead to greater projection of coronal femoral bowing in radiography, and seemingly, the RLFB appears to be larger. When both the RLFB angle and 3D measurement of the angle between the sagittal and arc plane are larger, the angle between the coronal and arc plane becomes smaller.

When flexion contracture and varus and valgus deformity are corrected through surgery, the average postoperative RLFB angle becomes significantly lower than

the preoperative RLFB angle. The RLFB disappears after surgery, which further confirms that the larger RLFB angle is caused by flexion contracture and varus and valgus deformity.

In six cases, the RLFB angle was >15° and the RLFB angle remained greater than 5° after surgery indicating that an RLFB angle greater 15° preoperatively prompts the existence of a real lateral femoral bowing angle, and the postoperative residual bowing observed on radiography will be ≥5°. Therefore, we believe that when the RLFB angle is >15°, the patient has real lateral femoral bowing.

The unique methods applied in this study are mainly embodied in the following three aspects. First, through 3D printing design technology, a coordinate system was established, in which a circle could be drawn on the basis of the centre line of the femoral marrow cavity. The size of the sagittal angle-arc plane was used to present femoral lateral bowing, which allows for

Table 1 Baseline characteristics between group A and group B

	Group A(<5°)	Group B(>5°)	p
Gender (m/fm)	4/21	2/13	1.000
Age (years)	64.95 ± 7.83	66.55 ± 6.52	0.231
Height (cm)	162.55 ± 6.67	159.60 ± 7.84	0.231
Weight (kg)	66.70 ± 8.70	65.02 ± 7.93	0.883
BMI (kg/cm^2)	25.33 ± 3.91	25.21 ± 2.95	0.889

A significant difference between groups was considered for $p < 0.05$

quantitative analysis of lateral femoral bowing and reflects the extent of the bow lateral femoral stereoscopic and related measurement. Second, through the comparison of the angle between the mechanical and anatomical axes with 3D measurement and traditional radiograph measurement, we judged whether the larger RLFB affects the preoperative surgery design. As a result of the high precision of measurement with the 3D model, which can fully reflect the real angle between the mechanical axis and anatomical axis, the degree of surgical correction can be planned more accurately. Finally, through the comparison of the preoperative and postoperative RLFB angle, the flexion contracture and varus and valgus deformity were corrected and the RLFB angle disappeared postoperatively, indicating that these two factors affect the RLFB angle which further verifies our findings.

The present study has some limitations. First, the sample size was small; however, the radiographic lateral bowing angle data were widely distributed; thus, enough cases with large radiographic lateral bowing were included. Second, this was a single-centre study. The conclusions of the present study should be confirmed in a multi-centre study with a larger sample size. Third, we only explored the main influencing factors such as flexion contracture deformity and varus and valgus deformity of the distal femur; other factors might be discovered through further study.

Table 2 Relationship of groups A and B according to arc plane and sagittal plane angle, flexion contracture and varus and valgus deformity

	Angle between arc plane and sagittal plane	Flexion contracture	Varus and valgus deformity
<5° group A	19.05 ± 7.85	9.59 ± 7.99	2.20 ± 1.83
>5° group B	24.39 ± 14.07	11.20 ± 6.97*	4.17 ± 2.20**
p	0.327	0.221	0.03

*A significant difference between groups was considered for $p < 0.05$. When the radiographic RLFB angle is greater than 5°, the flexion contracture angle has strong linear positive correlation with the RLFB angle ($r = 0.535$, $p < 0.05$) Comparing the angle of sagittal plane and arc plane, it is found that there is no statistical difference between the two groups ($p = 0.327$)
**When RLFB is greater than 5°, it has no linear correlation with the varus and valgus deformity, but there are statistical differences in the varus and valgus deformity between two groups ($p = 0.03$)

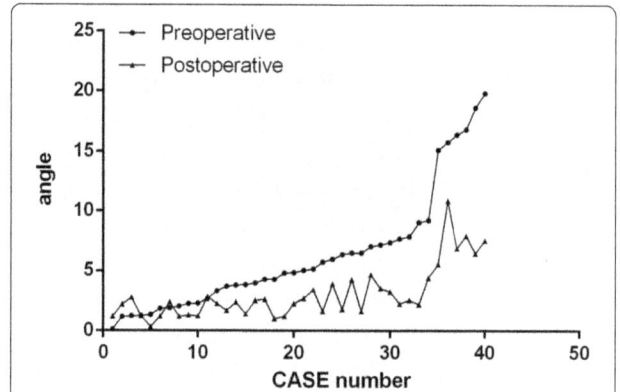

Fig. 5 Preoperative radiographic lateral femoral bowing angle is 5.52 ± 4.56, 4.57, while the postoperative radiographic lateral femoral bowing angle's average is 3.01 ± 1.99, 2.60. When flexion contracture and varus and valgus deformity are corrected through surgery, the average postoperative RLFB angle becomes significantly lower than the preoperative RLFB angle. The RLFB decreases after surgery, which further confirms that the larger RLFB angle is caused by flexion contracture and varus and valgus deformity

Conclusion

In conclusion, radiographic measurement cannot accurately reflect the size of the lateral femoral bowing angle. The RLFB angle is greatly affected by flexion contracture deformity as well as varus and valgus deformity of the distal femur. Although the RLFB angle is larger than that measured by 3D CT, it does not affect the angle between the mechanical and anatomical axes and the surgery design. A large RLFB angle and small sagittal and arc angle prompt femoral rotation, which can lead to greater projection of radiographic coronal femoral bowing and, seemingly, a larger lateral bowing angle. A large 3D lateral femoral bowing index and radiographic lateral femoral bowing angle indicate a real large lateral femur bowing angle. An RLFB angle >15° indicates real lateral femoral bowing.

Abbreviations
3D: Three-dimensional; CT: Computed tomography; RLFB: Radiographic lateral femoral bowing; TKA: Total knee arthroplasty

Acknowledgements
We extend sincere gratitude to the staff of the Department of Orthopaedic Surgery for their assistance during this study.

Funding
Funding information is not applicable.

Authors' contributions
XQ and JGL participated in the design of this study. YRL and YHG carried out the studies and performed the statistical analysis. YRL, SQL, LD, ZZ, CY, and XQ drafted the manuscript. All authors read and approved the final manuscript.

Competing interests
The authors declare that they have no competing interests.

References
1. Bäthis H, et al. Alignment in total knee arthroplasty. A comparison of computer-assisted surgery with the conventional technique. J Bone Joint Surg (Br). 2004;86(5):682–7.
2. Rand J, Coventry M. Ten-year evaluation of geometric total knee arthroplasty. Clin. Orthop. Relat. Res. 1988;232:168–73.
3. Mullaji AB, et al. Which factors increase risk of malalignment of the hip-knee-ankle axis in TKA? Clin Orthop Relat Res. 2013;471(1):134–41.
4. Yau W, et al. Coronal bowing of the femur and tibia in Chinese: its incidence and effects on total knee arthroplasty planning. J Orthop Surg (Hong Kong). 2007;15(1):32–6.
5. Lee SA, Choi SH, Chang MJ. How accurate is anatomic limb alignment in predicting mechanical limb alignment after total knee arthroplasty? BMC Musculoskelet Disord. 2015;16:323.
6. Kim JM, et al. Femoral shaft bowing in the coronal plane has more significant effect on the coronal alignment of TKA than proximal or distal variations of femoral shape. Knee Surg Sports Traumatol Arthrosc. 2015;23(7):1936–42.
7. Akamatsu Y, et al. Femoral shaft bowing in the coronal and sagittal planes on reconstructed computed tomography in women with medial compartment knee osteoarthritis: a comparison with radiograph and its predictive factors. Arch Orthop Trauma Surg. 2016;136(9):1227–32.
8. Sebastian AS, et al. Femoral bow predicts postoperative malalignment in revision total knee arthroplasty. J Arthroplasty. 2014;29(8):1605–9.
9. Buford W, et al. Three-dimensional computed tomography-based modeling of sagittal cadaveric femoral bowing and implications for intramedullary nailing. J Orthop Trauma. 2014;28(1):10–6.
10. Mullaji AB, Marawar SV, Mittal V. A comparison of coronal plane axial femoral relationships in Asian patients with varus osteoarthritic knees and healthy knees. J Arthroplasty. 2009;24(6):861–7.
11. Dutton AQ, Yeo SJ. Computer-assisted minimally invasive total knee arthroplasty compared with standard total knee arthroplasty. Surg Technique J Bone Joint Surg Am. 2009;91(Suppl 2 Pt 1):116–30.
12. Victor J, et al. How precise can bony landmarks be determined on a CT scan of the knee? Knee. 2009;16(5):358–65.
13. Yoshino N, et al. Computed tomography measurement of the surgical and clinical transepicondylar axis of the distal femur in osteoarthritic knees. J Arthroplasty. 2001;16(4):493–7.
14. Victor J, Hoste D. Image-based computer-assisted total knee arthroplasty leads to lower variability in coronal alignment. Clin. Orthop. Relat. Res. 2004;428:131–9.
15. Patil S, et al. Improving tibial component coronal alignment during total knee arthroplasty with use of a tibial planning device. J Bone Joint Surg Am. 2007;89(2):381–7.
16. Thippanna RK, Kumar MN. Lateralization of femoral entry point to improve the coronal alignment during total knee arthroplasty in patients with bowed femur. J Arthroplasty. 2016;31(9):1943–8.
17. Shi X, et al. Comparison of postoperative alignment using fixed vs individual valgus correction angle in primary total knee arthroplasty with lateral bowing femur. J Arthroplasty. 2016;31(5):976–83.

6

Thresholds for Oxford Knee Score after total knee replacement surgery: a novel approach to post-operative evaluation

Christian Lund Petersen[2*], Jonas Bruun Kjærsgaard[2], Nicolai Kjærgaard[2], Michael Ulrich Jensen[1] and Mogens Berg Laursen[1]

Abstract

Background: In a prospective cohort study, we wanted to detect thresholds distinguishing between patients with a satisfactory and an unsatisfactory outcome after total knee replacement (TKR) based on Patient-Reported Outcome Measures (PROMs), namely the Oxford Knee Score (OKS), using patient satisfaction and patient-perceived function as global transition items.

Methods: Seventy-three TKR patients completed the OKS questionnaire before surgery and were invited to complete the same questionnaire again 6 (4 to 9) months after surgery. Correlations between outcome measures and anchors were calculated using Pearson's correlation coefficient. Thresholds were established by receiver operating characteristics (ROC) analysis, using multiple anchor-based approaches.

Results: Patients showed a mean increase of 16.5 (SD 9.5) in OKS following TKR. Significant positive correlations were found between outcome measures and anchors. Six different thresholds were determined for outcome measures coupled with satisfaction, patient-perceived function and a combination thereof using a cut-off of 50 and 70.

Conclusions: This study has established a set of clinically meaningful thresholds for Oxford Knee scores that may help to detect TKR patients who might be in need of post-operative evaluation.

Keywords: PROM, Oxford Knee Score, OKS, Knee arthroplasty, Knee, Total knee replacement

Background

Traditionally, when evaluating the quality of total knee replacements (TKR), indicators such as survival of the prosthesis and revision rates have been used as standard measurements [1]. However, in recent years, Patient-Reported Outcome Measures (PROMs) have gained increased attention when evaluating outcomes of TKR [2, 3]. Joint-specific PROMs allow the assessment of the outcome from the perspective of the patient, including the level of pain and function of the specific joint.

One such PROM was devised in 1998. At the time of introduction of the Oxford Knee Score (OKS), the scoring system was developed as a measure of post-operative outcome for TKR [4]. Used in cohort studies and collected in national registries, such as in England and Wales, Sweden and New Zealand [5, 6], it has since been coupled to other patient-reported measures allowing a more comprehensive assessment of TKR outcomes [2, 6]. This simplifies the interpretation of the quantitative score into qualitatively meaningful information [7].

Thresholds can be established for OKS values above which patients are satisfied with surgery or have experienced improvement of function after surgery. Multiple methodological approaches to calculating such thresholds exist. One approach is called the minimal clinically important difference (MCID), which is defined as "the smallest change that is important to patients" [8]. Another approach is calculating a threshold of the post-operative OKS value, providing another perspective of patient-perceived outcome.

* Correspondence: christian.lund@rn.dk
[2]School of Medicine and Health, Aalborg University, Niels Jernes Vej 12 A5, 9220 Aalborg Ø, Denmark
Full list of author information is available at the end of the article

These approaches require the use of global transition items as anchors. Previous studies have used patient satisfaction with surgery and perceived change in function of the specific joint as anchors [2, 6–9].

Previous studies have identified OKS thresholds to aid the clinician in presenting the expected outcome of surgery in a meaningful way to the patient [6]. However, the thresholds may have other possible applications. As the use of Oxford scores provides a means of comparing preoperative and post-operative health status, they may be used as a tool in the process of determining which patients are in need of further post-operative treatment.

In Danish hospitals, there is no standardised method for identifying TKR patients in need of further post-operative treatment. Current methods range from yearly outpatient visits in the surgeon's office to nurse-performed structural phone interviews using a modified version of the American Knee Society Score (AKSS) with defined triggering responses [10]. This is very time consuming, and the proportion of patients in need of re-evaluation is relatively small and hence does not fully satisfy the time and resources spent.

A screening procedure using OKS as part of a web-based questionnaire is planned to be used as a tool to select patients for outpatient evaluation in the North Denmark Region. Thus, this paper is a pilot study intended to create an initial algorithm intended to choose which patients should be called in for outpatient evaluation 1 year after surgery.

Based on the above considerations, we hypothesise that it is possible to identify clinically meaningful thresholds for OKS determining which patients are in need of post-operative evaluation.

Methods

Data were obtained from a clinical quality database ("Jointbase") at the Department of Orthopaedic Surgery, Aalborg University Hospital. The purpose of this database is to prospectively monitor the results of hip and knee arthroplasty surgery. This is assessed through a questionnaire using a condition-specific instrument (OKS), a generic instrument (EQ-5D-3L) and pain measurements.

All patients who completed the questionnaire prior to their surgery and underwent TKR ($n = 73$) at Aalborg University Hospital in the period between May 1 and October 31, 2014, were included in the study. Patients were invited to a follow-up investigation during February and March 2015. At this visit, the preoperative questionnaire was repeated in order to identify changes in the aforementioned scores. Additionally, patients completed a post-operative form, which included two global transition items.

Outcome measures and global transition items

Joint-specific PROMs were collected using the Danish translation of OKS [11]. The OKS is a 12-item questionnaire assessing pain and function in the patient's knee during the last 4 weeks.

Current overall satisfaction with the outcome of surgery was evaluated by a bipolar visual analogue scale (VAS) from 0 (very unsatisfied) to 100 (very satisfied). Present patient-perceived function in the knee compared with before the surgery was assessed by a bipolar VAS from 0 (much worse) to 100 (much better).

Statistical analysis

Descriptive statistics were performed for attenders and non-attenders. The attenders were compared to the non-attenders by chi-squared tests for categorical variables and two-sample t tests for continuous variables. To support the conclusions of the two-sample t tests, permutation tests were conducted.

Correlations between satisfaction with surgery and post-operative OKS, change in OKS was calculated using Pearson's correlation coefficient. Correlations with patient-perceived function were calculated in the same manner.

Using a sensitivity- and specificity-based approach, [8] thresholds were calculated for change in OKS (ΔOKS) and absolute post-operative OKS by using two global transition items for constructing three anchors: patient satisfaction, patient-perceived function and a combination of the two former by using the most conservative value, i.e. the lowest value hereof.

Cut-off points of 50 and 70 for patient satisfaction with surgery were chosen, and thus define a binary outcome: patients with satisfaction values below the cut-off should be invited for out-patient evaluation and patients with values above the cut-off should not. Likewise, cut-off points of 50 and 70 for patient-perceived function in the knee in question were used. Finally, thresholds were calculated by defining the cut-off as 50 or 70 for the combined anchor. In other words, patients who scored below the cut-off in either one of the two global transition items were identified as patients who should be invited for out-patient evaluation. Thus, we do not seek to identify patients that are, e.g. 100% satisfied, but merely discriminate between the two groups of patients based on a score of either below or above the cut-off, i.e. 50 or 70.

Coupling the anchors to the outcome measures (ΔOKS, OKS), sensitivity and specificity for different threshold values were assessed by receiver operating characteristics (ROC) curves plotting sensitivity against specificity.

Thresholds were established for each outcome measure by identifying the point on the relevant ROC curve closest to the upper left corner, as this represents the most efficient threshold value with regard to specificity and sensitivity [7].

Furthermore, the area under the curve (AUC) was calculated. The AUC represents the probability that the outcome measure threshold value correctly discriminates between patients who do and do not reach the cut-off. An AUC between 0.7 and 0.8 is considered acceptable, and an AUC between 0.8 and 0.9 is considered excellent [8].

Statistical analysis was performed using R version 3.1.3 [12].

Results
Study population characteristics
A total number of 73 TKR patients were included in the study of which 57 patients (78%) attended the post-operative follow-up. Patients were seen at an average of 6.05 (SD 1.62) months after surgery.

Attenders and non-attenders were analysed for differences between groups. Analyses regarding gender, age, preoperative OKS and body mass index (BMI) revealed no statistically significant differences. Descriptive statistics and p values are shown in Table 1.

Post-operative improvements and correlation with global transition items
On average, patients showed an increase of 16.5 (SD 8.5) in OKS, demonstrating an improvement in knee function after TKR ($p < 0.01$). The mean OKS before surgery was 20.3 (SD 6.9) and 36.8 (SD 6.8) after surgery.

Significant correlations were found between global transition items (patient satisfaction or patient-perceived function) and outcomes (post-operative OKS, change in OKS) as assessed by simple linear regression and derived by Pearson's correlation coefficient.

Positive correlations were found between satisfaction and post-operative OKS ($r = 0.56$ (CI 0.35; 0.71)) and

between satisfaction and change in OKS ($r = 0.42$ (CI 0.17; 0.61)).

The same pattern is seen for correlations with function. Post-operative OKS ($r = 0.56$ (CI 0.35; 0.71)) and change in OKS ($r = 0.42$ (CI 0.17;0.61)) are positively correlated to function.

Anchors and cut-off values
Using a cut-off of 50 for satisfaction, the study identified 91.2% (52/57) TKR patients as being satisfied. 84.2% (48/57) were identified as satisfied when using a cut-off of 70.

Patient-perceived function cut-offs of 50 and 70 revealed function gain in 91.2% (52/57) and 78.9% (45/57) of patients, respectively.

The combined anchor cut-offs identified 86.0% (49/57) of patients as above 50 and 73.7% (42/57) of patients as above 70.

Thresholds for outcomes after surgery
Thresholds for various outcome measures identified by ROC-curves at cut-off values of 50 and 70 for satisfaction and patient-perceived function are presented in Tables 2 and 3.

As an example, when using a cut-off value of 50 for satisfaction, a threshold of 9.5 in ΔOKS provides a sensitivity of 0.8 and a specificity of 0.83, AUC = 0.86.

All AUC values are above 0.7.

Discussion
Post-operative improvements
The present study found TKR patients to undergo a mean improvement in OKS of 16.5, which is consistent with findings in other studies. Judge et al. reported a mean 6–month change of 14.5 [6], whilst Beard et al. reported a change of 14.7 [7]. This demonstrates a slightly larger change in our patient group, even though mean preoperative OKS was higher in our study with 20.3 compared to 19.9 [6] and 18.5 [7], respectively.

Thresholds
For each group, we found thresholds for two different outcome measures (post-operative OKS, change in OKS) using three different anchors (satisfaction, patient-perceived function and the combination anchor) and two different cut-offs (50 and 70). This provides additional perspectives and a better foundation for evaluating the different strengths and limitations of each threshold if they were to be used as thresholds for contacting patients. In line with previous studies [2, 6, 7], we were able to document significant correlations between the global transition items (satisfaction and patient-perceived function) and all outcome measures,

Table 1 Comparison of preoperative OKS, age, BMI and gender of attenders and non-attenders. P values from two-sample t test unless otherwise stated

	TKR patients		
	Attenders	Non-attenders	
	($n = 57$, 78.1%)	($n = 16$, 21.9%)	p value
Pre-operative OKS, mean (SD)	20.3 (6.9)	18.4 (7.6)	0.36
Age (years), mean (SD)	65.6 (11.5)	66.1 (12.0)	0.88
BMI, preoperative, mean (SD)	30.5 (5.6)	30.6 (5.0)	0.95
Gender (n, %)			1[a]
Male	20 (35.1)	6 (37.5)	
Female	37 (64.9)	10 (62.5)	

SD standard deviation
[a]Chi-squared test

Table 2 Thresholds, percentage of patients who will be called with the given threshold, specificity, sensitivity and area under curve (AUC) for OKS and ΔOKS anchored to patient-perceived satisfaction, function and either satisfaction or function with a cut-off of 50. True positives is the amount of patients who should be called according to the cut-off value

Anchor	Cut-off value 50				
	Threshold	Called (%)	Specificity	Sensitivity	AUC
Satisfaction (n = 5)					
Post-operative OKS	34.5	31.6	0.75	1.00	0.88
ΔOKS	9.5	22.8	0.83	0.80	0.86
Function (n = 5)					
Post-operative OKS	32.5	24.6	0.81	0.80	0.85
ΔOKS	9.5	22.8	0.83	0.80	0.89
Satisfaction or function (n = 9)					
Post-operative OKS	34.5	31.6	0.78	0.88	0.87
ΔOKS	9.5	22.8	0.86	0.75	0.88

n number of patients with anchor values below the cut-off

justifying the use of these as anchors when establishing thresholds for the outcome measures.

Using a cut-off of 50 for each anchor, we established thresholds for change in OKS and post-operative OKS. The thresholds found in this manner were shown to have reasonable levels of sensitivity and specificity and to be consistent with results presented by Judge et al., [6] thus supporting these findings.

It may be questioned whether a cut-off of 50 is appropriate when establishing thresholds for calling patients post-operatively. Choosing a cut-off of 50 to discriminate between patients satisfied and not satisfied implies the assumption that all patients who are more than indifferent, as indicated by a score of 50, are indeed satisfied. In this respect, one may argue that patients should be more than just above "indifferent" after having undergone TKR. Similarly, patients with a function perception of 50 are not experiencing a change in function. With that in

mind, we added to our analysis a higher cut-off (70) in order to detect patients who might have had a suboptimal surgery outcome. By introducing a cut-off of 70, another set of thresholds were calculated detecting a larger proportion of patients for out-patient evaluation.

Apart from applying an extra cut-off value, we transformed the two global transition items to form one combined anchor, as it is our belief that surgery cannot be considered successful if not both satisfaction and function reach the cut-off values.

Applicability of thresholds

Previous studies have focused on one global transition item and OKS, thus using a more simple approach to detect thresholds for satisfactory surgery outcomes. This may leave out potentially important perspectives, which this study aims to accommodate by including two different global transition items.

Table 3 Thresholds, percentage of patients who will be called with the given threshold, specificity, sensitivity and area under curve (AUC) for OKS and ΔOKS anchored to patient-perceived satisfaction, function and either satisfaction or function with a cut-off of 70. True positives is the amount of patients who should be called according to the cut-off value

TKR: Cut-off value 70					
Anchor	Threshold	Called (%)	Specificity	Sensitivity	AUC
Satisfaction (n = 9)					
Post-operative OKS	35.5	36.8	0.71	0.78	0.78
ΔOKS	13.5	42.1	0.65	0.78	0.76
Function (n = 12)					
Post-operative OKS	35.5	36.8	0.76	0.83	0.85
ΔOKS	13.5	42.1	0.69	0.83	0.84
Satisfaction or function (n = 15)					
Post-operative OKS	35.5	36.8	0.79	0.80	0.87
ΔOKS	14.5	49.1	0.67	0.93	0.83

n number of patients with anchor values below cut-off

The purpose of previous studies has been to provide clinicians with simple and meaningful information regarding outcome after surgery and at the same time allowing a more comprehensive interpretation of OKS. Our results may be used in the same fashion; although, this has not been the main aim of our study. Instead, our approach allows us to present a variety of thresholds, using various combinations of anchors and outcome measures. In this way, we provide a large body of limits potentially useful in the clinical process of choosing patients for post-operative evaluation.

In order to make up for the sub-optimal sensitivities of the established thresholds, and thereby decrease the probability of not including all patients who might have had sub-optimal outcomes, it may be beneficial to use thresholds for both outcome measures.

A concern regarding the implementation of our thresholds as stand-alone criterions for post-operative evaluation is the considerable number of patients not in need of post-operative evaluation who are identified by the established thresholds because of specificity values below 1. This could be accommodated by an additional filter, e.g. interviewing the identified patients by phone beforehand to minimise the number of unnecessary consultations.

Established thresholds

One of the thresholds most capable of discriminating patients into the correct group, i.e. has the highest AUC-value, is post-operative pain at rest coupled to the combination anchor. A cut-off of 50 gives a threshold of 21.5, whilst the 70-point cut-off defines a threshold of 8.5. Implementation of these thresholds would find 14 and 31.6% of all patients to be in need of out-patient evaluation, respectively. The specificity (0.90) and sensitivity (0.88) at cut-off 50 indicate that this could be a useful tool when electing patients for out-patient evaluation. At cut-off 70, specificity (0.83) and sensitivity (0.73) are lower, yielding a lower efficiency if applied in the process of electing patients for post-operative evaluation. However, this threshold may detect patients with sub-optimal improvements not identified by the threshold derived from the 50-point cut-off.

Strengths and limitations

The sample size of 57 TKR patients is relatively small compared to that of other studies including hundreds or thousands of patients [6, 7]. As addressed previously, there is consistency between our results and those of the previous studies. This supports the assumption that our results are representative of the population.

However, as a consequence of the relatively small cohort, adjusting for confounding factors between attenders and non-attenders was not found relevant.

Also, the absolute number of patients classified as eligible for evaluation is relatively low (5–15). Thus, small differences in outcome measures for these patients would have a large impact on the established thresholds. This made it impossible to yield meaningful results if patients were stratified according to age, preoperative scores, etc. This approach would be preferable, as it would have been possible to detect differentiated thresholds, e.g. based on the preoperative OKS. An alternative to stratification of patients according to preoperative scores is calculating thresholds for the percentage of potential change (PoPC) [3]. This takes into account the maximum increase possible for each patient.

As the scores range from 0 to 48, patients with a higher preoperative score have a lower potential of change than patients with a low preoperative score. As an example, if a threshold for change in OKS of 15.5 points is used as the only limit, patients with a preoperative score of 10 will not be called if their post-operative score is above 25 points. However, patients with a preoperative score of 30 points will be called even though scoring 45 points, which is close to the maximum score of 48. Furthermore, patients with a preoperative score of 34 or more will inevitably be called for evaluation, because their maximum possible improvement is 14 points. Thresholds for absolute OKS involve a similar problem, as patients with a relatively low preoperative OKS may have a big and satisfactory improvement but still not reach the threshold.

Judge et al. have shown a variance in thresholds for post-operative scores and change of OKS anchored to satisfaction when stratifying patients according to preoperative scores [6]. Further research on larger sample sizes may establish an array of thresholds based on patient groups stratified by preoperative OKS and other possible variables. This may allow the use of these thresholds as decisive for calling patients for evaluation, thus eliminating the need for the additional filter proposed previously.

Another possible limitation of the study is the follow-up period of 6 months. Previous research has shown clinical improvements in TKR patients up to 1 year after surgery, but these changes have been shown to be minor [13, 14]. Also, previous research comparable to the present study has used a 6-month follow-up to estimate clinically meaningful changes in OKS after TKR [7]. We acknowledge that a 12-month follow-up would have been preferable, but as the purpose of this study has been to develop an initial algorithm for use in a novel approach to post-operative evaluation, we believe that the 6-month follow-up is a justifiable measure in the context of this study. Thus, based on these studies, we believe that the 6-month post-operative status is a reliable indicator of long-term outcome after surgery.

In addition, it is our hope that the results of our study can be implemented as part of a post-operative battery sent to patients either by e-mail or regular mail. Therefore, a certain delay is very possible to occur from the time the forms are initially sent out until they have been answered and patients are seen in the clinic for their potential post-operative evaluation, which will then be closer to a full year after surgery.

Adding up these circumstances, we find the follow-up period of 6 months to be adequate within the aim and scope of this study.

Conclusions

In line with the objectives of this paper, we have established a set of thresholds for the Oxford Knee Score that can be used to identify patients in need of post-operative evaluation. These clinically meaningful thresholds discriminate between patients that are satisfied with TKR surgery 6 months post-operatively and patients that are not and a similar set of thresholds differentiates between patients who have and have not experienced a gain in function after surgery.

The thresholds presented in this paper may be used when choosing limits in an at-home, web-based system comprised of questionnaires including Oxford scores, which determines whether or not to call patients for post-operative evaluation. These thresholds may require the use of an additional filter to detect patients not in need for evaluation depending on the specificity of the threshold chosen.

To establish thresholds applicable as sole determinants of which patients should be offered post-operative evaluation, we advise further research on larger sample sizes, allowing stratification of patients.

Abbreviations
AKSS: American Knee Society Score; AUC: Area under the curve; BMI: Body mass index; CI: Confidence interval; OKS: Oxford Knee Score; PoPC: Percentage of potential change; PROMs: Patient-Reported Outcome Measures; ROC: Receiver operating characteristics; SD: Standard deviation; TKR: Total knee replacement; VAS: Visual analogue scale

Acknowledgements
No acknowledgements.

Funding
No funding was received for this study.

Authors' contributions
JBK, NK and CLP contributed to the study design, data collection, data management, data analysis and writing of the manuscript. MUJ contributed to the study design, project management, project advisor, manuscript review. MBL contributed to the approvals, protocol, study design, project advisor, logistics and manuscript review. All authors read and approved the final manuscript.

Competing interests
The authors declare that they have no competing interests.

Author details
[1]Department of Orthopaedic Surgery, Aalborg University Hospital, Hobrovej 18-22, 9000 Aalborg, Denmark. [2]School of Medicine and Health, Aalborg University, Niels Jernes Vej 12 A5, 9220 Aalborg Ø, Denmark.

References
1. Kompetencecenter for Klinisk Kvalitet og Sundhedsinformatik Vest (2013) Dansk Knæalloplastikregister - Årsrapport 2013. Den Ortopædiske Fællesdatabase.
2. Keurentjes JC, Van Tol FR, Fiocco M, et al. Patient acceptable symptom states after total hip or knee replacement at mid-term follow-up. Bone Jt Res. 2014;3:7–13.
3. Kiran A, Hunter DJ, Judge A, et al. A novel methodological approach for measuring symptomatic change following total joint arthroplasty. J Arthroplasty. 2014;29:2140–5.
4. Dawson J, Fitzpatrick R, Murray D, Carr A. Questionnaire on the perceptions of patients about total knee replacement. J Bone Joint Surg (Br). 1998;80:63–9.
5. Murray DW, Fitzpatrick R, Rogers K, et al. The use of the Oxford hip and knee scores. J Bone Joint Surg (Br). 2007;89:1010–4. doi:10.1302/0301-620X. 89B8.19424.
6. Judge A, Arden NK, Kiran A, et al. Interpretation of patient-reported outcomes for hip and knee replacement surgery: identification of thresholds associated with satisfaction with surgery. J Bone Joint Surg (Br). 2012;94:412–8.
7. Beard DJ, Harris K, Dawson J, et al. Meaningful changes for the Oxford hip and knee scores after joint replacement surgery. J Clin Epidemiol. 2015;68: 73–9. doi:10.1016/j.jclinepi.2014.08.009.
8. Copay AG, Subach BR, Glassman SD, et al. Understanding the minimum clinically important difference: a review of concepts and methods. Spine J. 2007;7:541–6. doi:10.1016/j.spinee.2007.01.008.
9. Paulsen A, Roos EM, Pedersen AB, Overgaard S. Minimal clinically important improvement (MCII) and patient-acceptable symptom state (PASS) in total hip arthroplasty (THA) patients 1 year postoperatively. Acta Orthop. 2014;85: 39–48. doi:10.3109/17453674.2013.867782.
10. Grønhøj E 1 års telefoninterview af total hofte- og knæalloplastik. https://pri. rn.dk/Sider/19751.aspx. Accessed 16 Apr 2015.
11. Odgaard A. Paulsen A Translation and Cross-Cultural Adaptation of the Danish Version of Oxford Knee Score (OKS); 2009.
12. R Core Team. R: A Language and Environment for Statistical Computing. 2015.
13. Brander V a, Stulberg SD, Adams AD, et al. (2003) Predicting total knee replacement pain: a prospective, observational study. Clin Orthop Relat Res 27–36. doi: 10.1097/01.blo.0000092983.12414.e9
14. Browne JP, Bastaki H, Dawson J. What is the optimal time point to assess patient-reported recovery after hip and knee replacement? A systematic review and analysis of routinely reported outcome data from the English patient-reported outcome measures programme. Health Qual Life Outcomes. 2013;11:128.

7

Genetic effects of rs3740199 polymorphism in *ADAM12* gene on knee osteoarthritis

Zheng Hao[1†], Xin Li[2†], Jin Dai[3,4], Baocheng Zhao[1*] and Qing Jiang[3,4*]
†Equal contributors

Abstract

Background: Knee osteoarthritis (OA) is a complex arthritic condition in which genetic factors play an important role. *ADAM12* gene is one of the recognized candidate genes although the results are conflicting. To derive a more precise estimation of the association between rs3740199 polymorphism in *ADAM12* gene and risk of knee OA, we performed a meta-analysis based on six related studies, including a total of 2185 cases and 3716 controls.

Methods: A comprehensive search was performed to identify related studies up to April 14, 2017. We used odds ratios (ORs) with 95% confidence intervals (CIs) to assess the strength of the association. Different genetic models were used to assess the pooled and stratified data.

Results: Overall, no significant association was found in all genetic models (C vs. G, OR = 0.983, 95% CI = 0.910–1.061; CC vs. GG, OR = 1.033, 95% CI = 0.851–1.255; CG vs. GG, OR = 1.030, 95% CI = 0.877–1.209; CC/CG vs. GG, OR = 1.031, 95% CI = 0.886–1.201; CC vs. CG/GG, OR = 1.017, 95% CI = 0.868–1.190). When stratified by ethnicity, no significant association was found.

Conclusions: This meta-analysis suggested that the rs3740199 polymorphism does not contribute to the development of knee OA. Additional well-designed large studies are required to confirm these findings in different populations.

Keywords: Osteoarthritis, *ADAM12*, rs3740199, Polymorphism, Meta-analysis

Background

Osteoarthritis (OA) is a complex arthritic condition characterized by progressive cartilage loss, synovitis, osteophyte formation, and subchondral sclerosis. It is a cause of important handicap among the elderly [1, 2]. It has been reported that there were nearly 85 million OA patients in the world in 2009, and it might increase to 122 million in 2017. Hence, it is an enormous burden on the national economy and healthcare system [3, 4]. OA is a multifactorial disease resulting from the combined influence of environmental factors and genes [5]. Age,

joint injury, and obesity are the major risk factors [6, 7]. Several studies have identified some genetic factors such as *ASPN* [8], *FRZB* [9], and *GDF5* [10]. These three genes are involved in controlling growth and differentiation pathways [11]. Many other polymorphisms have shown association to OA although the results are inconsistent. Further research is needed to replicate these findings and identify some new genetic factors [12].

A disintegrin and metalloprotease (ADAM), a member of the Zn-dependent metzincin superfamily, is associated with many complex diseases such as heart disease, rheumatoid arthritis, Alzheimer's disease, and cancer [13, 14]. *ADAM12* may play an important role in chondrocyte proliferation, maturation, bone formation, and osteoclast differentiation [15–18]. ADAM12 is up-regulated in multinucleated giant cells surrounding loose hip implants and OA cartilage [19, 20]. Recently, promising but contradictory data have been published for the association of *ADAM12* with OA [21–25]. Poonpet et al. [24] and Kerna et al.

* Correspondence: drzhaobaocheng@outlook.com;
jiangqing112@hotmail.com
†Equal contributors
¹Center of Diagnosis and Treatment for Developmental Dysplasia of the Hip, Nanjing Zhongyangmen Community Health Service Center, Kang'ai Hospital, Nanjing 210037, Jiangsu, People's Republic of China
³Department of Sports Medicine and Adult Reconstructive Surgery, Drum Tower Hospital, School of Medicine, Nanjing University, 321 Zhongshan Road, Nanjing 210008, Jiangsu, People's Republic of China
Full list of author information is available at the end of the article

[25] found that rs3740199 in *ADAM12* was associated with knee OA risk although the results were conflicting rather than conclusion [12, 23, 26, 27].

In the present study, a meta-analysis was performed to determine the overall association between *ADAM12* rs3740199 polymorphism and knee OA susceptibility and whether the association varies by ethnicity.

Methods

Literature search strategy

To identify all relevant reports on rs3740199 polymorphism and knee OA risk, we performed a systematic search for all English language papers from PubMed (the last search update was April 14, 2017), using the key words "rs3740199" or "*ADAM12*," "polymorphism" or "polymorphisms" or "SNP," "osteoarthritis" or "OA". Additional eligible studies were identified by a manual search of the references of retrieved studies and review articles.

According to the following criteria, six studies were included in this meta-analysis: (1) was a cohort or case-control study; (2) was a study of the *ADAM12* rs3740199 polymorphism and knee OA risk; and (3) contained available genotype or allele frequency of rs3740199.

Data extraction

Two of the investigators extracted all data independently according to the criteria described above. We developed a data extraction sheet including year of publication, the first author's name, OA type, country of origin, ethnicity, assessment of OA, genotyping method, source of control groups, genotype, and allele frequency. For studies contain the results from different knee OA types, each type was treated independently. Any controversies of the data were discussed within our research team and the authors reached a consensus on all items.

Statistical methods

Allele frequencies of the *ADAM12* rs3740199 polymorphism from the six eligible studies were calculated by the allele counting method respectively. Hardy–Weinberg equilibrium (HWE) was used to evaluate the deviation of data associated with the *ADAM12* rs3740199 SNP in the control groups using χ^2 test. The strength of association between the *ADAM12* rs3740199 polymorphism and knee OA susceptibility was evaluated by pooled odds ratios (ORs) and their 95% confidence intervals (CIs). The significance of the ORs and 95% CIs was determined by Z test. The pooled ORs and 95% CIs were performed for additive model (C vs. G), co-dominant model (CC vs. GG; CG vs. GG), dominant model (CC/CG vs. GG), and recessive model (CC vs. CG/GG). Stratified analysis was also performed by ethnicity.

We assessed the between-study heterogeneity using chi-square-based Q test. If the P value was less than 0.10, the heterogeneity was considered significant. We also used the I^2 statistic $(I^2 = 100\% \times (Q - df)/Q)$ to quantify heterogeneity. I^2 greater than 50% indicated the presence of heterogeneity among studies. The fixed-effects model based on the Mantel–Haenszel method and the random-effects model based on the Dersimonian and Laird method were used to pool the data [28]. The random-effects model was more appropriate in the presence of heterogeneity; otherwise, the two methods provide similar results.

In meta-analysis, publication bias is also a concern. To test for publication bias, both Egger's and Begg's test are commonly used [29]. In this study, publication bias was evaluated by funnel plot and the linear regression asymmetry test.

All analyses were carried out using Stata software version 8.2 (Stata Corporation, College Station, TX, USA). All tests were two-sided.

Results

Characteristics of the included studies

Eleven relevant studies identified and screened. Four studies were added through manual search of the reference lists of retrieved studies. Nine of the 15 studies were excluded: three not polymorphism, one not for OA research, and five no useable data reported. A total of six reports were identified [12, 23–27]. Among these, Rodriguez-Lopez et al. reported six sample collections [12] while Kerna et al. included subjects with tibiofemoral knee OA (TFOA) and patellofemoral knee OA (PFOA) [25], they were considered as independent studies. Finally, nine studies with 2185 cases and 3716 controls were included in the present meta-analysis. The detailed study flow chart was illustrated in Fig. 1. Characteristics of the nine studies were listed in Tables 1 and 2. Of eligible studies, four and five studies were conducted in Asian and European populations respectively.

Quantitative synthesis

The details of meta-analysis for *ADAM12* rs3740199 polymorphism with knee OA risk are shown in Table 3.

Overall population

Nine separate studies with a total sample size of 2185 cases and 3716 controls had available data for analyzing the association of *ADAM12* rs3740199 polymorphism and knee OA risk. No significant association was found in all genetic models (C vs. G, OR = 0.983, 95% CI = 0.910–1.061; CC vs. GG, OR = 1.033, 95% CI = 0.851–1.255; CG vs. GG, OR = 1.030, 95% CI = 0.877–1.209; CC/CG vs. GG, OR = 1.031, 95% CI = 0.886–1.201; CC vs. qECG/GG, OR = 1.017, 95% CI = 0.868–1.190) (Table 3).

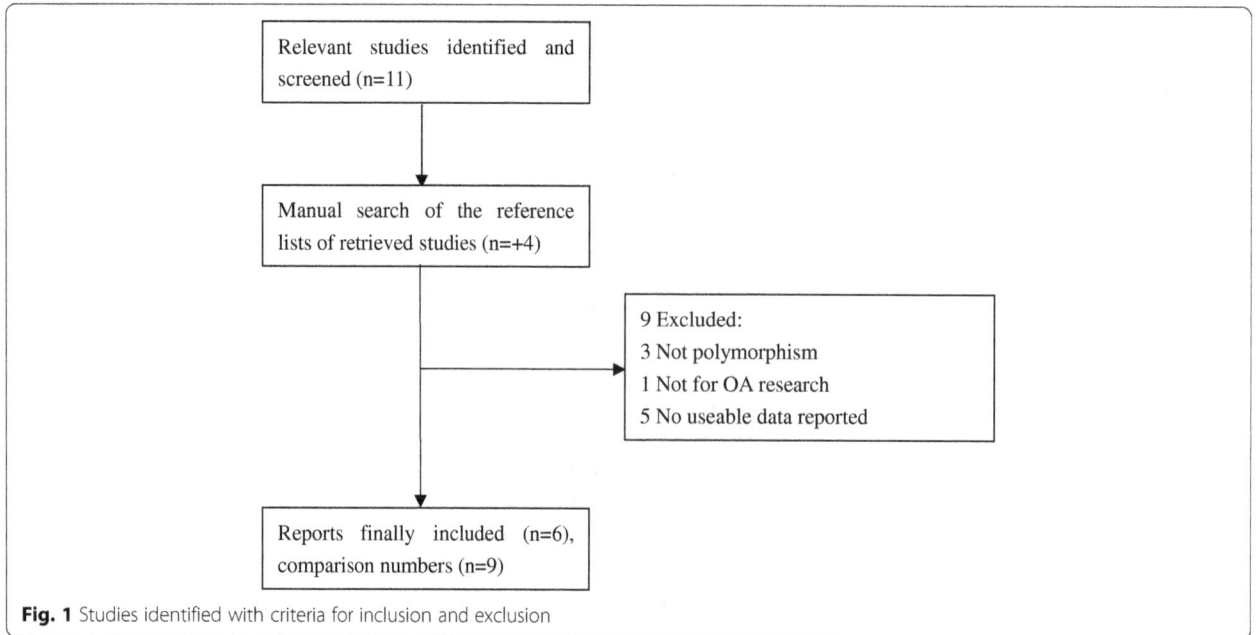

Fig. 1 Studies identified with criteria for inclusion and exclusion

Subgroup analysis by ethnicity

No significant association was found in all genetic models among Asian population (C vs. G, OR = 1.020, 95% CI = 0.924–1.127; CC vs. GG, OR = 1.040, 95% CI = 0.850–1.272; CG vs. GG, OR = 1.035, CI = 0.878–1.221; CC/CG vs. GG, OR = 1.036, CI = 0.887–1.211; CC vs. CG/GG, OR = 1.017, 95% CI = 0.858–1.207). No significant association was found in European population either.

Heterogeneity and publication bias

The between-study heterogeneity of the *ADAM12* rs3740199 polymorphism was not found in all subjects, and thus, the meta-analysis of the *ADAM12* rs3740199 polymorphism was performed using a fixed-effects model for all subjects except for the recessive model in European population, which was analyzed using a random-effects model (I^2 = 73.4%) (Table 3).

In this study, publication bias was evaluated by funnel plot and the linear regression asymmetry test. As shown in Fig. 2, the shape of the funnel did not reveal obvious asymmetry. Then, Egger's test was then performed to estimate the funnel plot symmetry. The results still did not show any evidence of publication bias (t = –0.40, P = 0.699 for C vs. G).

Discussion

OA is well recognized as a multifactorial disease. In addition to age, sex, trauma, and body weight, genetic factors are also strong determinants of this disease [30]. More than 50% of the OA cases can be attributed to genetic factors, demonstrated by twins and family studies [31]. It is suggested that OA of the hand, spine, hip, and knee are all heritable [32]. Recently, genetic studies have found many genes are contributing to OA, although with relatively modest effect [33]. These observations have

Table 1 Characteristics of literatures included in this meta-analysis

Year	First author	OA type	Country	Ethnicity	Assessment of OA	Genotyping	Source of controls	Cases	Controls
2009	J. Rodriguez-Lopez	TKR	Spain	European	K/L score	Multiplex single-base extension	PB	262	294
		TKR	UK	European	K/L score	Multiplex single-base extension	PB	360	698
		TKR	Greece	European	K/L score	Multiplex single-base extension	PB	159	193
2009	I. Kerna	TFOA	Estonian	European	OA score	PCR-RFLP	PB	66	123
		PFOA	Estonian	European	OA score	PCR-RFLP	PB	97	92
2012	Min-Ho Shin	Knee OA	Korea	Asian	K/L score	TaqMan	PB	725	1737
2014	Suliang Lou	Knee OA	China	Asian	K/L score	TaqMan	PB	152	179
2015	LinWang	Knee OA	China	Asian	K/L score	iMLDR	PB	164	200
2016	Thitiya Poonpet	Knee OA	Thai	Asian	K/L score	HRM analysis	PB	200	200

K/L score Kellgren–Lawrence score, *PB* population based, *TKR* total knee replacement, *TFOA* tibiofemoral knee OA, *PCR-RFLP* polymerase chain reaction-restriction fragment length polymorphism, *PFOA* patellofemoral knee OA, *iMLDR* improved multiplex ligase detection reaction, *HRM* high resolution melting

Table 2 Distributions of ADAM2 rs3740199 genotypes and alleles among cases and controls

Year	First author	Case			Control			Case		Control		HWE in control
		CC	GC	GG	CC	GC	GG	C	G	C	G	
2009	J. Rodriguez-Lopez[a]	NA	NA	NA	NA	NA	NA	290	234	327	261	NA
2009	J. Rodriguez-Lopez[a]	NA	NA	NA	NA	NA	NA	370	350	744	652	NA
2009	J. Rodriguez-Lopez[a]	NA	NA	NA	NA	NA	NA	180	138	239	147	NA
2009	I. Kerna[a]	28	32	6	65	46	12	88	44	176	70	0.366
2009	I. Kerna[a]	53	34	10	41	43	8	140	54	125	59	0.485
2012	Min-Ho Shin	147	364	214	350	863	524	658	792	1563	1911	0.876
2014	Suliang Lou	32	78	42	42	93	44	142	162	177	181	0.6
2015	LinWang	36	84	44	47	102	51	156	172	196	204	0.773
2016	Thitiya Poonpet	56	102	42	46	100	54	214	186	192	208	0.982

HWE Hardy–Weinberg equilibrium, *NA* data not available
[a]An independent study in one article

encouraged us to search for more responsible genes. Many genes have been studied and the *ADAM12* gene is one of the possible candidate genes for OA [12, 23–27]. Some investigations suggested a regulatory role of *ADAM12* in chondrocyte proliferation, maturation, bone formation, and osteoclast differentiation [15–18]. Association studies have been arranged to investigate the role of a nonsynonymous polymorphism (rs3740199) in the second exon of *ADAM12* in knee OA risk that has been reported to date [12, 21, 25, 26, 34]. However, these findings have been inconsistent and contradictory.

Meta-analysis is a suitable method to combine the results of individual studies, overcome the disadvantages of a single study, and increase the statistical power. The present study was to investigate and update the results associating the *ADAM12* rs3740199 polymorphism with knee OA risk in different ethnic populations. To our knowledge, the present study is the first meta-analysis which estimated the association between *ADAM12* rs3740199 and knee OA susceptibility. No significant association of *ADAM12* rs3740199 polymorphisms with knee OA risk was demonstrated in our study. We also failed to find the association between knee OA and the

Table 3 Meta-analysis for the ADAM2 rs3740199 polymorphism and knee OA risk

Population	Comparison (*N*[a])	Test of association		Test of heterogeneity	
		OR (95% CI)	*p*[b]	*p*[c]	*I*[2] (%)
Overall	C vs. G (12)	0.983 (0.910–1.061)	0.657	0.490	0.0
	CC vs. GG (6)	1.033 (0.851–1.255)	0.740	0.681	0.0
	CG vs. GG (6)	1.030 (0.877–1.209)	0.721	0.770	0.0
	CC/CG vs. GG (6)	1.031 (0.886–1.201)	0.690	0.768	0.0
	CC vs. CG/GG (6)	1.017 (0.868–1.190)	0.837	0.364	8.1
Ethnicity					
Asian	C vs. G (4)	1.020 (0.924–1.127)	0.689	0.398	0.0
	CC vs. GG (4)	1.040 (0.850–1.272)	0.703	0.390	0.4
	CG vs. GG (4)	1.035 (0.878–1.221)	0.681	0.709	0.0
	CC/CG vs. GG (4)	1.036 (0.887–1.211)	0.656	0.502	0.0
	CC vs. CG/GG (4)	1.017 (0.858–1.207)	0.843	0.642	0.0
European	C vs. G (8)	0.930 (0.825–1.049)	0.239	0.538	0.0
	CC vs. GG (2)	0.950 (0.453–1.992)	0.891	0.809	0.0
	CG vs. GG (2)	0.927 (0.446–1.930)	0.840	0.301	6.6
	CC/CG vs. GG (2)	0.940 (0.465–1.901)	0.864	0.713	0.0
	CC vs. CG/GG (2)	0.998 (0.445–2.237)	0.996	0.052	73.4

OR odds ratio, *CI* confidence interval
[a]Number of comparison
[b]*P* values for within group differences were determined by *Z* test
[c]*P* value of *Q* test for heterogeneity test

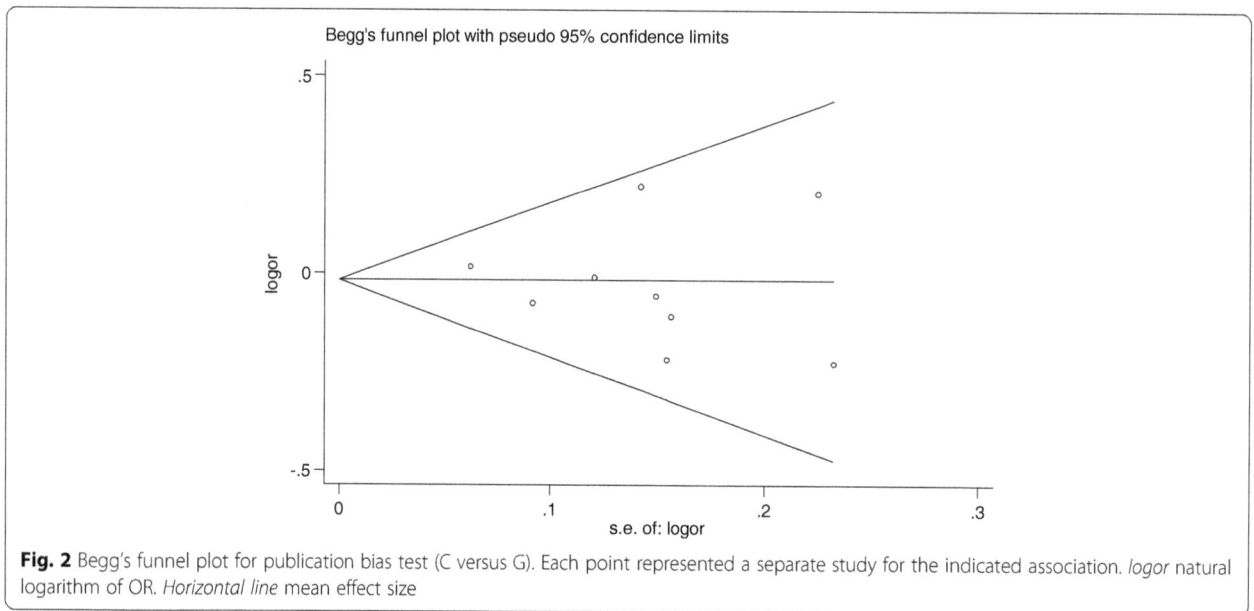

Fig. 2 Begg's funnel plot for publication bias test (C versus G). Each point represented a separate study for the indicated association. *logor* natural logarithm of OR. *Horizontal line* mean effect size

ADAM12 polymorphism in Asian and European population. No heterogeneity was found in overall population and Asian population, while high heterogeneity was seen in the recessive model in European population.

Association studies with complex outcomes for detecting genetic variants must be considered with caution because the results may be influenced by many factors. Our present study showed a lack of association between the *ADAM12* rs3740199 polymorphism and knee OA risk, which is not consistent with the association or functional studies of the *ADAM12* polymorphism. However, epidemiologic results are always different from the functional studies because OA is a multifactorial disease influenced by different genetic backgrounds, multiple genes, and environmental factors. Our negative results of the *ADAM12* polymorphism may also be due to type II error. In recent years, some genome-wide association studies (GWAS) have already reported *GDF5*, *BTNL2*, *DUS4L*, *COG5*, *SENP6*, and *FILIP1* as OA candidate genes [35, 36]. However, the *ADAM12* polymorphism has not been confirmed in these GWAS [35, 36].

Our results are consistent with some studies that also failed to detect association between rs3740199 and OA susceptibility in either male or female patients [12, 23, 26, 27]. On the other hand, Poonpet et al. reported the rs3740199 polymorphism was associated with knee OA risk, while the effect was only found in Thai male patients [24]. The C allele of rs3740199 was found to be associated with OA in female patients in the UK [21]. Kerna et al. found significant association between *ADAM12* rs3740199 and PFOA in male patients [25]. The reason for the contradictory results remain unclear, but the differences in study populations including age, gender, sample size, and disease severity may play an

important role. In the meanwhile, the environmental factors in each sample such as lifestyles, diets, and selected physical activity may also affect the association between rs3740199 polymorphism and OA risk. Lastly, each population has their own gene pool, so it is not surprising that there are differences in the distributions of *ADAM12* rs3740199 genotypes and alleles from subjects with different ethnicities.

Some limitations of this meta-analysis should also be noted. First, the potential confounding factors (such as age, gender) were not adjusted in the present study. Second, the gene-environment interactions and the effect of gene-gene should also be considered because they might influence the biological effects of the polymorphisms of the *ADAM12* gene. Third, because it was difficult to get all full papers published in different languages, we only included six studies published in English language. Fourth, the included subjects were not adequate to confirm a robust conclusion and the association should be resolved by larger studies.

Conclusions

In conclusion, this meta-analysis did not reveal any association between the *ADAM12* rs3740199 polymorphism and knee OA risk. Additional larger studies are needed to confirm our findings in the future.

Abbreviations
ADAM: A disintegrin and metalloprotease; CIs: Confidence intervals; GWAS: Genome-wide association studies; HRM: High resolution melting; HWE: Hardy–Weinberg equilibrium; iMLDR: Improved multiplex ligase detection reaction; K/L score: Kellgren–Lawrence score; OA: Osteoarthritis; ORs: Odds ratios; PB: Population based; PCR-RFLP: Polymerase chain reaction-restriction fragment length polymorphism; PFOA: Patellofemoral knee OA; TFOA: Tibiofemoral knee OA; TKR: Total knee replacement

Acknowledgements
This work was supported by the Projects of International Cooperation and Exchanges NSFC (81420108021), National Key Technology Support Program (2015BAI08B02), Excellent Young Scholars NSFC (81622033), Jiangsu Provincial Key Medical Center Foundation, Jiangsu Provincial Medical Talent Foundation, and Jiangsu Provincial Medical Outstanding Talent Foundation. We thank the patients and their families who donated their blood samples for this study.

Funding
Not applicable.

Authors' contributions
BZ, QJ contributed to the critical revision of the article. ZH, XL conceived of the design of the study. ZH, XL and JD performed and collected the data and contributed to the design of the study. ZH, XL and JD prepared and revised the manuscript. All authors read and approved the final content of the manuscript.

Competing interests
The authors declare that they have no competing interests.

Author details
[1]Center of Diagnosis and Treatment for Developmental Dysplasia of the Hip, Nanjing Zhongyangmen Community Health Service Center, Kang'ai Hospital, Nanjing 210037, Jiangsu, People's Republic of China. [2]Department of HIV/AIDS/STI Prevention and Control, Nanjing Municipal Center for Diseases Control and Prevention, Nanjing 210009, Jiangsu, People's Republic of China. [3]Department of Sports Medicine and Adult Reconstructive Surgery, Drum Tower Hospital, School of Medicine, Nanjing University, 321 Zhongshan Road, Nanjing 210008, Jiangsu, People's Republic of China. [4]Laboratory for Bone and Joint Disease, Model Animal Research Center (MARC), Nanjing University, Nanjing 210093, Jiangsu, China.

References
1. Zhuo Q, Yang W, Chen J, Wang Y. Metabolic syndrome meets osteoarthritis. Nat Rev Rheumatol. 2012;8:729–37.
2. Felson DT. Developments in the clinical understanding of osteoarthritis. Arthritis Res Ther. 2009;11:203.
3. Litwic A, Edwards MH, Dennison EM, Cooper C. Epidemiology and burden of osteoarthritis. Br Med Bull. 2013;105:185–99.
4. Cross M, Smith E, Hoy D, Nolte S, Ackerman I, Fransen M, et al. The global burden of hip and knee osteoarthritis: estimates from the global burden of disease 2010 study. Ann Rheum Dis. 2014;73:1323–30.
5. Johnson VL, Hunter DJ. The epidemiology of osteoarthritis. Best Pract Res Clin Rheumatol. 2014;28:5–15.
6. Guilak F. Biomechanical factors in osteoarthritis. Best Pract Res Clin Rheumatol. 2011;25:815–23.
7. van Tunen JA, Dell'Isola A, Juhl C, Dekker J, Steultjens M, Lund H. Biomechanical factors associated with the development of tibiofemoral knee osteoarthritis: protocol for a systematic review and meta-analysis. BMJ Open. 2016;6:e11066.
8. Kizawa H, Kou I, Iida A, Sudo A, Miyamoto Y, Fukuda A, et al. An aspartic acid repeat polymorphism in asporin inhibits chondrogenesis and increases susceptibility to osteoarthritis. Nat Genet. 2005;37:138–44.
9. Loughlin J, Dowling B, Chapman K, Marcelline L, Mustafa Z, Southam L, et al. Functional variants within the secreted frizzled-related protein 3 gene are associated with hip osteoarthritis in females. Proc Natl Acad Sci U S A. 2004; 101:9757–62.
10. Miyamoto Y, Mabuchi A, Shi D, Kubo T, Takatori Y, Saito S, et al. A functional polymorphism in the 5' UTR of GDF5 is associated with susceptibility to osteoarthritis. Nat Genet. 2007;39:529–33.
11. Nakajima M, Kizawa H, Saitoh M, Kou I, Miyazono K, Ikegawa S. Mechanisms for asporin function and regulation in articular cartilage. J Biol Chem. 2007; 282:32185–92.
12. Rodriguez-Lopez J, Pombo-Suarez M, Loughlin J, Tsezou A, Blanco FJ,

13. Meulenbelt I, et al. Association of a nsSNP in ADAMTS14 to some osteoarthritis phenotypes. Osteoarthritis Cartilage. 2009;17:321–7.
13. Kveiborg M, Albrechtsen R, Couchman JR, Wewer UM. Cellular roles of ADAM12 in health and disease. Int J Biochem Cell Biol. 2008;40:1685–702.
14. Mochizuki S, Okada Y. ADAMs in cancer cell proliferation and progression. Cancer Sci. 2007;98:621–8.
15. Verrier S, Hogan A, McKie N, Horton M. ADAM gene expression and regulation during human osteoclast formation. Bone. 2004;35:34–46.
16. Abe E, Mocharla H, Yamate T, Taguchi Y, Manolagas SC. Meltrin-alpha, a fusion protein involved in multinucleated giant cell and osteoclast formation. Calcif Tissue Int. 1999;64:508–15.
17. Kveiborg M, Albrechtsen R, Rudkjaer L, Wen G, Damgaard-Pedersen K, Wewer UM. ADAM12-S stimulates bone growth in transgenic mice by modulating chondrocyte proliferation and maturation. J Bone Miner Res. 2006;21:1288–96.
18. Okada A, Mochizuki S, Yatabe T, Kimura T, Shiomi T, Fujita Y, et al. ADAM-12 (meltrin alpha) is involved in chondrocyte proliferation via cleavage of insulin-like growth factor binding protein 5 in osteoarthritic cartilage. Arthritis Rheum. 2008;58:778–89.
19. Sato T, Konomi K, Yamasaki S, Aratani S, Tsuchimochi K, Yokouchi M, et al. Comparative analysis of gene expression profiles in intact and damaged regions of human osteoarthritic cartilage. Arthritis Rheum. 2006;54:808–17.
20. Ma G, Ainola M, Liljestrom M, Santavirta S, Poduval P, Zhao D, et al. Increased expression and processing of ADAM 12 (meltrin-alpha) in osteolysis associated with aseptic loosening of total hip replacement implants. J Rheumatol. 2005;32:1943–50.
21. Valdes AM, Hart DJ, Jones KA, Surdulescu G, Swarbrick P, Doyle DV, et al. Association study of candidate genes for the prevalence and progression of knee osteoarthritis. Arthritis Rheum. 2004;50:2497–507.
22. Limer KL, Tosh K, Bujac SR, McConnell R, Doherty S, Nyberg F, et al. Attempt to replicate published genetic associations in a large, well-defined osteoarthritis case-control population (the GOAL study). Osteoarthritis Cartilage. 2009;17:782–9.
23. Lou S, Zhao Z, Qian J, Zhao K, Wang R. Association of single nucleotide polymorphisms in ADAM12 gene with susceptibility to knee osteoarthritis: a case-control study in a Chinese Han population. Int J Clin Exp Pathol. 2014; 7:5154–9.
24. Poonpet T, Tammachote R, Tammachote N, Kanitnate S, Honsawek S. Association between ADAM12 polymorphism and knee osteoarthritis in Thai population. Knee. 2016;23:357–61.
25. Kerna I, Kisand K, Tamm AE, Lintrop M, Veske K, Tamm AO. Missense single nucleotide polymorphism of the ADAM12 gene is associated with radiographic knee osteoarthritis in middle-aged Estonian cohort. Osteoarthritis Cartilage. 2009;17:1093–8.
26. Shin MH, Lee SJ, Kee SJ, Song SK, Kweon SS, Park DJ, et al. Genetic association analysis of GDF5 and ADAM12 for knee osteoarthritis. Joint Bone Spine. 2012;79:488–91.
27. Wang L, Guo L, Tian F, Hao R, Yang T. Analysis of single nucleotide polymorphisms within ADAM12 and risk of knee osteoarthritis in a Chinese Han population. Biomed Res Int. 2015;2015:518643.
28. MANTEL N, HAENSZEL W. Statistical aspects of the analysis of data from retrospective studies of disease. J Natl Cancer Inst. 1959;22:719–48.
29. Egger M, Davey SG, Schneider M, Minder C. Bias in meta-analysis detected by a simple, graphical test. BMJ. 1997;315:629–34.
30. Lee YH, Rho YH, Choi SJ, Ji JD, Song GG. Osteoarthritis susceptibility loci defined by genome scan meta-analysis. Rheumatol Int. 2006;26:959–63.
31. MacGregor AJ, Spector TD. Twins and the genetic architecture of osteoarthritis. Rheumatology (Oxford). 1999;38:583–8.
32. Bijkerk C, Houwing-Duistermaat JJ, Valkenburg HA, Meulenbelt I, Hofman A, Breedveld FC, et al. Heritabilities of radiologic osteoarthritis in peripheral joints and of disc degeneration of the spine. Arthritis Rheum. 1999;42:1729–35.
33. Valdes AM, Doherty M, Spector TD. The additive effect of individual genes in predicting risk of knee osteoarthritis. Ann Rheum Dis. 2008;67:124–7.
34. Valdes AM, Van Oene M, Hart DJ, Surdulescu GL, Loughlin J, Doherty M, et al. Reproducible genetic associations between candidate genes and clinical knee osteoarthritis in men and women. Arthritis Rheum. 2006;54:533–9.
35. Zeggini E, Panoutsopoulou K, Southam L, Rayner NW, Day-Williams AG, Lopes MC, et al. Identification of new susceptibility loci for osteoarthritis (arcOGEN): a genome-wide association study. Lancet. 2012;380:815–23.

8

Relationship between knee osteoarthritis and meniscal shape in observation of Japanese patients by using magnetic resonance imaging

Tsuneo Kawahara[1,2*], Takahisa Sasho[3,4], Joe Katsuragi[5], Takashi Ohnishi[6] and Hideaki Haneishi[6]

Abstract

Background: The aims of this study were to reveal the characteristics of the meniscal shape at each knee osteoarthritis (OA) severity level and to predict trends or patterns of the meniscal shape change as associated with knee OA progression.

Methods: Fifty-one patients diagnosed with knee OA based on X-ray and magnetic resonance (MR) images were evaluated. They were divided into three groups based on the Kellgren–Lawrence (KL) grade: normal group (KL grade of 0 or 1), mild group (KL grade of 2 or 3), and severe group (KL grade of 4). We measured the patients' meniscal size and meniscal extrusion using MR images. In addition, semiquantitative measurement was performed using MR images to determine the arthritic status of the corresponding compartment using a whole-organ magnetic resonance imaging score (WORMS).

Results: The longitudinal diameter and posterior wedge angle of the medial meniscus were significantly larger, and the posterior wedge width of the medial meniscus was significantly smaller in the severe group than in the normal group. The WORMS scores for cartilage and osteophytes in the medial region were significantly different among the groups. The WORMS score of each region was strongly correlated with the longitudinal diameter. The WORMS scores of the lateral region were lower than those of the medial region.

Conclusion: Our observation of the shape change of the medial meniscus in the posterior region was roughly consistent with that in many previous studies of meniscal degeneration. On the other hand, we saw that the most relevant relation between the progression of the knee OA and the deformation of the meniscus was in the longitudinal direction.

Keywords: Meniscus, Knee osteoarthritis, Shape measurement, Deformation pattern, WORMS

Background

The number of patients with knee osteoarthritis (OA) has been increasing yearly. Approximately 25.3 million Japanese individuals aged >40 years reportedly had knee OA in 2009 [1]. In recent years, although many reports have described the detection of articular cartilage degeneration on magnetic resonance (MR) imaging for early detection of knee OA [2], the meniscus has received little attention. The meniscus is a fibrocartilage organization that plays several important roles, including load balancing and shock absorbance in the knee joint. However, few papers have focused on the meniscal shape in patients with knee OA [3–6]. The relationship between meniscal deformation and knee OA remains unclear. Although attention has been given to medial meniscal extrusion, other changes also require examination. We considered that morphological changes occur in accordance with medial meniscal extrusion.

* Correspondence: tsunekawahara007@gmail.com
[1]Graduate School of Engineering, Chiba University, 1-33 Yayoi-cho, Inage-ku, Chiba 263-8522, Japan
[2]Medical Corporation Jinseikai, Togane, Japan
Full list of author information is available at the end of the article

The purposes of this study were to reveal the characteristics of the meniscal shape in patients with knee OA at each severity level by measuring several quantitative geometric parameters on MR images and to reveal the pattern of meniscal deformation with the progression of knee OA.

Methods

Patients

Fifty-one patients who had been diagnosed with medial type knee OA based on X-ray and MR images were evaluated. The patients were divided into three groups in Table 1 according to their knee OA severity level using the Kellgren–Lawrence (KL) method [7].

MR images and segmentation

MR images were obtained with a 3.0-T DISCOVERY MR750 (GE Healthcare, UK). T1rho-weighted MR images (512×512 pixels, 88 slices) were used to segment the meniscus. Using a three-dimensional MR image, two sagittal slices were extracted: one including the longest diameter of the lateral meniscus and the other including the longest diameter of the medial meniscus. Figure 1 shows the segmentation procedure [8]. First, the sagittal slice was selected as shown in Fig. 1a. The binarization process was then performed to isolate the meniscus from the surrounding tissue. The mode method was used for this purpose [9]. This method automatically identifies a valley between two peaks in the histogram and uses it as a threshold for binarization. Figure 1b represents the binarization result of the original image shown in Fig. 1a. Finally, by manual segmentation, the meniscal region was determined from the binary image as shown in Fig. 1c.

Quantitative measurement

The following quantities as illustrated in Fig. 2 were measured from both medial and lateral slices:

– Maximum size of longitudinal diameter (LD)
– Anterior wedge thickness

– Anterior wedge width
– Posterior wedge width
– Posterior wedge thickness
– Anterior wedge angle
– Posterior wedge angle

The measurements were conducted with the free image analysis software ImageJ 1.47v. As knee OA progresses, the fibers of the meniscal inner edge become frayed. Highly irregular edges are difficult to extract; thus, such edges were excluded from the measurement object. We modeled the cross section of the meniscus by two wedge-shaped triangles, measured each geometric quantity four times, excluded the maximum and minimum values, and adopted the average of the remaining two values. Each measurement value was normalized by the patient's height.

The amount of medial meniscal extrusion was measured on an MR coronal image. Using a volume image composed of a set of sagittal images, a coronal image was produced (512×528 pixels, 512 slices) by 0-th order interpolation. The amount of meniscal extrusion was defined as the distance from the end of the tibia to the meniscal edge in a slice (Fig. 2, right).

Semiquantitative measurement

The orthopedic surgeons performed semiquantitative measurement of MR imaging using whole-organ magnetic resonance imaging score (WORMS) [10]. WORMS incorporates 14 features. Among them, this paper adopted five features that were related to the articular surface: articular cartilage integrity, subarticular bone marrow abnormality, subarticular cysts, subarticular bone attrition, and marginal osteophytes. These features were evaluated in different regions subdivided by anatomical landmarks in the fully extended knee (Fig. 3). The articular cartilage integrity and marginal osteophytes were evaluated and scored into any of eight levels in each region; the other parts were scored into any of four levels. The resultant value indicated the severity of knee OA. Zero indicated a normal condition, and larger values indicated a more severe condition.

Table 1 Statistics of patient groups

	Number	Age	Height (mm)	Weight (kg)
Normal (KL grades 0–1)	14	27.4 ± 12.6	167.6 ± 9.7	63.4 ± 10.6
	9 males/5 females			
Mild (KL grades 2–3)	15	57.3 ± 17.9	158.6 ± 7.1	62.5 ± 6.4
	4 males/11 females			
Severe (KL grade 4)	22	72.9 ± 7.6	152.0 ± 7.7	58.8 ± 10.5
	2 males/20 females			

The patients were divided into three groups according to their knee OA severity level using the Kellgren–Lawrence (KL) method

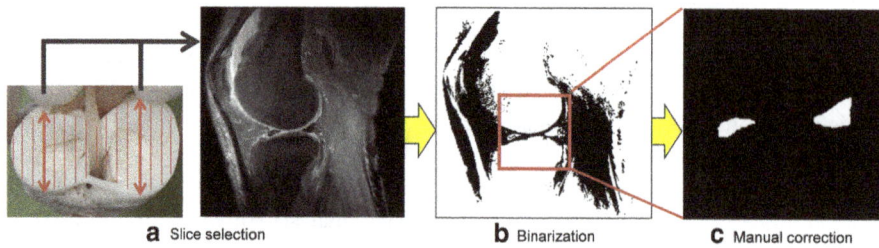

Fig. 1 Meniscal segmentation procedure. **a** Schematic illustration of slice selection. **b** Binarization of the image in **a** with a proper threshold. **c** Manually segmented meniscus

Statistical analysis

Significant differences in the mean values among the groups were verified using one-way analysis of variance. Multiple comparisons were performed by the Bonferroni method ($p < 0.05$). Correlations between groups were examined using Pearson's correlation coefficient.

Results

The meniscal measurement results are shown in Table 2 and Fig. 4. The deformations with significant difference are also summarized in Fig. 5. The medial LD, medial posterior wedge width, medial posterior wedge angle, and lateral LD were significantly different between the normal and severe groups. The medial LD and posterior wedge angle in the severe group were 19.3% and 52.7% greater than the respective values in the normal group. The medial posterior wedge width in the severe group was 15.5% smaller than that in the normal group. The lateral LD in the severe group was 9.9% greater than that in the normal group. The standard deviation of each measured quantity in the severe group was markedly high.

Table 3 shows the WORMS scores of the medial region and the significant differences in each group and region. The WORMS score for the cartilage and osteophytes in the medial meniscus was significantly different between the groups. In the normal group, the cartilage score of the medial femoral central (MFC) was larger than that of the medial femoral posterior (MFP) and medial tibial posterior (MTP). In the severe group, the cartilage score of the MTP was smaller than that of the MFC and medial femoral central (MTC). In all groups, bone attrition score was largest for the MTC. In the normal group, the osteophytes score of the MTP was smaller than that of the MFC and MFP. In the severe group, the osteophytes score of the MFP was larger than that of the medial tibial anterior (MTA), MTC, and MFP.

Table 4 shows the same components in the lateral region. The WORMS scores in the lateral region were lower than those in the medial region. The marrow abnormality and bone cyst scores showed no significant differences in each group. In the mild group, the bone attrition score of the lateral femoral central (LFC) was larger than that of the lateral femoral posterior (LFP), lateral tibial anterior (LTA), and lateral femoral central (LTC). In normal and mild groups, the femoral osteophytes score (LFC and LFP) was larger than the tibial osteophytes score (LTA, LTC, and LTP).

Table 5 shows the amount of medial meniscal extrusion. There was a significant difference between the normal and severe groups ($p = 0.0136$).

This paper adopted the WORMS score of cartilage and osteophytes, which exhibited a significant difference among the groups. Tables 6 and 7 show the correlation

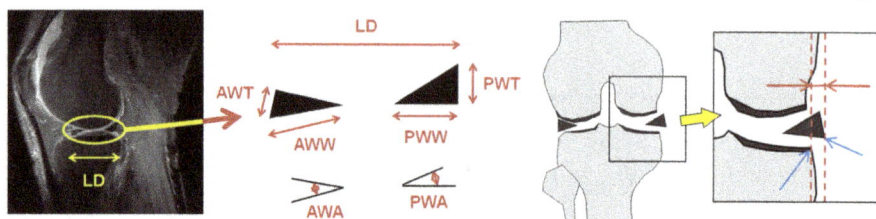

Fig. 2 Quantitative measurement of the meniscus. (*left*) Geometric quantities for analysis of meniscal shape. *LD* maximum size of longitudinal diameter, *AWT* anterior wedge thickness, *AWW* anterior wedge width, *PWW* posterior wedge width, *PWT* posterior wedge thickness, *AWA* anterior wedge angle, *PWA* posterior wedge angle. (*right*) Illustration of the amount of meniscal extrusion. The end of the tibia and the meniscal edge are manually identified from an MR coronal slice (*blue arrows*), and the horizontal distance between them (*red arrows*) is defined as the amount of meniscal extrusion

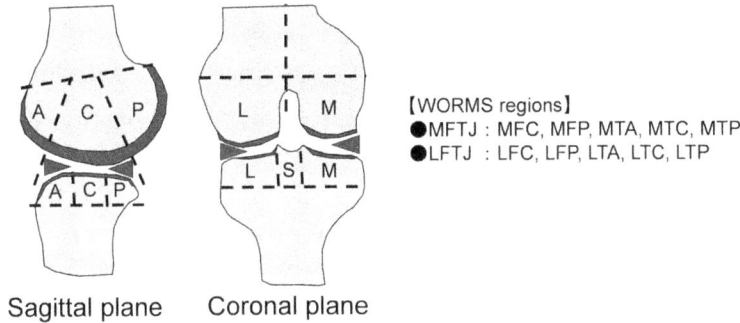

Fig. 3 WORMS regions. The femur and tibia are divided into anterior (*A*), central (*C*), and posterior (*P*) regions in the sagittal plane. Both bones are further divided into medial (*M*) and lateral (*L*) regions in the coronal plane. Region *S* refers to the intercondylar eminence of the tibia. The abbreviations for the WORMS regions in the figure include the portion and bone name. For example, MFC refers to the medial femoral central region. MFTJ refers to the medial femorotibial joint, which includes five regions (MFC, MFP, MTA, MTC, and MTP)

coefficients between the WORMS scores of cartilage and osteophytes and the medial meniscal size. The WORMS scores of each region indicated a strong correlation, and the LD showed a strong correlation as well ($r = 0.59–0.68$).

Discussion

Many authors have reported the presence of degeneration in the posterior region of the medial meniscus in patients with knee OA [11–13]. We considered that Japanese patients with knee OA are likely to have

Table 2 Meniscal measurement on medial and lateral slices

a-1. Medial meniscal size (raw data)

	LD (mm)	AWT (mm)	AWW (mm)	PWW (mm)	PWT (mm)	AWA (degree)	PWA (degree)
Normal KL grade 0–1	44.2 ± 4.2	6.3 ± 1.6	10.1 ± 1.5	13.6 ± 2.1	5.9 ± 1.0	34.5 ± 7.0	24.2 ± 5.7
Mild KL grade 2–3	44.8 ± 3.9	6.6 ± 1.1	10.0 ± 1.2	11.1 ± 2.5	6.0 ± 1.5	40.3 ± 7.7	31.9 ± 9.4
Severe KL grade 4	47.8 ± 4.7	5.7 ± 2.1	9.8 ± 2.9	10.3 ± 1.9	6.9 ± 2.9	37.0 ± 9.7	37.0 ± 13.3

a-2. Medial meniscal size (normalized data)

	LD (mm)	AWT (mm)	AWW (mm)	PWW (mm)	PWT (mm)	AWA (degree)	PWA (degree)
Normal KL grade 0–1	$(26.5 ± 3.2) × 10^{-3}$ **	$(3.8 ± 1.0) × 10^{-3}$	$(6.1 ± 1.0) × 10^{-3}$	$(8.1 ± 1.3) × 10^{-3}$ **	$(3.6 ± 0.6) × 10^{-3}$	34.5 ± 7.0	24.2 ± 5.7 **
Mild KL grade 2–3	$(28.2 ± 2.1) × 10^{-3}$	$(4.2 ± 0.7) × 10^{-3}$	$(6.3 ± 0.8) × 10^{-3}$	$(7.0 ± 1.6) × 10^{-3}$	$(3.8 ± 0.9) × 10^{-3}$	40.3 ± 7.7	31.9 ± 9.4
Severe KL grade 4	$(31.6 ± 3.3) × 10^{-3}$	$(3.8 ± 1.4) × 10^{-3}$	$(6.5 ± 2.0) × 10^{-3}$	$(6.9 ± 1.4) × 10^{-3}$	$(4.5 ± 2.0) × 10^{-3}$	37.0 ± 9.7	37.0 ± 13.3

b-1. Lateral meniscal size (raw data)

	LD (mm)	AWT (mm)	AWW (mm)	PWW (mm)	PWT (mm)	AWA (degree)	PWA (degree)
Normal KL grade 0–1	34.5 ± 4.4	4.4 ± 0.8	10.4 ± 1.4	9.1 ± 1.8	6.1 ± 0.9	27.5 ± 4.4	33.5 ± 6.8
Mild KL grade 2–3	32.9 ± 2.5	4.3 ± 0.7	9.9 ± 1.5	8.2 ± 1.2	6.4 ± 1.0	27.1 ± 5.9	37.1 ± 7.1
Severe KL grade 4	34.2 ± 4.5	5.0 ± 1.2	10.2 ± 2.1	8.8 ± 1.6	6.4 ± 1.1	30.4 ± 6.5	36.2 ± 9.0

b-2. Lateral meniscal size (normalized data)

	LD (mm)	AWT (mm)	AWW (mm)	PWW (mm)	PWT (mm)	AWA (degree)	PWA (degree)
Normal KL grade 0–1	$(20.5 ± 1.9) × 10^{-3}$ *	$(2.6 ± 0.5) × 10^{-3}$	$(6.2 ± 0.9) × 10^{-3}$	$(5.4 ± 0.9) × 10^{-3}$	$(3.7 ± 0.6) × 10^{-3}$	27.5 ± 4.4	33.5 ± 6.8
Mild KL grade 2–3	$(20.7 ± 0.9) × 10^{-3}$	$(2.7 ± 0.4) × 10^{-3}$	$(6.2 ± 0.9) × 10^{-3}$	$(5.2 ± 0.6) × 10^{-3}$	$(4.1 ± 0.6) × 10^{-3}$	27.1 ± 5.9	37.1 ± 7.1
Severe KL grade 4	$(22.5 ± 3.1) × 10^{-3}$	$(3.3 ± 0.9) × 10^{-3}$	$(6.7 ± 1.5) × 10^{-3}$	$(5.8 ± 1.1) × 10^{-3}$	$(4.2 ± 0.7) × 10^{-3}$	30.4 ± 6.5	36.2 ± 9.0

This table shows the average value ± standard deviation of medial (a) and lateral (b) meniscal slices. "a-1" and "b-1" indicate the measurement value (raw data), and "a-2" and "b-2" indicate the number normalized by the each patient's height. Two groups showing significant differences are indicated by one or two asterisks. The normalized values were evaluated in the comparison of length

LD maximum size of longitudinal diameter, *AWT* anterior wedge thickness, *AWW* anterior wedge width, *PWW* posterior wedge width, *PWT* posterior wedge thickness, *AWA* anterior wedge angle, *PWA* posterior wedge angle

($*p < 0.05$, $**p < 0.01$)

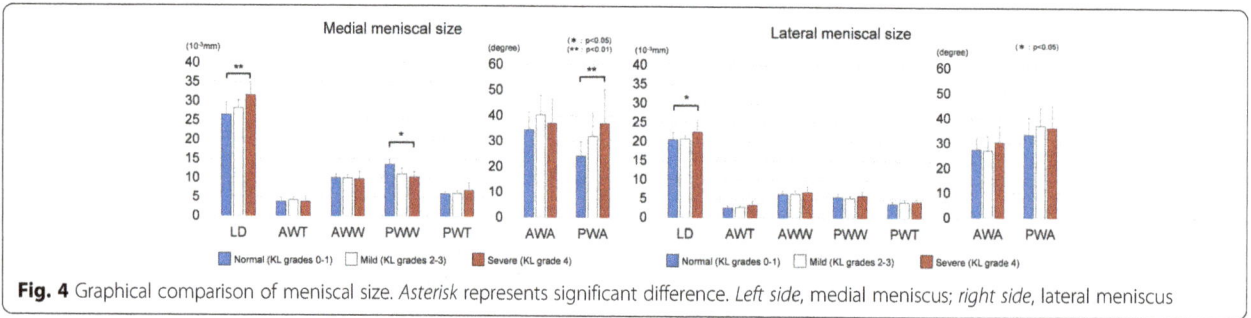

Fig. 4 Graphical comparison of meniscal size. *Asterisk* represents significant difference. *Left side*, medial meniscus; *right side*, lateral meniscus

different characteristics than Westerners because of the differences in lifestyles and body types between these two populations. Therefore, this paper has herein included a discussion of previously published Japanese reports. Fukuda et al. [14] and Nagata et al. [15] stated that degeneration occurred in the posterior region of the medial meniscus with a high probability and expanded from posterior to anterior. In the present study, we found that the LD and posterior region of the medial meniscus of the severe group changed in size compared with those in the normal group. These results support the findings of previous reports. The location of meniscal degeneration more or less corresponded to the position at which the meniscal size changed. Lee et al. [16] stated that the posterior region of the medial meniscus had a characteristic fiber array, and Kwak et al. [17] reported that the same region had high strength. Markris et al. [18] stated that meniscal cells with degeneration were larger in diameter than normal meniscal cells. Based on these previous reports and our results, we conclude that thickening due to degeneration occurs in the medial posterior region.

A few studies on the lateral meniscus have been reported. In Japan, Kitamura et al. [19] reported that lateral meniscal degeneration occurred in the middle and posterior regions. Hirotsu et al. [20] reported that such degeneration occurred in the anterior region. Thus, no consensus has been reached. In the present study, the LD of the lateral meniscus in the severe group was larger than that in the normal group. However, this paper obtained no information that supported the findings of previous studies. The lateral meniscus has a wider range of movements than does the medial meniscus because it has no adhesion to the surrounding tissue; therefore, we considered that the lateral meniscus is able to deflect mechanical stress and that this deflection leads to less degeneration.

In this study, we used the KL method to group the patients. The validity of this grouping method is supported by the fact that the WORMS scores were significantly different among the groups. In the medial region, the cartilage and osteophytes scores were markedly correlated with the characteristics of knee OA progression. The cartilage score reflected the characteristics of this region. The central region tended to be more severe than the posterior region; for example, the MTC was significantly greater

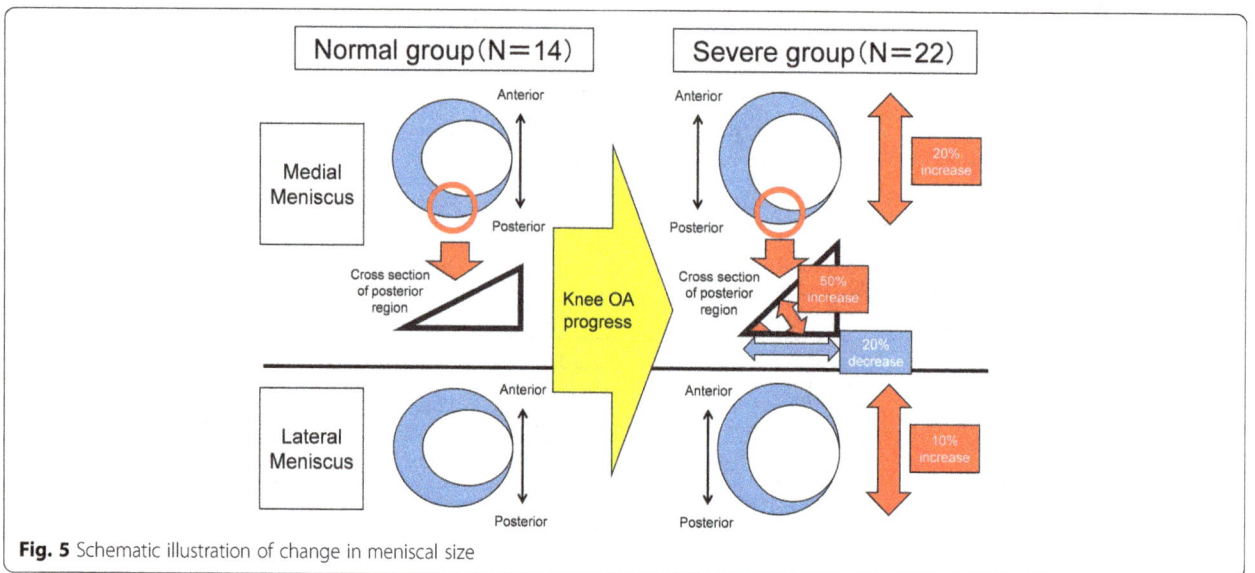

Fig. 5 Schematic illustration of change in meniscal size

Table 3 WORMS scores of medial region and significant differences

| Cartilage | MFTJ | Femur | | Tibia | | |
		MFC	MFP	MTA	MTC	MTP
Normal	5.21 ± 4.32	1.79 ± 1.76	0.57 ± 0.85	1.00 ± 0.88	1.21 ± 1.12	0.64 ± 0.50
Mild	16.80 ± 8.60	4.07 ± 1.83	2.80 ± 1.42	3.47 ± 2.23	3.80 ± 2.11	2.67 ± 1.72
Severe	27.91 ± 2.47	5.96 ± 0.21	5.41 ± 0.91	5.55 ± 0.96	5.91 ± 0.43	5.09 ± 0.92

| Marrow abnormality | MFTJ | Femur | | Tibia | | |
		MFC	MFP	MTA	MTC	MTP
Normal	0.29 ± 0.61	0.21 ± 0.58	0.07 ± 0.27	0.00 ± 0.00	0.00 ± 0.00	0.00 ± 0.00
Mild	1.20 ± 2.04	0.20 ± 0.78	0.07 ± 0.26	0.60 ± 1.12	0.33 ± 0.90	0.00 ± 0.00
Severe	4.23 ± 4.35	1.18 ± 1.26	0.41 ± 0.85	0.64 ± 1.14	1.27 ± 1.42	0.73 ± 1.28

| Bone cysts | MFTJ | Femur | | Tibia | | |
		MFC	MFP	MTA	MTC	MTP
Normal	0.00 ± 0.00	0.00 ± 0.00	0.00 ± 0.00	0.00 ± 0.00	0.00 ± 0.00	0.00 ± 0.00
Mild	0.20 ± 0.56	0.13 ± 0.52	0.00 ± 0.00	0.07 ± 0.26	0.00 ± 0.00	0.00 ± 0.00
Severe	1.86 ± 3.12	0.64 ± 1.00	0.18 ± 0.40	0.41 ± 0.80	0.46 ± 1.01	0.18 ± 0.66

| Bone attrition | MFTJ | Femur | | Tibia | | |
		MFC	MFP	MTA	MTC	MTP
Normal	0.79 ± 1.37	0.00 ± 0.00	0.00 ± 0.00	0.21 ± 0.58	0.43 ± 0.65	0.14 ± 0.36
Mild	1.93 ± 2.05	0.47 ± 0.83	0.00 ± 0.00	0.20 ± 0.41	0.87 ± 0.74	0.40 ± 0.51
Severe	2.59 ± 2.06	0.32 ± 0.72	0.09 ± 0.29	0.36 ± 0.66	1.23 ± 0.81	0.59 ± 0.85

| Osteophytes | MFTJ | Femur | | Tibia | | |
		MFC	MFP	MTA	MTC	MTP
Normal	3.71 ± 2.64	1.00 ± 0.68	1.14 ± 0.36	0.71 ± 0.73	0.57 ± 0.94	0.29 ± 0.47
Mild	10.67 ± 4.25	2.20 ± 0.94	2.60 ± 0.99	1.87 ± 0.92	2.00 ± 0.85	2.00 ± 1.20
Severe	22.77 ± 7.44	5.14 ± 1.42	5.46 ± 1.60	4.09 ± 1.72	4.09 ± 1.54	4.00 ± 1.90

Data are presented as average ± standard deviation. MFTJ refers to the medial femorotibial joint, which includes the MFC, MFP, MTA, MTC, and MTP regions as shown in Fig. 3. Significant differences in each group and region are indicated by an asterisk
*$p < 0.05$, **$p < 0.01$

than the MTP in the severe group. In the lateral region, the scores of all categories were lower than those in the medial region.

The WORMS score, which represents OA progression, showed a stronger correlation with LD ($r = 0.59–0.68$) than with the other geometric parameters of the meniscus. This suggests that meniscal changes associated with OA progression were greater in the longitudinal direction than in the inner and outer directions. It is well known that OA progression involves varus deformation and a smaller range of motion. However, patients with OA often have flexion contracture that leads to a limited range of motion. Therefore, we considered that OA progression may be strongly associated with a meniscal longitudinal element. Although some studies have shown a relationship between posterior horn tears

Table 4 WORMS scores of lateral region and significant differences

Cartilage	LFTJ	Femur		Tibia		
		LFC	LFP	LTA	LTC	LTP
Normal	2.86 ± 2.63	0.93 ± 0.47	0.50 ± 1.09	0.36 ± 0.50	0.71 ± 0.61	0.36 ± 0.63
Mild	13.67 ± 6.15	3.00 ± 1.20	3.00 ± 1.13	2.60 ± 1.68	2.60 ± 1.68	2.47 ± 1.51
Severe	16.55 ± 3.92	3.45 ± 0.67	3.59 ± 0.80	3.36 ± 1.09	2.95 ± 1.25	3.18 ± 1.05

Marrow abnormality	LFTJ	Femur		Tibia		
		LFC	LFP	LTA	LTC	LTP
Normal	0.00 ± 0.00	0.00 ± 0.00	0.00 ± 0.00	0.00 ± 0.00	0.00 ± 0.00	0.00 ± 0.00
Mild	0.13 ± 0.52	0.13 ± 0.52	0.00 ± 0.00	0.00 ± 0.00	0.00 ± 0.00	0.00 ± 0.00
Severe	0.14 ± 0.47	0.05 ± 0.21	0.09 ± 0.43	0.00 ± 0.00	0.00 ± 0.00	0.00 ± 0.00

Bone cysts	LFTJ	Femur		Tibia		
		LFC	LFP	LTA	LTC	LTP
Normal	0.00 ± 0.00	0.00 ± 0.00	0.00 ± 0.00	0.00 ± 0.00	0.00 ± 0.00	0.00 ± 0.00
Mild	0.00 ± 0.00	0.00 ± 0.00	0.00 ± 0.00	0.00 ± 0.00	0.00 ± 0.00	0.00 ± 0.00
Severe	0.09 ± 0.29	0.00 ± 0.00	0.00 ± 0.00	0.09 ± 0.29	0.00 ± 0.00	0.00 ± 0.00

Bone attrition	LFTJ	Femur		Tibia		
		LFC	LFP	LTA	LTC	LTP
Normal	0.36 ± 0.50	0.14 ± 0.36	0.00 ± 0.00	0.00 ± 0.00	0.21 ± 0.43	0.00 ± 0.00
Mild	0.60 ± 0.91	0.40 ± 0.51	0.07 ± 0.26	0.00 ± 0.00	0.13 ± 0.35	0.00 ± 0.00
Severe	0.82 ± 2.20	0.27 ± 0.55	0.14 ± 0.47	0.14 ± 0.47	0.14 ± 0.47	0.14 ± 0.47

Osteophytes	LFTJ	Femur		Tibia		
		LFC	LFP	LTA	LTC	LTP
Normal	2.64 ±1.65	1.07± 0.47	1.14 ± 0.53	0.14 ± 0.36	0.14 ± 0.36	0.14 ± 0.36
Mild	7.60 ± 3.74	2.47 ± 0.83	2.20 ± 0.94	1.33 ± 0.82	1.00 ± 1.07	0.60 ± 0.91
Severe	14.09 ± 5.93	3.55 ± 1.41	3.27 ± 1.58	2.77 ± 1.41	2.32 ± 1.29	2.18 ± 1.33

Data are presented as average ± standard deviation. LFTJ refers to the lateral femorotibial joint, which includes the LFC, LFP, LTA, LTC, and LTP regions as shown in Fig. 3. Significant differences in each group and region are indicated by an asterisk ($*p < 0.05$, $**p < 0.01$)

and medial meniscal extrusion [16, 21], the present study revealed a low correlation coefficient between the WORMS scores and meniscal extrusion (WORMS score of cartilage and extrusion, $r = 0.36–0.45$; WORMS score of osteophytes and extrusion, $r = 0.22–0.26$). Although it is well known that the medial meniscal extrusion caused by degeneration occurs medially, this study showed that the posterior extrusion was more

remarkable. Considering that no patients had posterior root tears in this study, the medial meniscus appeared to expand in all directions in a posterior-dominant fashion. Consequently, this result did not support those of previous studies.

A limitation of the present study is that we did not compare the measured meniscal size with the presence of meniscal tears. It is well known that the

Table 5 Amount of medial meniscal extrusion

	Extrusion (mm)
Normal KL Grade 0–1	1.89 ± 1.80 ⎤
Mild KL Grade 2–3	2.56 ± 1.75 ⎬ *
Severe KL Grade 4	4.36 ± 3.00 ⎦

The amount of meniscal extrusion was defined as the distance from the end of the tibia to the meniscal edge in the imaging slice (Fig. 2, right). Significant differences in each group and region are indicated by an asterisk (*$p < 0.05$)

meniscal size depends on the type of meniscal injury. The second limitation is that the MR images used in this study were taken in a non-weight-bearing position. There is a possibility that weight bearing would change the results. The third limitation is that although observation of MR images using WORMS scores is very useful to understand the progression of knee OA, it shows only one aspect of the pathology. In clinical practice, it is necessary to compare other parameters such as pain and joint range of motion. These points will be studied in future work.

Table 6 Correlation coefficient between the WORMS scores of cartilage and the medial meniscal size, and meniscal extrusion

(a)

	MFC	MFP	MTP	MTC	MTP	MTFJ	LD	AWT	AWW	PWW	PWT	AWA	PWA	Extrusion
MFC	1													
MFP	0.87	1												
MTA	0.87	0.87	1											
MTC	0.94	0.89	0.92	1										
MTP	0.86	0.90	0.93	0.89	1									
MTFJ	0.95	0.95	0.96	0.97	0.96	1								
LD	0.63	0.68	0.59	0.65	0.63	0.66	1							
AWT	0.05	0.10	0.07	0.06	0.15	0.09	0.20	1						
AWW	0.10	0.23	0.13	0.14	0.22	0.17	0.42	0.55	1					
PWW	−0.18	−0.22	−0.15	−0.19	−0.17	−0.19	0.01	0.17	0.16	1				
PWT	0.26	0.33	0.30	0.31	0.26	0.31	0.58	0.35	0.48	0.25	1			
AWA	0.33	0.25	0.29	0.29	0.25	0.30	0.23	0.37	−0.22	−0.07	0.11	1		
PWA	0.47	0.46	0.46	0.50	0.39	0.48	0.57	0.11	0.19	−0.26	0.73	0.27	1	
Extrusion	0.36	0.35	0.41	0.40	0.45	0.41	0.33	−0.14	−0.05	−0.28	0.31	0.12	0.55	1

(b)

	MFC	MFP	MTP	MTC	MTP	MTFJ	LD	AWT	AWW	PWW	PWT	AWA	PWA	Extrusion
MFC	–													
MFP	0.00	–												
MTA	0.00	0.00	–											
MTC	0.00	0.00	0.00	–										
MTP	0.00	0.00	0.00	0.00	–									
MTFJ	0.00	0.00	0.00	0.00	0.00	–								
LD	0.00	0.00	0.00	0.00	0.00	0.00	–							
AWT	0.60	0.30	0.46	0.00	0.14	0.36	0.04	–						
AWW	0.30	0.02	0.18	0.15	0.03	0.08	0.00	0.00	–					
PWW	0.07	0.03	0.12	0.06	0.09	0.06	0.92	0.09	0.10	–				
PWT	0.01	0.00	0.00	0.00	0.01	0.00	0.00	0.00	0.00	0.01	–			
AWA	0.00	0.01	0.00	0.00	0.01	0.00	0.02	0.00	0.02	0.50	0.26	–		
PWA	0.00	0.00	0.00	0.00	0.00	0.00	0.00	0.25	0.05	0.01	0.00	0.01	–	
Extrusion	0.00	0.00	0.00	0.00	0.00	0.00	0.00	0.15	0.62	0.00	0.00	0.24	0.00	–

(a) Values indicate the correlation coefficient between each region. MFTJ refers to the medial femorotibial joint, which includes the MFC, MFP, MTA, MTC, and MTP (see Fig. 3). (b) Probability in each region
High correlation values and corresponding probabilities that should be focused were shown in italics for quick recognition

Table 7 Correlation coefficient between the WORMS scores of osteophytes and the medial meniscal size, and meniscal extrusion

(a)

	MFC	MFP	MTP	MTC	MTP	MTFJ	LD	AWT	AWW	PWW	PWT	AWA	PWA	Extrusion
MFC	1													
MFP	0.95	1												
MTA	0.90	0.91	1											
MTC	0.89	0.92	0.93	1										
MTP	0.87	0.87	0.87	0.89	1									
MTFJ	0.96	0.97	0.96	0.96	0.94	1								
LD	*0.67*	*0.65*	*0.63*	*0.66*	*0.67*	*0.68*	1							
AWT	−0.05	−0.08	−0.13	−0.04	−0.02	−0.07	0.20	1						
AWW	0.25	0.24	0.28	0.25	0.20	0.25	0.42	0.55	1					
PWW	−0.10	−0.11	−0.13	−0.07	−0.13	−0.11	0.01	0.17	0.16	1				
PWT	0.32	0.30	0.34	0.36	0.37	0.35	0.58	0.35	0.48	0.25	1			
AWA	−0.06	−0.13	−0.18	−0.06	−0.10	−0.11	0.23	0.37	−0.22	−0.07	0.11	1		
PWA	0.35	0.31	0.35	0.32	0.35	0.35	0.57	0.11	0.19	−0.26	0.73	0.27	1	
Extrusion	0.26	0.22	0.24	0.22	0.24	0.25	0.33	−0.14	−0.05	−0.28	0.31	0.12	0.55	1

(b)

	MFC	MFP	MTP	MTC	MTP	MTFJ	LD	AWT	AWW	PWW	PWT	AWA	PWA	Extrusion
MFC	–													
MFP	0.00	–												
MTA	0.00	0.00	–											
MTC	0.00	0.00	0.00	–										
MTP	0.00	0.00	0.00	0.00	–									
MTFJ	0.00	0.00	0.00	0.00	0.00	–								
LD	*0.00*	*0.00*	*0.00*	*0.00*	*0.00*	*0.00*	–							
AWT	0.60	0.40	0.19	0.65	0.83	0.49	0.04	–						
AWW	0.01	0.01	0.00	0.01	0.05	0.01	0.00	0.00	–					
PWW	0.30	0.27	0.19	0.49	0.18	0.25	0.92	0.09	0.10	–				
PWT	0.00	0.00	0.00	0.00	0.00	0.00	0.00	0.00	0.00	0.01	–			
AWA	0.56	0.19	0.07	0.54	0.30	0.27	0.02	0.00	0.02	0.50	0.26	–		
PWA	0.00	0.00	0.00	0.00	0.00	0.00	0.00	0.25	0.05	0.01	0.00	0.01	–	
Extrusion	0.01	0.03	0.01	0.03	0.01	0.01	0.00	0.15	0.62	0.00	0.00	0.24	0.00	–

(a) Values indicate the correlation coefficient between each region. MFTJ refers to the medial femorotibial joint, which includes the MFC, MFP, MTA, MTC, and MTP (see Fig. 3). (b) Probability in each region
High correlation values and corresponding probabilities that should be focused were shown in italics for quick recognition

Conclusion

This is the first report on the relationship between the progression of knee OA and the meniscal size in Japanese patients with OA. The finding that the change in the posterior region of the medial meniscus was roughly consistent with the meniscal degeneration is in agreement with many previous studies. On the other hand, it is a new finding that the most relevant relation between the progression of the knee OA and the deformation of the meniscus was in the longitudinal direction. In addition, although meniscal deformation and meniscal extrusion can be found in many patients, the severities of these changes differ among individual patients. We need more detailed analyses of the individual biomechanical impact of the progression of knee OA on the meniscus.

Abbreviations
AWA: Anterior wedge angle; AWT: Anterior wedge thickness; AWW: Anterior wedge width; KL: Kellgren–Lawrence; LD: Longitudinal diameter; LFC: Lateral femoral central; LFP: Lateral femoral posterior; LTA: Lateral tibial anterior; LTC: Lateral femoral central; LTP: Lateral tibial posterior; MFC: Medial femoral central; MFP: Medial femoral posterior; MR: Magnetic resonance; MTA: Medial tibial anterior; MTC: Medial femoral central; MTP: Medial tibial posterior; OA: Osteoarthritis; PWA: Posterior wedge angle; PWT: Posterior wedge thickness; PWW: Posterior wedge width; WORMS: Whole-organ magnetic resonance imaging score

Acknowledgements
None.

Funding
None.

Authors' contributions
TK conceived and designed this study. TS, TO, HH cooperated in designing this study. TS created the WORMS scores. JK collected MR images and organized information. TK charged segmentation of the meniscus and extracted and analyzed the data. TK, TS, TO, HH wrote and revised the manuscript. All authors read and approved the final manuscript.

Competing interests
The authors declare that they have no competing interests.

Author details
[1]Graduate School of Engineering, Chiba University, 1-33 Yayoi-cho, Inage-ku, Chiba 263-8522, Japan. [2]Medical Corporation Jinseikai, Togane, Japan. [3]Center for Preventive Medicine, Musculoskeletal disease and pain, Chiba University, Chiba, Japan. [4]Department of Orthopaedic Surgery, School of Medicine, Chiba University, Chiba, Japan. [5]Department of Orthopaedic Surgery, Local Incorporated Administrative Agency, Sanmu Medical Center, Sanmu, Japan. [6]Center for Frontier Medical Engineering, Chiba University, Chiba, Japan.

References
1. Yoshimura N, Muraki S, Oka H, Mabuchi A, En-Yo Y, Yoshida M, et al. Prevalence of knee osteoarthritis, lumbar spondylosis, and osteoporosis in Japanese men and women: the research on osteoarthritis/osteoporosis against disability study. J Bone Miner Metab. 2009;27:620–8.
2. Wang L, Vieira RLR, Rybak LD, Babb JS, Chang G, Krasnokutsky S, et al. Relationship between knee alignment and T1ρvalues of articular cartilage and menisci in patient with knee osteoarthritis. Eur J Radiol. 2013;82:1946–52.
3. Bloecker K, Guermazi A, Wirth W, Kwoh CK, Resch H, Hunter DJ, et al. Correlation of semiquantitative vs quantitative MRI meniscus measures in osteoarthritic knees: results from the Osteoarthritis Initiative. Skeletal Radiol. 2014;43:227–32.
4. Bloecker K, Guermazi A, Wirth W, Benichou O, Kwoh CK, Hunter DJ, et al. Tibial coverage, meniscus position, size and damage in knees discordant for joint space narrowing—data from the Osteoarthritis Initiative. Osteoarthritis Cartilage. 2013;21:419–27.
5. Wenger A, Wirth W, Hudelmaier M, Noebauer-Huhmann I, Trattnig S, Bloecker K, et al. Meniscus body position, size, and shape in persons with and persons without radiographic knee osteoarthritis: quantitative analyses of knee magnetic resonance images from the osteoarthritis initiative. Arthritis & Rheumatism. 2013;65:1804–11.
6. Wirth W, Frobell RB, Souza RB, Li X, Wyman BT, Le Graverand MP, et al. A three-dimensional quantitative method to measure meniscus shape, position, and signal intensity using MR images: a pilot study and preliminary results in knee osteoarthritis. Magn Reson Med. 2010;63:1162–71.
7. Kellgren JH, Lawrence JS. Radiological assessment of osteoarthrosis. Ann Rheum Dis. 1957;16:494–502.
8. Swanson MS, Prescott JW, Best TM, Powell K, Jackson RD, Haq F, et al. Semi-automated segmentation to assess the lateral meniscus in normal and osteoarthritic knees. Osteoarthritis and Cartilage. 2010;18:344–53.
9. Rosenfeld A, Kak AC. Digital picture processing second edition. 1982; Vol.1: 61–66.
10. Peterfy CG, Guermazi A, Zaim S, Tirman PF, Miaux Y, White D, et al. Whole-organ magnetic resonance imaging score (WORMS) of the knee in osteoarthritis. Osteoarthritis Cartilage. 2004;12:177–90.
11. Petersen W, Forkel P, Feucht MJ, Zantop T, Imhoff AB, Brucker PU. Posterior root tear of the medial and lateral meniscus. Arch Orthop Trauma Surg. 2015;134:237–55.
12. Choi JY, Chang EY, Cunha GM, Tafur M, Statum S, Chung CB. Posterior medial meniscus root ligament lesion: MRI classification and associated findings. Am J Roentgenol. 2014;203:1286–92.
13. LaPrade RF, Ho CP, James E, Crespo B, Laprade CM, Matheny LM. Diagnostic accuracy of 3.0 T magnetic resonance imaging for the detection of meniscus posterior root pathology. Knee Surg Sports Traumatol Arthrosc. 2015;23:152–7.
14. Fukuta S, Masaki K, Korai F. Prevalence of abnormal findings in magnetic resonance images of asymptomatic knees. J Orthop Sci. 2002;7:287–91.
15. Nagata N, Koshino T, Saito T, Sakai N, Takagi T, Takeuchi R. Typing of MRI in medial meniscus degeneration in relation to radiological grade in medial compartmental osteoarthritis of the knee. Japanese journal of rheumatism and joint surgery. 1998;17(2):139–44.
16. Lee DW, Ha JK, Kim JG. Medial meniscus posterior root tear: a comprehensive review. Knee Surgery & Related Research. 2014;26:125–34.
17. Kwak DS, Bae JY, Kim SY, Jeon I, Lu TJ. Evaluation of pre-stress in the menisci of human knee joint using microindentation. J Eng Med. 2014;228(1):11–8.
18. Markris EA, Hadidi P, Athanasiou KA. The knee meniscus: structure-function, pathophysiology, current repair techniques, and prospects for regeneration. Biomaterials. 2011;32:7411–31.
19. Kitamura A, Fujii K, Marumo K, Tanaka T, Nagafuchi T, Yoshimatu C. Meniscus tears in osteoarthritis of the knee; comparison between MRI and arthroscopic findings. Orthopedic Surgery. 1998;49(13):1659–62.
20. Hirotsu M, et al. Analyses of degeneration of lateral meniscus in medial compartmental osteoarthritis of the knee (OA) with MRI. Orthopedic Surgery and Traumatology. 2001;50:412–6.
21. Ohishi T, Suzuki D, Yamamoto K, Banno T, Shimizu Y, Matsuyama Y. Medial extrusion of the posterior segment of medial meniscus is a sensitive sign for posterior horn tears. The Knee. 2014;21:112–8.

9

Iopromide- and gadopentetic acid-derived preparates used in MR arthrography may be harmful to chondrocytes

Kadir Oznam[1], Duygu Yasar Sirin[2], Ibrahim Yilmaz[3*], Yasin Emre Kaya[4], Mehmet Isyar[5], Seyit Ali Gumustas[6], Hanefi Ozbek[3], Semih Akkaya[7], Arda Kayhan[8] and Mahir Mahirogullari[9]

Abstract

Background: Magnetic resonance arthrography, a procedure through which contrast agents containing gadolinium and/or iopromide are administered intra-articularly, has become a useful tool in musculoskeletal diagnosis. Nevertheless, despite being considered safe for systemic use, certain tissue toxicities have been identified for both drugs. In this study, the effects of short-term exposure of human primary chondrocyte cell cultures to gadolinium and/or iopromide contrast agents were examined by assaying for stage-specific embryonic antigen-1 (SSEA-1) protein expression (a chondrogenic differentiation marker), cell viability, toxicity, and proliferation.

Methods: Human articular chondrocytes were grown in monolayer culture and were exposed to iopromide and/or gadolinium diethylenetriamine-pentaacetate (Gd-DPT) for 2 and 6 h. Cell cultures with no drug exposure were used as the control group. Cell differentiation status was assessed according to SSEA-1 protein expression. Contrast agent effects on cell viability and proliferation were analyzed using MTT analysis. Further, changes in cell morphology in relation to the control group were evaluated using inverted light microscopy, environmental scanning electron microscopy (ESEM), and 3-tesla magnetic resonance imaging. The obtained data were statistically compared.

Results: When compared with the control group, both SSEA-1 protein expression and cell proliferation were lowest in the Gd-DPT group ($P = 0.000$). There was a statistically significant correlation between SSEA-1 expression and MTT results (rho = 0.351; $P = 0.003$).

Conclusions: Nevertheless, the data obtained from in vitro experiments may not directly correspond to clinical applications. However, the mere fact that a drug used solely for diagnostic purposes may repress chondrocyte cell proliferation should be carefully considered by clinicians.

Keywords: MR-arthrography, Gadopentetic acid, Iopromide, Chondrotoxicity, Primary cell culture, Stage-specific embryonic antigen-1

Background

Arthrographic contrast agents are commonly used to determine free intra-articular objects and to diagnose shoulder labroligament abnormalities, rotator cuff tendon damage, partial and full-thickness elbow tears, hip joint labral tears, residual or recurrent knee tears following meniscectomy, triangle fibrocartilage and ligamentary damage in carpus, and impingement syndrome in the ankle [1, 2].

Arthography induces swelling of the joint capsule through an increase in the intra-articular liquid volume following the injection of contrast agents, thus enabling more accurate imaging of intra-articular structures [1]. Intra-articular imaging performed by magnetic resonance (MR) imaging and computed tomography employs various pharmaceutical contrast agents [3]. Iopromide (IPM), a low osmolality non-ionic contrast medium, and gadolinium diethylenetriaminepentaacetate (Gd-DPT), which has a high magnetocaloric effect in acyclic IIIB group are routinely used arthography contrast agents [4–6].

* Correspondence: ibrahimyilmaz77@yahoo.com
[3]Department of Medical Pharmacology, Istanbul Medipol University School of Medicine, 34810 Istanbul, Turkey
Full list of author information is available at the end of the article

Nevertheless, despite their wide use, previous studies have reported side effects following the use of several contrast agents in clinical settings [7–10]. Various multidisciplinary pharmacogenetic and pharmacogenomic studies have been performed to address damaged tissue repair without causing side/adverse effects [11, 12]. Indeed, recent studies have developed customizable biological treatment models for the regeneration of articular cartilage tissues [10, 13–17].

The purpose of the present study is to assess the possible cytotoxic effects of IPM and Gd-DPT on chondrocytes by blindly comparing the use of these agents in human primer cell cultures at the molecular level in vitro.

Methods
Materials
Collagenase type II enzyme (1 mg/mL; Invitrogen Corporation), Hank's Balanced Salt Solution (HBSS)-1X (Cat. 14025, Gibco), penicillin-streptomycin, fetal calf serum, Dulbecco's modified Eagle's medium (DMEM, 1000 mg glucose/L), and an agarose solution (Cat. A9539) used to fix the cells for MR imaging, were all supplied from Sigma Chemicals, USA. Sodium dodecyl sulfate (SDS; cat. L4522), insulin-transferrin-selenous acid premix, and DMEM were supplied from Sigma-Aldrich Gmbh Germany. IPM (300/100 mL) was purchased from Bayer, whereas Gd-DPT was supplied from Schering Corporation. 3-(4,5-dimethylthiazol-2-yl)-2,5-diphenyltetrazolium bromide (MTT) commercial kit (Vybrant MTT cell Proliferation assay, cat. V-13154) was purchased from Cell Biolabs, USA. Stage-specific embryonic antigen-1 (SSEA-1) and the Human Mesenchymal Stem Cell Characterization Kit (Cat. K36094-21A) were obtained from Celprogen, USA.

A laminar current cabinet (cat. NF–800 R) and incubator (cat. 06750) were purchased from Nuve, Turkey. Inverted light microscopy was performed on an Olympus camera (cat. CKX41). The images were evaluated using Olympus Cell Soft Imaging System program. The enzyme-linked immunosorbent assay (ELISA) reader used to measure cytotoxicity and SSEA-1 gene expression was purchased from Mindray MR 96 A, PRC. Environmental scanning electron microscopy (ESEM) was performed on a Quanta 250 FEG (Fei Company, USA). MR was performed on a Siemens Magnetom Skyra 3-tesla (Germany).

Study design
The researchers were blind to the active ingredient content of the contrast agents added to the cell cultures. In order to minimize bias, all analyses were carried out by the same researcher. All the experiments were performed in triplicate.

Pure human primer chondrocyte cultures were used as the control (group I). Cells in groups II and III were treated with IPM and Gd-DPT, respectively. Finally, group IV cells were treated with Gd-DPT 0.9% physiological saline solution at a 1:250 gadolinium dilution rate, IPM, and a mixed lidocaine solution.

A total of 180 wells were prepared for each group and the five sub-groups, allowing experiments to be performed in triplicate.

Cultures were allowed to progress for 0, 2, and 6 h, at which times the SSEA-1 protein expression, MTT cell viability, toxicity, and proliferation, as well as prechondrocyte formation, were compared. Synchronously, the cell surface morphologies of all samples were scanned using inverted light microscopy and ESEM, and with MR imaging at the macroscopic level.

Eligibility criteria
Osteochondral tissues taken from patients ($n = 9$) surgically treated for knee arthroplasty at the Orthopedics and Traumatology Clinic due to gonarthrosis were included in the study. However, tissues of patients with a hypersensitivity to IPM and Gd-DPT contrast agents ($n = 1$), abnormal thyroid function ($n = 1$), or nephrologic problems ($n = 1$), were excluded from the study. Following the exclusion process, primer chondrocyte cultures were performed in six samples.

Isolation and cell culture of primary human chondrocytes
Osteochondral tissues from the proximal and distal ends of tibia and femur were resected during total knee arthroplasty. Tissues were transferred to the laboratory using culture medium (Fig. 1) and were placed in laminar cabinets, were washed with 0.9% isotonic sodium chloride solution, and were separated from the red blood cells. Chondral tissues were separated from osteochondral tissues.

Tissue samples were dispersed with a rongeur and were transferred to falcon tubes. Collagenase type II enzyme solubilized in HBSS in accordance with the drug bulletin then added on tissue samples and samples were placed in an incubator overnight at 37.4 °C and a 5% CO_2 atmosphere. Samples were then centrifuged for 10 min at 120 rpm in a cooled centrifuge. The cell pellet was resuspended in DMEM fresh culture medium, was transferred to a petri dish, and was left for a further 72-h incubation. Following incubation, cells were trypsinized with trypsin-ethylenediaminetetraacetic acid (0.25%). Cells were counted by trypan blue using a Thoma slide, and were placed in 96-well plates at 1.5×10^4 cells/well, in 24-well plates at 3.3×10^4 cells/well, and in 10-mm petri dishes at 4.4×10^6 cells/dish. Cell which were replaced in every 2 days were taken into the incubator for 24 h. With the help of trypsinization and

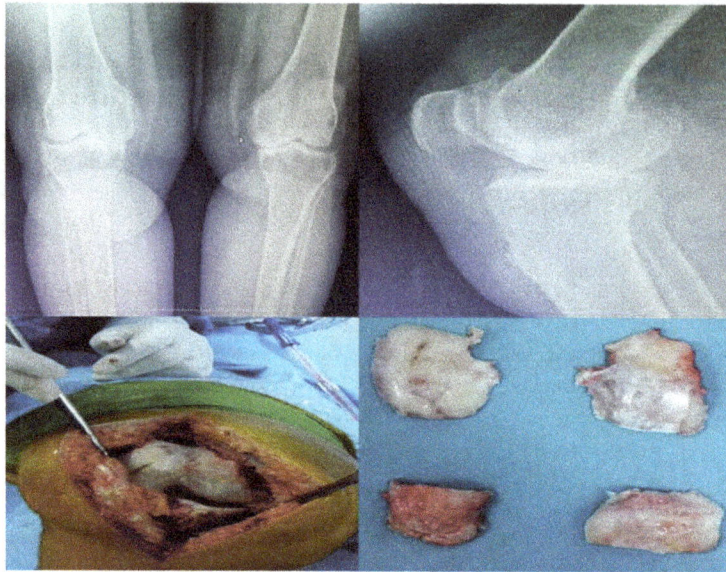

Fig. 1 Osteochondral tissue obtained during total knee replacement surgery

scraper, they were transferred into well plates from petri dishes [1, 8]. Contrast agent addition was commenced as of the second culture passage.

Preparation and application of drugs in chondrocyte culture samples

Samples in group I was cultured with no contrast agent addition. Main stock solutions were prepared in 50 mL volumes with 0.623 g IPM, 20 mL with 469.01 mg Gd-DPT in each 1 mL aqueous solution, respectively. IPM (15.6 mg/mL) and Gd-DPT (18.7 mg/mL) were applied to the culture samples in groups II and III by dilution with medium. The dose concentrations applied were calculated according to toxicity results from drugs containing similar active ingredients [2].

A mixed contrast agent solution was also prepared by adding 0.8 mL of Gd-DPT solution to 100 mL 0.9% sodium chlorur; 10 mL of this mixture was then mixed with 5 mL IPM and 5 mL lidocaine, diluted by gadolinium at the rate of 1:250. Such a solution is commonly injected into intra-articular joints [2]. Herein, the mixture (18.7 mg/mL) prepared as 1:250 Gd-DPT dilution was added to the wells in group IV (Table 1).

Solutions were prepared and stored in light-proof letter coded bottles and delivered to researchers blind to the content of each bottle. The contrast medium was added to the samples, except for the control group, using an automatic pipette with a calculated volume.

Inverted light microscopy

Micro images of cell organizations belonging to cartilaginous tissue were recorded confocally at ×4, ×10, ×20, and ×40 magnification under phase-contrast microscopy

before and after plating in petri dishes. The images were analyzed using Olympus Cell Soft Imaging program.

ESEM analysis

ESEM analysis was performed to obtain information about surface topography and sample compositions. The cell culture medium and contents were retrieved using a gun pipettor. A cacodylate and glutaraldehyde mixture was used for fixation. The fixation solution was then removed, and samples were left at room temperature for 2 h. Samples were then washed three times with pure cacodylate and were analyzed [10, 13, 15, 18].

FEG ion pumps were used to achieve a high vacuum. The images were recorded at a pressure of 219–231 Pa in ESEM vacuum mode, at ×5000 magnification and 82.9 μm resolution depths (HFW), at an operating

Table 1 Agents, commercial stock solution concentrations, and final concentrations

Pharmacological agents	Commercial stock solution concentration (mg/mL)	Final concentration (mg/mL)	Groups
–	–	–	Group I (untreated control group)
Gd-DPT	469.01	18.7	Group II
IPM	623	15.6	Group III
0.9% saline	–	Diluent	Group IV (mixture)
Gd-DPT	469.01	18.7	
IPM	623	15.6	
Lidocaine	100	2.5	

Gd-DPT gadolinium-diethylenetriaminepentaacetate, *IPM* iopropamide

voltage of 5.00 kV, and at a working distance of 9.4–10.7 mm.

MTT-ELISA viability and toxicity proliferation analyses

The viability tests were carried out using an MTT kit (3-[4,5-dimethyltiazol-2-yl]-2,5-diphenyltetrazolium bromide; Thiazolyl blue), which inhibits formazan crystal formation in dead cells [10, 14, 15, 18].

Analyses were performed prior to and at 0, 2, and 6 h following agent addition. The cell culture medium was removed and replaced with a fresh MTT tetrazolium solution (100 µL of stock solution 5 mg–12 mM/6 mL, 1 mL DMEM, and 1 mL sterile PBS; pH = 7.4). A 0.01 M HCl and 1 g/10 mL SDS mixture was also added. Following a 150 min incubation period at 37 °C in a dark environment, 500 µL of medium was removed from the samples. DMSO was then added and the samples were incubated for 10 min at 37 °C. The wave length absorbance was recorded at 540 nm.

By adding 500 µL SDS-HCl solution in the cells left for proliferation tests, they were incubated at 37 °C at 0, 2, 6, and 18 h. Then, absorbances at 570 nm were recorded, thus evaluating cell proliferation [10, 14].

The viability of the control group prior to contrast agent addition was accepted as 100%. Cell viability absorbances were recorded at 2 and 6 h.

SSEA-1 chondrocytic activity assay

During the differentiation of human mesenchymal stem cells containing embryonic stem cells, SSEA-1 protein expression is upregulated, whereas in cells that do not undergo differentiation expression is downregulated. A pre-chondrocytic human characterization ELISA kit was used to assess whether cells in chondrocyte cultures underwent differentiation, undifferentiation, stimulation, or inhibition by determining changes in SSEA-1 expression in the cultured cells [19-21]. Analyses were performed at 540 nm absorbance in an ELISA reader at 0, 2, and 6 h.

The evaluation of cell morphology by MR scanning

The samples were prepared through chondrocyte culture at 4.4×10^6 cells/dish in 10-mm petri dishes. At 2 and 6 h following agent application, cells were washed thoroughly with 0.01 M PBS in order to eliminate the volume of agents not taken up by the cells. Cells were covered with 1% agarose gel, which solidified at room temperature, to immobilize them [22].

MR protocol

All samples were imaged on a 3 T MR scanner. The samples were imaged with T2-weighted haste sequence. The protocol consisted of an spin echo-SE acquisition with a repetition time of 800 ms and echo times of 92 ms. The field of view was 260×260 mm, the pixel matrix was 256×256 mm, and slice thickness was 2 mm.

Statistical analyses

Descriptive statistics were shown as mean ± standard deviation. In the analyses of the obtained data, results were evaluated by cell number, proliferation, and SSEA-1 protein expression. The Minitab R16 program was used for statistical evaluation. Evaluations were made at 95% confidence interval.

The results were evaluated using analysis of variance (ANOVA) to assess whether there were significant differences across groups. When differences across groups were observed, Tukey's honest significant difference (HSD) test, a post-hoc multiple pairwise comparison test, was used to determine the difference and to investigate the false positive, thus evaluating the various averages across experimental groups.

Since there were many measures, and the data were comprised of sub-groups, the Pearson correlation test was used to assess whether there was a direct relation between SSEA-1 and MTT cell proliferation variables.

Results

Evaluation through inverted light microscopy and ESEM

When the inverted light microscopy and ESEM images were examined, a change in cell morphology was found to be correlated with MTT data (Figs. 2 and 3).

In group III, in which Gd-DPT was used exclusively, shrinkage, typical of a reaction of cells to cytotoxic agents, was observed after 2–6 h. The formation of extracellular matrix was substantially decreased. Chondrocyte cells were detached from the culture vessel and had a round shape, which is an indicator of cytotoxicity.

Interpretation of 3-tesla MRI

MRI performed in all experimental groups including the control group. Chondrocytes, where Gd-DPT and the mixture solution have been applied, absorbed the contrast agents and monitorized (Fig. 4).

In groups II and III, where IPM and Gd-DPT were applied, loss of cell integrity, and cavity formation was observed after 2 h (red arrow). Considerably more loss of cell integrity and further cell damage was observed after 6 h.

Statistical analysis of the toxic effects of contrast agents on chondrocytes as MTT-proliferation and SSEA-1 protein expression

The Tukey's test resulted in a yes/no response to the hypothesis (e.g., are there significant differences between the wells with $P < 0.05$). $P < 0.01$ was considered to be highly significant. Differences across the groups were found through Tukey's HSD evaluation after ANOVA, and these were statistically significant (Tables 2 and 3).

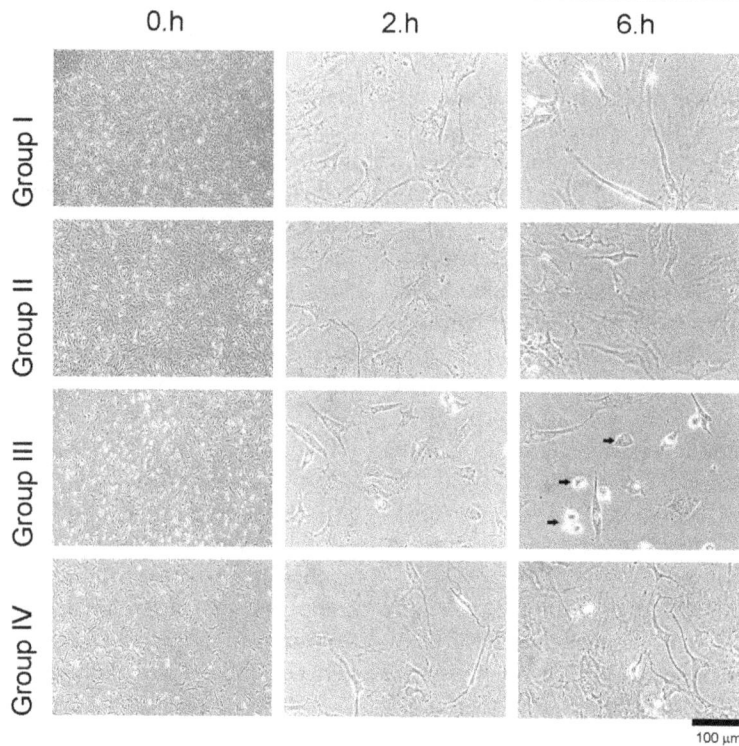

Fig. 2 Evaluation of round-shaped chondrocytes through inverted light microscopy

When compared with the control group, the lowest chondrogenic differentiation activity was observed in group III at 2 and 6 h, among all agents applied. Cell viability, toxicity, and proliferation were evaluated with MTT analysis and were compared with the non-drug control group. Likewise, the lowest number of cells was observed in group III, where IPM was applied for 6 h (Fig. 5).

SSEA-1 protein expression in a word chondrogenic activity was slightly lower in group IV where a mixed solution was applied than group II, both in 2 and 6 h applications. But decrease in cell viability and proliferation was obvious in group IV at 6 h when compared with group II and control ($P < 0.001$). These differences were statistically significant (Table 2).

A statistically significant correlation between SSEA-1 protein expression and MTT cell viability, toxicity, and proliferation was observed (Pearson correlation sig. (2-tailed); rho = 0.351; $P = 0.003$).

Discussion

In all areas of medicine, orthopedic surgery addresses the repair of damaged tissues, especially articular cartilage. On the other hand, the protection of healthy tissues is also an important issue [10, 14, 18]. Therefore, studies assessing the toxicity of frequently prescribed drugs on articular cartilage at the molecular level have gained recent popularity [10, 14]. The present study aimed to

evaluate the chondrotoxic effects of IPM and Gd-DPT, which are widely applied intra-articular contrast agents in arthrography.

As is well known, destruction in articular cartilage occurs in degenerative diseases such as osteoarthritis, as a result of traumatic, mechanical, genetic, metabolic, and biochemical factors [22]. Further, cartilage tissue and/or cells may be damaged by clinically prescribed pharmaceutical preparations [10, 14, 23–25].

A recent study assessed the cytotoxicity of drugs such as rituximab, adalimumab, abatacept, etanercept, and infliximab in primer cell in vitro cultures isolated from gonarthrosis cases and found that the least damaging biological agents were rituximab and adalimumab, whereas the remaining drugs were seen to negatively affect chondrocytes [10, 26]. A similar study assessed the chondrotoxicity of drugs widely used before and after surgery, such as vancomycin, linezolid, and teicoplanin, was assessed and concluded that these drugs were not chondrotoxic [14]. However, in both studies, the number of cells and proliferation analyses were only statistically evaluated based on mitochondrial activity as from the application of the drugs in a culture environment. A similar in vitro experimental setup was used herein; however, in addition to mitochondrial activity analyses, the proliferation and viability of chondrocytes, the toxicity of IPM, Gd-DPT, and their mixture, and SSEA-1 protein expression were evaluated with spectrophotometer. Thus, whether

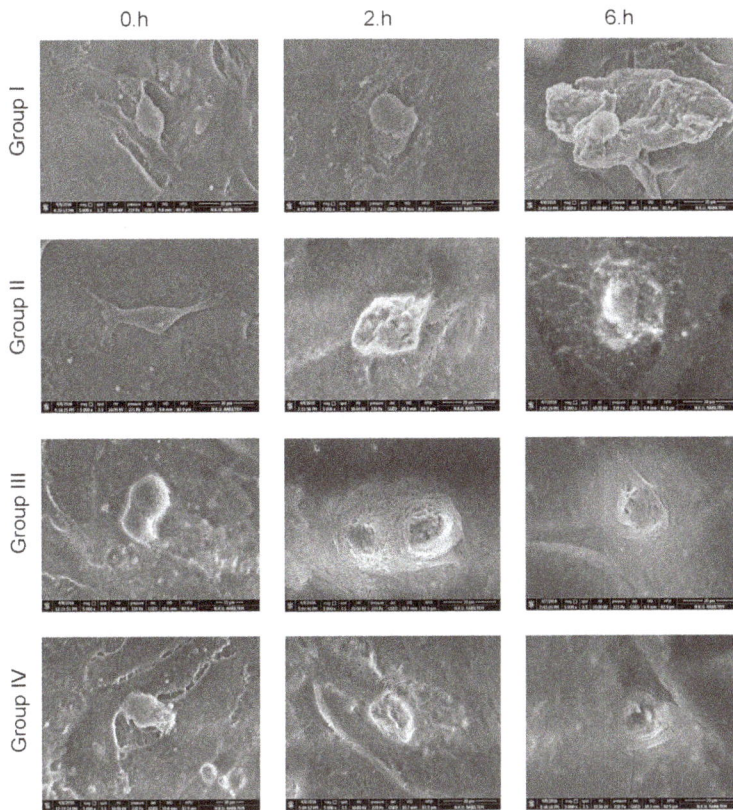

Fig. 3 Evaluation of chondrocyte surface morphology through environmental scanning electron microscopy

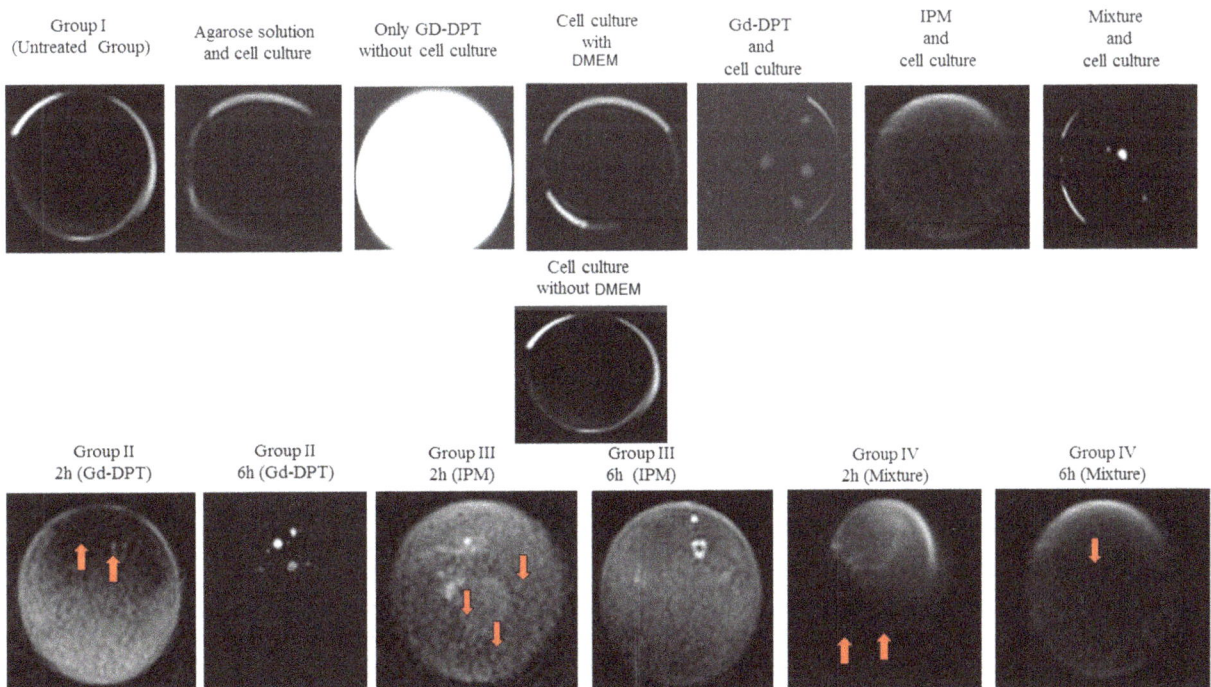

Fig. 4 Evaluation of chondrocytes through 3-tesla magnetic resonance imaging

Table 2 Comparison of differences between groups

SSEA-1 versus for analysis of variance

Source	DF	Adj SS	Adj MS	F value	P value
Method	11	0.127148	0.011559	505.82	<0.001
Error	60	0.001371	0.000023		
Total	71	0.128519			

MTT-cell proliferation versus for analysis of variance

Source	DF	Adj SS	Adj MS	F value	P value
Method	11	0.012400	0.001127	8903.31	<0.001
Error	60	0.000008	0.000023		
Total	71	0.012407	0.000000		

Table 3 Statistical analyses. Tukey's pairwise comparisons for SSEA-1 protein and MTT cell proliferation

	N	Mean ± St. Dv.	Grouping

Tukey's pairwise comparisons for SSEA-1 protein (grouping information using the Tukey's method and 95% confidence interval)

	N	Mean ± St. Dv.	Grouping
Group I (control 6 h)	6	0.489500 ± 0.000379	(A)
Group I (control 2 h)	6	0.477067 ± 0.000489	(B)
Group IV (mixture 0 h)	6	0.476467 ± 0.000052	(B)
Group III (Gd-DPT 0 h)	6	0.476450 ± 0.000084	(B)
Group II (IPM 0 h)	6	0.476450 ± 0.000084	(B)
Group I (control 0 h)	6	0.476450 ± 0.000105	(B)
Group II (IPM 2 h)	6	0.464500 ± 0.000000	(C)
Group II (IPM 6 h)	6	0.462500 ± 0.000000	(C)
Group IV (mixture 6 h)	6	0.451667 ± 0.000816	(D)
Group IV (mixture 2 h)	6	0.450167 ± 0.000983	(D)
Group III (Gd-DPT 2 h)	6	0.444133 ± 0.000103	(D)
Group III (Gd-DPT 6 h)	6	0.323167 ± 0.01650	(E)

Tukey's pairwise comparisons for MTT-cell proliferation (grouping information using the Tukey's method and 95% confidence interval)

	N	Mean ± St. Dv.	Grouping
Group I (control 6 h)	6	0.159017 ± 0.000130	(A)
Group I (control 2 h)	6	0.157450 ± 0.000418	(B)
Group I (control 0 h)	6	0.155900 ± 0.000420	(C)
Group II (IPM 0 h)	6	0.155800 ± 0.000438	(C)
Group III (Gd-DPT 0 h)	6	0.155767 ± 0.000532	(C)
Group IV (mixture 0 h)	6	0.155753 ± 0.000513	(C)
Group III (Gd-DPT 2 h)	6	0.147450 ± 0.000472	(D)
Group II (IPM 2 h)	6	0.141317 ± 0.000293	(E)
Group II (IPM 6 h)	6	0.140817 ± 0.000041	(E)
Group IV (mixture 2 h)	6	0.140667 ± 0.000082	(E) (F)
Group IV (mixture 6 h)	6	0.140117 ± 0.000103	(F)
Group III (Gd-DPT 6 h)	6	0.110333 ± 0.000075	(G)

chondrocyte cells in culture were exposed to differentiation, undifferentitation, stimulation, or inhibition was assessed in addition to an evaluation of drug toxicity and proliferation; these aspects represent the strengths of the present study.

In 2007, the toxicity of iodinated contrast medium was analyzed in various cell cultures in vitro [27]. Further, studies examining the toxicity of contrast substances indicated that ixotitalamate, used in discography or percutaneous endoscopic lumbar discectomy, induced toxicity in the disc nucleus pulposus and not on cartilage cells [28, 29].

A literature search revealed only one study assessing in vitro cell toxicity of cartilage-targeted low-generation dendrimer-linked nitroxide MR contrast agents and gadopentetate dimeglumine using a long-term Swarm rat chondrosarcoma chondrocyte-like cell line [30]. The study evaluated spectrophotometric assays of metabolic activity and cell proliferation and concluded that long-term exposure to either diaminobutyl-linked nitroxides citrate or gadolinium-*d*iethylene*t*riamine*penta*cetate had no detectable toxicity, with the results being equivalent to untreated cultures.

No studies were retrieved in which the use of IPM contrast agent itself or with Gd-DPT was compared. Further, the limited number of studies in which cartilage tissues or the chondrocyte-directed toxicity were analyzed were carried out on animal models. However, as the physiological structure and/or sensitivity may differ from that of humans, it was reported that the results may not be reliable. In similar studies where animal tissues were not used, commercial cell-lines, known to have lost the in vivo phenotypic and genotypic features, were used instead [10, 14, 18, 21, 28, 31].

In the present study, the cartilage tissue used belonged to patients with knee prosthesis in the course of routine clinical practice. Thus, primer chondrocyte cultures were prepared from undamaged chondral tissues of the resected articular surface, allowing analyses in the natural cell environment, including the extracellular matrix. Further, the present study evaluates both Gd-DPT and IPM contrast agents and the chondrotoxicity of the mixture of these in an in vitro culture environment derived from human tissue.

In control group, regular cell morphology and intact extracellular matrix formation observed with inverted light microscopy. Contrarily, none of the chondrocyte cultures which arthrography agents applied reached confluency. Besides, lose of cell morphology and deterioration of extracellular matrix was observed. Further, ESEM analyses indicated that, in healthy chondrocytes, all natural surface characteristics were visible in the control group, thus supporting inverted light microscopy. Cell viability analysis, quantitative ELISA, and MR imaging also support these morphological data.

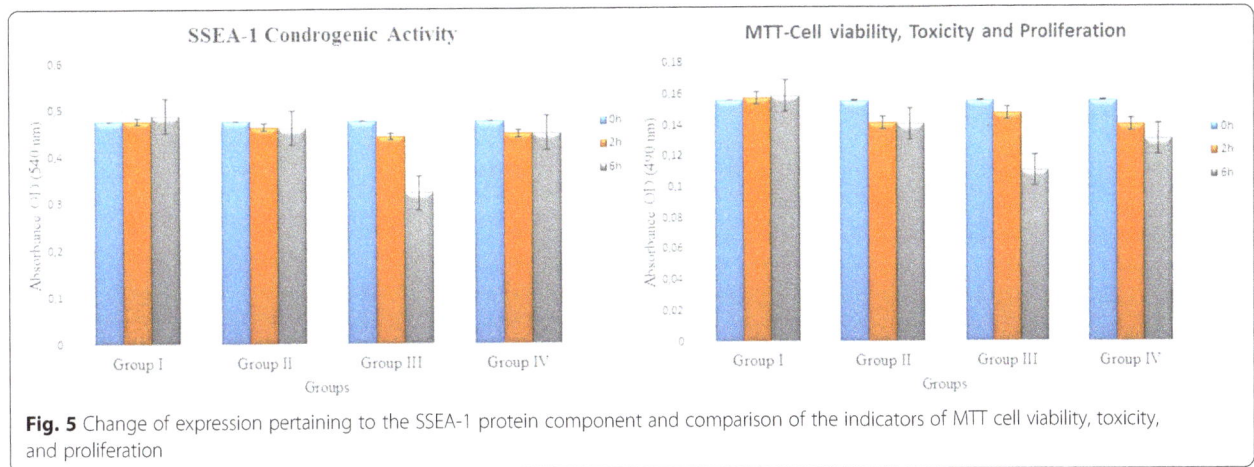

Fig. 5 Change of expression pertaining to the SSEA-1 protein component and comparison of the indicators of MTT cell viability, toxicity, and proliferation

Compared with the control group, IPM treatment had the lowest SSEA-1 expression after 6 h of culture followed by the mixed solution and Gd-DPT treatments. The same pattern was observed in the MTT proliferation, cell viability, and toxicity assays–IPM treatment was the most cytotoxic. The differences observed were statistically significant ($P < 0.001$). Further, a statistically significant correlation between SSEA-1 and MTT values and cell proliferation was observed (Pearson product moment correlation sig. (2-tailed); rho = 0.351; $P = 0.003$). These results support those obtained through imaging techniques, whereby round-shaped cells were observed, indicating cytotoxicity. Thus, the present study shows that contrast agents commonly used in intra-articular imaging are toxic to human primer articular chondrocytes, albeit Gd-DPT to lower degree than IPM.

As known, cartilage tissues are avascular and aneuronal and they are deprived of lymph tissues. For this very reason, cartilage cells are fed via synovial liquid which washes articulation surfaces in certain areas without perichondrium or perichondrium layer in vascular shape. Since the outer layer of the synovial fluid is thicker, drugs and/or nutrition diffuse from synovial tissue to the synovial liquid. Afterwards, they pass through pores to the synovial fluid and reach chondrocytes, which results in a second diffusion [32, 33].

It is known that drugs accumulate in the synovial fluid whether they are taken orally or parenterally. Many drugs taken into the body accumulate in the synovial fluid compartment [32, 33].

Even though we carried out our study in primary human chondrocyte cultures but not in the synovial liquid, we doubt that toxification occurs due to accumulation of drugs in the synovial liquid.

We suggest that agents used in this diagnostic methods, which allows for detailed imaging of intra-articular structures, should be administered, if possible, without addition of the local anesthetic agents. It should be remembered that chelated agents when used in combination form may be more harmful to cartilage tissue especially to chondrocytes and extracellular matrix and/or associated tissues when administered intra-articularly in the clinic.

Conclusions

The present study performed in vitro chondrocyte cultures and compared the detrimental effects of Gd-DPT and/or IPM at low concentrations on cartilage tissue cells and extracellular matrix in terms of cell size in the short term. Further evaluation of Gd-DPT and/or IPM with clinically appropriate long-term exposure times is required to determine the maximum useful concentration. Despite its valuable in vitro results, the present study is limited by its insufficient clinical relevance; therefore, studies evaluating the clinical outcomes in vivo are required.

Abbreviations
ESEM: Environmental scanning electron microscope; FEG: Field emission guns; HBSS: Hank's balanced salt solution; HSD: Honest significant difference; MTT: 3-(4,5-dimethylthiazol-2-yl)-2,5-diphenyltetrazolium bromide; NSAIDs: Non-steroidal anti-inflammatory drugs; OD: Optical density; SDS: Sodium dodecyl sulfate; SSEA-1: Stage-specific embryonic antigen-1.7; WD: Wavelength-dispersive

Acknowledgements
We are thankful to radiographers Huseyin Tunahan KAYA of the Istanbul Kanuni Sultan Training and Research Hospital, Turkey, and Sertan YALCIN of the Istanbul Acibadem Hospital, Turkey, for their help with radiological image.

Funding
None.

Authors' contributions
KO contributed to the study concept and design, acquisition of subjects and/or data, analysis and interpretation of data, and preparation of manuscript. DYS contributed to the preparation of human primer chondrocyte culture, inverted light microscopy, ESEM microscopy, performance and evaluation of ELISA analyses. IY contributed to the preparation of human primer chondrocyte culture, inverted light microscopy, ESEM microscopy, performance and evaluation of magnetic resonance imaging protocol and ELISA analyses,

preparation and storage of culture drugs. YEK and MI contributed to the removal of tissues from the cases and transfer to the laboratory, statistical evaluation of findings, and writing of the manuscript. SAG contributed to the removal of the tissues from the cases and transfer to the laboratory, selection of patients who met the inclusion criteria. SA contributed to the removal of the tissues from the cases and transfer to the laboratory, and critical revision of the manuscript for important intellectual content. AK contributed to the evaluation and preparation of cells for magnetic resonance imaging protocols and writing of the discussion section. HO and MM contributed to the preparation of the manuscript and critical revision of the manuscript for important intellectual content. All authors have read and approved the final version of the manuscript.

Competing interests

The authors declare that they have no competing interests.

Author details

[1]Department of Orthopaedic and Traumatology, Istanbul Medipol University School of Medicine, 34214 Istanbul, Turkey. [2]Department of Molecular Biology and Genetic, Namik Kemal University Faculty of Arts and Sciences, 59100 Tekirdag, Turkey. [3]Department of Medical Pharmacology, Istanbul Medipol University School of Medicine, 34810 Istanbul, Turkey. [4]Republic of Turkey, Ministry of Health, Department of Orthopaedic and Traumatology, Corlu State Hospital, 59100 Tekirdag, Turkey. [5]Department of Orthopaedic and Traumatology, Acibadem Hospitals Group, 34180 Istanbul, Turkey. [6]Republic of Turkey, Ministry of Health, Dr. Lutfi Kirdar Research and Training Hospital, 34890 Istanbul, Turkey. [7]Department of Orthopaedic and Traumatology, Denizli Private Surgery Hospital, 20070 Denizli, Turkey. [8]Department of Radiology, Istanbul Kanuni Sultan Suleyman Training and Research Hospital, 34303 Istanbul, Turkey. [9]Department of Orthopaedic and Traumatology, Memorial Health Group, 34384 Istanbul, Turkey.

References

1. Steinbach LS, Palmer WE, Schweitzer. MR arthrography. Radiographics. 2002; 22:1223–46.
2. Elentuck D, Palmer WE. Direct magnetic resonance arthrography. Eur Radiol. 2004;14:1956–67.
3. Greisberg JK, Wolf JM, Wyman J, Zou L, Terek RM. Gadolinium inhibits thymidine incorporation and induces apoptosis in chondrocytes. J Orthop Res. 2001;19:797–801.
4. Algotsson J, Forsman J, Topgaard D, Söderman O. Electrostatic interactions are for the distrubution of Gd(DTPA) < sup > 2-</sup > in articular cartilage. Magn Reson Med. 2016;76(2):500–9.
5. Shafieyan Y, Khosravi N, Moeini M, Quinn TM. Diffusion of MRI and CT contrast agents in articular cartilage under static compression. Biophys J. 2014;107:485–92.
6. Guggenberger R, Fischer MA, Hodler J, Pfammatter T, Andreisek G. Flat-panel CT arthrography: feasibility study and comparison to multidetector CT arthrography. Invest Radiol. 2012;47:312–8.
7. Van Bree H, Van Rijssen B, Tshamala M, Maenhout T. Comparison of the nonionic contrast agents, iopromide and iotrolan, for positive-contrast arthrography of the scapulohumeral joint in dogs. Am J Vet Res. 1992;53: 1622–6.
8. Saupe N, Zanetti M, Pfirrmann CW, Wels T, Schwenke C, Hodler J. Pain and other side effects after MR arthrography: prospective evaluation in 1085 patients. Radiology. 2009;250:830–8.
9. Wang K, Xu J, Hunter DJ, Ding C. Inverstigational drugs fort he treatment of osteoarthritis. Expert Opin Investig Drugs. 2015;24:1539–56.
10. Isyar M, Bilir B, Yilmaz I, Cakmak S, Sirin DY, Guzelant AY, Mahirogullari M. Are biological agents toxic to human chondrocytes and osteocytes? J Orthop Surg Res. 2015;10:118.
11. Iida A, Kizawa H, Nakamura Y, Ikegawa S. High-resolution SNP map of ASPN, a susceptibility gene for osteoarthritis. J Hum Genet. 2006;51:151–4.
12. Zhu H, Deng FY, Mo XB, Qiu YH, Lei SF. Pharmacogenetics and pharmacogenomics for rheumatoid arthritis responsiveness to methotrexate treatment: the 2013 update. Pharmacogenomics. 2013;15: 551–66.
13. Gökçe A, Yılmaz I, Gökay NS, Can L, Gökçe C. Does insulin, transferrin and

14. selenous acid preparation effect chondrocyte proliferation? Acta Orthop Traumatol Turc. 2014;48:313–9.
14. Dogan M, Isyar M, Yilmaz I, et al. Are the leading drugs against Staphylococcus aureus really toxic to cartilage? J Infect Public Health. 2016;9:251–8.
15. Gokce A, Yilmaz I, Bircan R, Tonbul M, Gokay NS, Gokce C. Synergistic effect of TGF-β1 and BMP-7 on chondrogenesis and extracellular matrix synthesis: an in vitro study. Open Orthop J. 2012;6:406–13.
16. Yilmaz I, Gokay NS, Gokce A, Tonbul M, Gokce C. A novel designed chitosan based hydrogel which is capable of consecutively controlled release of TGF-Beta 1 and BMP-7. Turkiye Klinikleri J Med Sci. 2013;33:18–32.
17. Yilmaz I, Gokay NS, Bircan R, Saracoglu GV, Dervisoglu S, Gokce A. How different methodologies of harvesting and analysing the samples affect the test results in determining joint mediators. Arthritis. 2013;2013:631959.
18. Isyar M, Yilmaz I, Sirin DY, Yalcin S, Guler O, Mahirogullari M. A practical way to prepare primer human chondrocyte culture. J Orthop. 2016;13:162–7.
19. Cellprogen Commercial kit monograph. http://www.celprogen.com/details. php?pid=10765. Accessed 26 April 2017.
20. Li YQ, Tang Y, Fu R, Menq QH, Zhou X, Ling ZM, et al. Efficient labeling in vitro with non-ionic gadolinium magnetic resonance imagingcontrast agent and fluorescent transfection agent in bone marrow stromal cells of neonatal rats. Mol Med Rep. 2015;12:913–20.
21. Gumustas F, Yilmaz I, Sirin DY, Gumustas SA, Batmaz AG, Isyar M, Akkaya S, Mahirogullari M. Chondrocyte proliferation, viability and differentiation is declined following administration of methylphenidate utilized for the treatment of attention-deficit/hyperactivity disorder. Hum Exp Toxicol. 2016. [Epub ahead of print].
22. Jasin HE. Immune mechanisms in osteoarthritis. Semin Arthritis Rheum. 1989;18:89–90.
23. Stueber T, Karsten J, Stoetzer C, Leffler A. Differential cytotoxic properties of drugs used for intra-articular injection on human chondrocytes: an experimental in-vitro study. Eur J Anaesthesiol. 2014;31:640–5.
24. Wyles CC, Houdek MT, Wyles SP, Wagner ER, Behfar A, Sierra RJ. Differentia lcytotoxicity of corticosteroids on human mesenchymal stem cells. Clin Orthop Relat Res. 2015;473:1155–64.
25. Goto K, Imaoka M, Goto M, Kilkuchi I, Suzuki T, Jindo T, Takasaki W. Effect of body-weight loading on to the articular cartilage on the occurrence of quinolone-induced chondrotoxicity in juvenile rats. Toxicol Lett. 2013;16: 124–9.
26. Guzelant AY, Isyar M, Yilmaz I, Sirin DY, Cakmak S, Mahirogullari M. Are chondrocytes damaged when rheumatologic inflammation is suppressed? Drug Chem Toxicol. 2017;40:13–23.
27. Heinrich M, Scheer M, Heckmann M, Bautz W, Uder M. Reversibility and time-dependency of contrast medium induced inhibition of 3-(4,5-dimethylthiazol-2-yl)-2,5-diphenyl-tetrazolium bromide (MTT) conversion in renal proximal tubular cells in vitro: comparison of a monomeric and a dimeric nonionic iodinated contrast medium. Invest Radiol. 2007;42:732–8.
28. Kim KH, Kim YS, Kuh SU, Park HS, Park JY, Chin DK, Kim KS, Cho YE. Time- and dose-dependent cytotoxicities of ioxitalamate and indigocarmine in human nucleus pulposus cells. Spine J. 2013;13:564–71.
29. Kim KH, Park JY, Park HS, Kuh SU, Chin DK, Kim KS, Cho YE. Which iodinated contrast media is the least cytotoxic to human disc cells? Spine J. 2015;15: 1021–7.
30. Midura S, Schneider E, Sakamoto FA, Rosen GM, Winalski CS, Midura RJ. In vitro toxicity in long-term cell culture of MR contrast agents targeted to cartilage evaluation. Osteoarthritis Cartilage. 2014;22:1337–45.
31. Isyar M, Gumsutas SA, Yilmaz I, Sirin DY, Tosun HB, Mahirogullari M. Are we economically efficient enough to increase the potential of in vitro proliferation of osteoblasts by means of pharmacochemical agents? Open Orthop J. 2016; 10:420–30.
32. Gumustas SA, Yilmaz İ, Isyar M, Sirin DY, Batmaz AG, Ugras AA, Oznam K, Ciftci Z, Mahirogullari M. Assessing the negative impact of phenyl alkanoic acid derivative, a frequently prescribed drug for the suppression of pain and inflammation, on the differentiation and proliferation of chondrocytes. J Orthop Surg Res. 2016;11(1):70.
33. Gumustas F, Yilmaz I, Sirin DY, Gumustas SA, Batmaz AG, Isyar M, Akkaya S, Mahirogullari M. Chondrocyte proliferation, viability and differentiation is declined following administration of methylphenidate utilized for the treatment of attention-deficit/hyperactivity disorder. Hum Exp Toxicol. 2016. PMID: 27837176. doi:10.1177/0960327116678294.

10

Do small changes in rotation affect measurements of lower extremity limb alignment?

Amir A. Jamali[1*], John P. Meehan[2], Nathan M. Moroski[3], Matthew J. Anderson[4], Ramit Lamba[5] and Carol Parise[6]

Abstract

Background: The alignment of the lower extremity has important implications in the development of knee arthritis. The effect of incremental rotations of the limb on common parameters of alignment has not been studied. The purpose of the study was to (1) determine the standardized neutral position measurements of alignment and (2) determine the effect of rotation on commonly used measurements of alignment.

Methods: Eighty-seven full length CT angiography studies (49 males and 38 females, average age 66 years old) were included. Three-dimensional models were created using a rendering software program and placed on a virtual plane. An image of the extremity was obtained. Thirty scans were randomly selected, and those models were rotated in 3° intervals around the longitudinal axis and additional images were obtained.

Results: In the neutral position, the mechanical lateral distal femoral articular angle (mLDFA) was 85.6 ± 2.3°, medial proximal tibial angle (MPTA) was 86.1 ± 2.8°, and mechanical tibiofemoral angle (mTFA) was −0.7 ± 3.1°. Females had a more valgus alignment with a mTFA of 0.5 ± 2.9° while males had a more varus alignment with a mTFA of −1.7 ± 2.9°. The anatomic tibiofemoral angle (aTFA) was 4.8 ± 2.6°, the anatomic lateral distal femoral angle (aLDFA) measured 80.2 ± 2.2°, and the anatomical-mechanical angle (AMA) was 5.4 ± 0.7°. The prevalence of constitutional varus was 18%.
The effect of rotation on the rotated scans led to statistically significant differences relative to the 0° measurement for all measurements. These effects may be small, and their clinical importance is unknown.

Conclusions: This study provides new information on standardized measures of lower extremity alignment and the relationship between discreet axial rotations of the entire lower extremity and these parameters.

Keywords: Alignment, Lower extremity, Osteotomy, Rotation, Constitutional varus, Total knee replacement

Background

The alignment of the lower extremity has been an area of ongoing study for decades. Standard radiographs have been used to determine the "normal" parameters of alignment of the lower extremity. These are prone to technical errors based on distance from the cassette and rotation of the lower extremity around the longitudinal axis. Deviations from "normal" have been broadly categorized at malalignment although a clear definition of "normal alignment" has not been established. One can define "normal" on a statistical basis as lying within some arbitrarily defined range relative to the mean or on a pathological basis according to the risk of the joint undergoing degeneration secondary to the deformity. Malalignment of the native lower extremity has been associated in previous studies with a higher risk of osteoarthritis [1–4]. Accurate preoperative and postoperative alignment parameters are required for planning and prediction of outcome for both osteotomies and total knee replacement [5–11]. Thus, the assessments of both the lower extremity alignment in native knees and those that have undergone replacement depend on an accurate definition of native lower extremity alignment [12, 13].

In spite of increased sophistication in imaging and computer generated reconstructions, most surgeons still depend on two-dimensional radiographs in planning

* Correspondence: contact@hipandknee.net
[1] Joint Preservation Institute, 2825 J Street, Suite 440, Sacramento, CA 95816, USA
Full list of author information is available at the end of the article

operations such as osteotomy, unicompartmental knee replacement, or total knee replacement.

The objectives of this study were twofold. We sought to (1) determine the standardized neutral position measurements of alignment and (2) determine the effect of rotation on commonly used measurements of alignment. We prepared three-dimensional models of the lower extremity in a standardized position and rotated the models in 3° increments in each direction, taking digital photographs in each position.

Methods

A total of 221 full lower extremity CT angiography studies for vascular disease workup were performed at our institute between July 8, 2008, and May 14, 2010. Of these, 87 patients (49 males and 38 females) were included in the present study. The average age was 66 years old (range 28–91 years old) Exclusion criteria included advanced osteoarthritis of the hip, knee, or ankle, radiographic evidence of previous realignment surgery or fracture, irregular positioning in the scanner, or any type of lower extremity joint prosthesis.

Normal values of coronal alignment of the lower extremities with the femur placed on a virtual flat table

The first portion of the study was the determination of the normal values of coronal alignment of the lower extremity without the effect of rotation and in a neutral position. Three-dimensional models were created from the CT data using a commercially available and previously validated three-dimensional rendering software program (Mimics, Materialise, Ann Arbor, MI) [14]. These models were then placed on a virtual flat table in the computer environment. The femora rested with the virtual table plane passing through the posterior most point of the greater trochanter and the posterior most points of both the medial and lateral femoral condyles. In this neutral position, a high resolution image of the femur and the tibia from anterior to posterior was obtained. Next, 30 scans were randomly selected, and using the software, the entire lower extremity model was rotated in discreet 3° intervals in both internal and external rotation around the virtual axis from the femoral head to the center of distal femur up to 12° in each direction. After each rotation, a new anterior to posterior image of the now rotated lower extremity was obtained. The image files were then analyzed using a custom measurement analysis program written in Matlab (Mathworks, Natick, MA, USA). The analysis was performed in this fashion to optimize speed and precision and minimize risk of observer bias. The independent variable was the degree of rotation. The dependent variables were the alignment parameters measured.

Definitions for image analysis, points, axes, and angular measurements

Points

The convention used by Moreland et al. was utilized to define the center of the femoral trochlea as the center point of the knee [15]. Moreland et al. had described taking a visual midpoint among a total of five points to define the center of the knee. These included the center of the femoral notch (trochlea), center of tibial spines, center of femoral condyles, center of soft tissue, and center of the tibia. They found that all points were within 5 mm of one another. Based on the high consistency of the center of the femoral trochlea, we chose that point as the center of the knee. The center of the ankle was defined visually as the center of the distal tibial articular surface. The other points selected on lower extremity images obtained were the center of the femoral head, the most distal points of the distal medial and lateral femoral condyles, and the most proximal point of the medial and lateral tibial plateaus.

The proximal femoral shaft center (PFSC) was defined by selecting two lateral points and two medial points in the subtrochanteric region of the femur and allowing the software to calculate the geometric center of those four points located centrally within the femoral shaft in the subtrochanteric region.

Axes

Mechanical axes

The mechanical axis of the femur was defined as a line drawn from the center of the femoral head to the center of the knee. The mechanical and anatomical axes of the tibia were both defined in an identical fashion as the line connecting the center of the knee and the center of the ankle.

Anatomical axes

The line connecting the PFSC and the center of the femoral trochlea was used to define the anatomical axis of the femur. The line connecting the center of the femoral trochlea and the center of the ankle was used to define the anatomical and mechanical axes of the tibia as noted above.

Articular axes

The distal femoral articular axis was defined by the line connecting the distal most points of the medial and lateral femoral condyles. The proximal tibial articular axis was defined as the line connecting the two most proximal points of the tibial plateaus.

Angular measurements

Mechanical angle measurements

The mechanical lateral distal femoral articular angle (mLDFA) was defined as the lateral angle between the femoral mechanical axis and the distal femoral articular axis [16] (Fig. 1a). The medial proximal tibial angle (MPTA) was unique among the measurements in that it was included in both the mechanical parameters and the anatomical parameters and was defined as the medial angle between the mechanical (as well as anatomical) axis of the tibia and the proximal tibial articular axis (Fig. 1b). The mechanical tibiofemoral angle (mTFA) [16] was defined as the angle between the femoral mechanical axis and the tibial mechanical axis with a positive value indicative of a valgus alignment and a negative value indicative of a varus alignment of the lower extremity (Fig. 1c). The joint line convergence angle (JLCA) was defined as the angle between the proximal tibial and distal femoral articular axes with a negative value indicative of convergence laterally and a positive value indicative of convergence medially (Fig. 1d).

Anatomical angle measurements

The anatomic tibiofemoral angle (aTFA) [16] was defined as the angle between the anatomical axis of the femur and the anatomical-mechanical axis of the tibia (Fig. 1e). Once again, a positive value was indicative of a valgus and a negative value indicative of a varus

alignment of the lower extremity. The angle between the mechanical and anatomical axes of the femur was defined as the anatomical-mechanical angle (AMA) [16] (Fig. 1f). The anatomical lateral distal femoral angle (aLDFA) was defined as the angle between the anatomical axis of the femur and the distal femoral articular axis [16] (Fig. 1g).

The anatomical medial proximal tibial angle was by convention defined to be equivalent to the medial proximal tibial angle (MPTA) due to the equivalence of the mechanical and anatomical tibial axes as noted above.

Effect of 3° rotational intervals on coronal alignment

The rotated anterior to posterior (AP) images of the 3D models of 30 randomly selected specimens were analyzed in the same fashion as the neutral AP images described above. By convention, negative measurements indicated the lower extremity to be internally rotated and positive measurements externally rotated around the longitudinal axis of the femur.

Statistical analysis

Inter- and intraobserver reliability analysis was performed for each parameter using intraclass correlation coefficients (ICC) for intraobserver reliability analysis for observer 1 (AAJ) at two time points 4 weeks apart and interobserver reliability between the two observers (AAJ and MA) for a total of 20 of subjects. All ICCs were

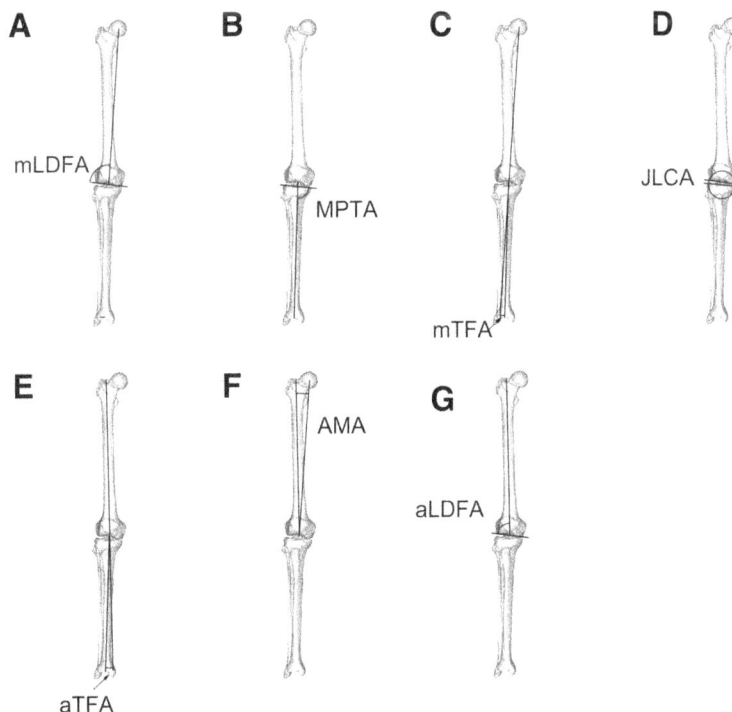

Fig. 1 Measurement methods of common parameters of lower extremity alignment studied in this paper. **a** mLDFA. **b** MPTA. **c** mTFA. **d** JLCA. **e** aTFA. **f** AMA. **g** aLDFA

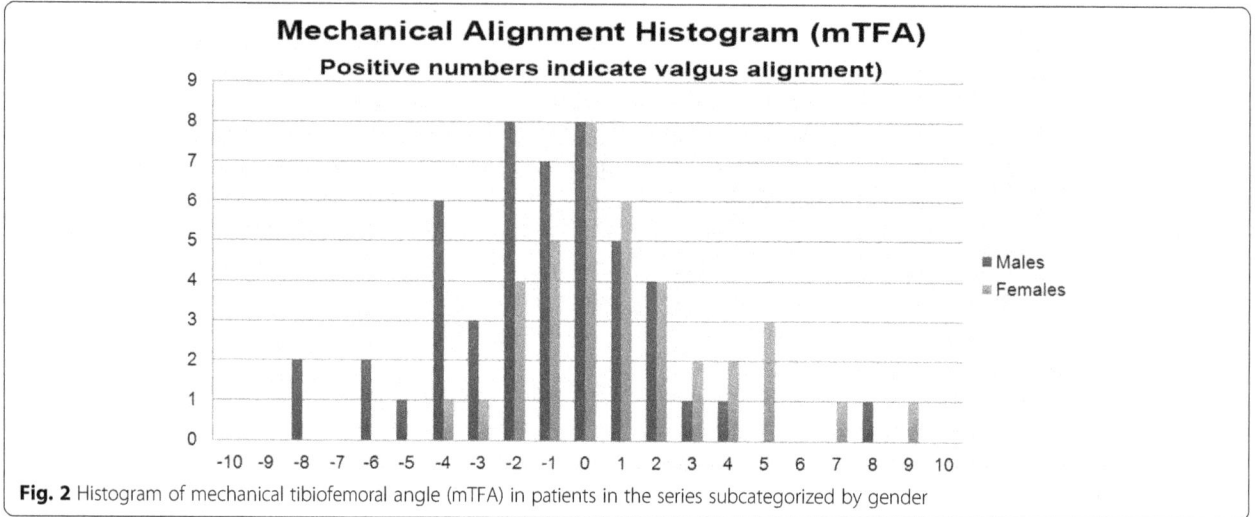

Fig. 2 Histogram of mechanical tibiofemoral angle (mTFA) in patients in the series subcategorized by gender

greater than 0.94 indicating excellent reliability with the exception of the measurements of JLCA with ICC of 0.18 and 0.68 for inter- and intraobserver reliability respectively. The effect of rotation of each parameter was analyzed using repeated measures analysis of variance (RMANOVA) with Bonferroni correction as appropriate. The prevalence of constitutional varus based on gender was analyzed using the chi-squared test. All analyses were performed with SPSS (IBM, Chicago, IL), Excel (Microsoft, Redmond, WA), and StatView software (SAS, Cary, NC). Statistical significance was set at $p < 0.05$.

Results

Mechanical measurements

The mLDFA was $85.6 \pm 2.3°$. The MPTA was $86.1 \pm 2.8°$. The JLCA angle was $-1.2 \pm 1.7°$. The mechanical tibiofemoral angle (mTFA) was $-0.7 \pm 3.1°$. Females had a more valgus alignment with a mTFA of $0.5 \pm 2.9°$ while males had a more varus alignment with a mTFA of $-1.7 \pm 2.9°$ (Fig. 2) (Table 1).

Constitutional varus

The prevalence of constitutional varus defined as mTFA of more than 3° varus was 16/87, or 18%. There was a statistically significant difference ($p = 0.005$) in the prevalence based on gender with 2/38, or 5% of females, and 14/49, or 29% for males, being classified as constitutional varus.

Anatomical measurements

The anatomic tibiofemoral angle (aTFA) was $4.8 \pm 2.6°$. The anatomic lateral distal femoral angle (aLDFA) measured $80.2 \pm 2.2°$. The medial proximal tibial angle (MPTA) was $86.1 \pm 2.8°$. The anatomical-mechanical angle (AMA) was $5.4 \pm 0.7°$.

Effect of rotation

The effect of rotation in 3° increments led to a statistically significant difference in measurements for all measurements except for aLDFA and mLDFA. For aLDFA and mLDFA, there was no significant difference in spite of rotation of the images. For the remaining parameters, the effect of rotation varied. Measurements taken with the lower extremity rotated as little as 3° leading to significant differences (Fig. 3). For the mTFA, aTFA, and AMA measurements, pairwise comparisons indicated that all rotated measurements were significantly different from the neutral, 0°, rotational position. This indicated that even a 3° rotational variation in these parameters leads to a statistically significant difference in the measured value. For MPTA, measurements at the –3° and –6° positions were not significantly different than those at the neutral position while all others were significantly different than the neutral position value. JLCA was not analyzed due to the low interobserver reliability of that measurement.

Table 1 Summary of lower extremity alignment measurements from this study (n=87)

Mechanical alignment parameters	
Mechanical lateral distal femoral articular angle (mLDFA)	$85.6 \pm 2.3°$
Medial proximal tibial angle (MPTA)	$86.1 \pm 2.8°$
Mechanical tibiofemoral angle	$-0.7 \pm 3.1°$
The joint line convergence angle (JLCA)	$-1.2 \pm 1.7°$
Anatomical alignment parameters	
Anatomic tibiofemoral angle (aTFA)	$4.8 \pm 2.6°$
Lateral distal femoral angle (aLDFA)	$80.2 \pm 2.2°$
Medial proximal tibial angle (MPTA)	$86.1 \pm 2.8°$
Other	
Anatomical-mechanical angle (AMA).	$5.4 \pm 0.7°$

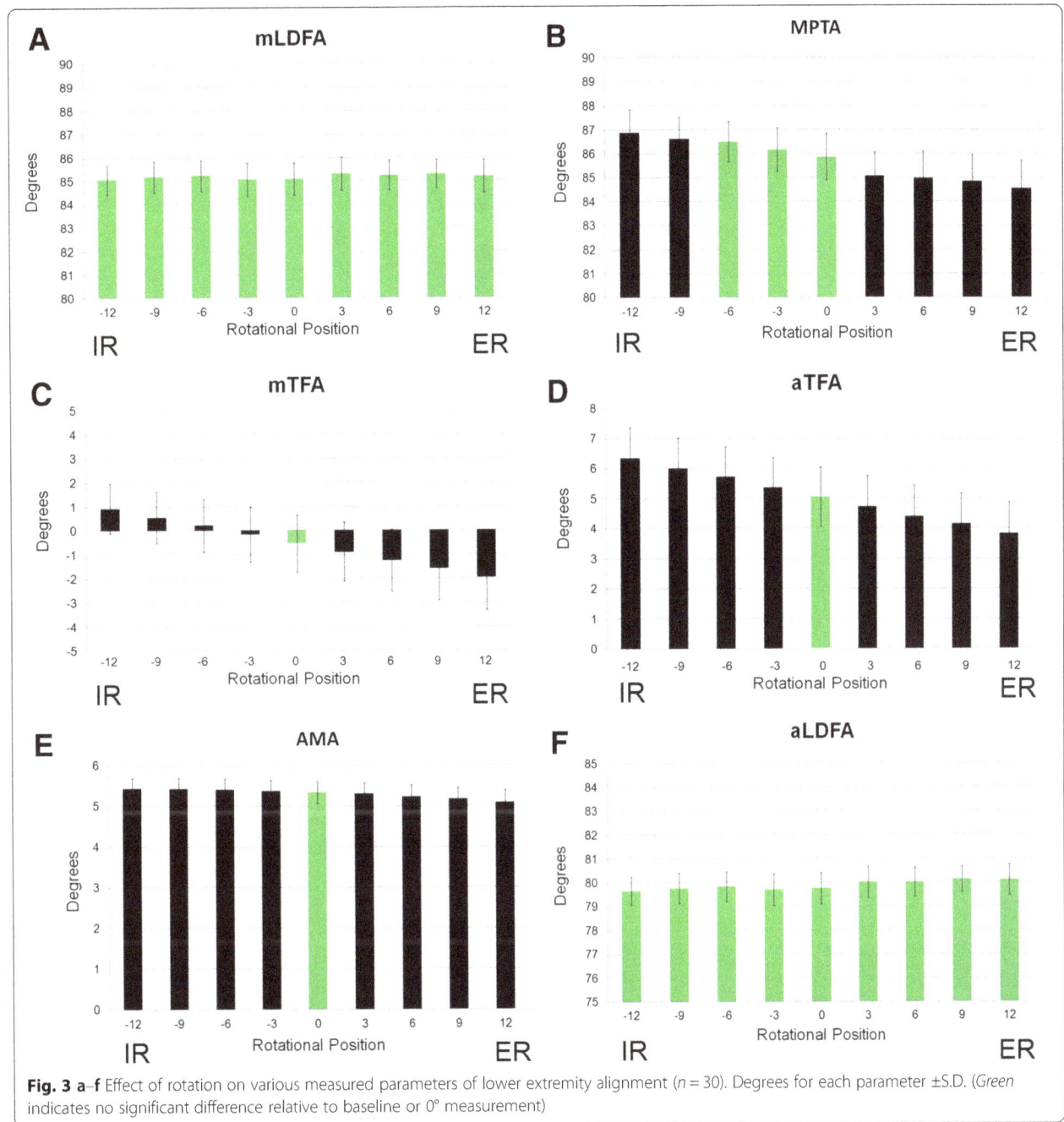

Fig. 3 a–f Effect of rotation on various measured parameters of lower extremity alignment ($n = 30$). Degrees for each parameter ±S.D. (*Green* indicates no significant difference relative to baseline or 0° measurement)

Discussion

The objective of this study was to twofold. The first goal was to obtain commonly performed measurements of alignment using standardized three-dimensional lower extremity models in a neutral position and to compare those values to data previously reported in the literature. Based on our analysis of the available literature, the measurements obtained in the study were comparable to those of the previous literature (Table 2) [1, 15, 17–20]. Our second goal was to determine the effect of rotation of the lower extremity, even in as little as 3° intervals, on

these commonly performed measurements of alignment. We found that small amounts of rotation did lead to statistically significant differences for a number of parameters analyzed including mTFA, aTFA, and AMA and to a limited degree for MPTA.

Bellemans et al. performed a study using standard radiographs positioned according to the methodology of Paley [16]. The study consisted of 250 volunteers, 125 male and 125 female. They measured many of the same parameters as in our study. Their main finding of their study was that 32% of males and 17% of females fit the

Table 2 Literature review

Reference	Number of normal subjects	Mean age	Gender	Technique	aLDFA	mLDFA	MPTA	AMA	mTFA	JLCA
Present study	87 patients undergoing CT angiography	N/A	49M, 38F	3D CT reconstructions with computer assisted analysis	80.24 ± 2.16°	85.59 ± 2.26°	86.09 ± 2.77°	5.35 ± 0.68°	−0.71 ± 3.07°	−1.21 ± 1.73°
3	119 healthy volunteers	38	52M, 67F	Standard full length radiographs	N/A	86.04−2.33°	86.92 ± 2.33°	N/A	−0.97 ± 2.86°	−1.85 ± 1.61°
15	25 male volunteers	30	25M, 0F	Standard full length radiographs	N/A	N/A	87.2°	4.05°	−1.3°(varus)	N/A
18	50 healthy Chinese adult volunteers	23-year-old females, 24-year-old males	25M, 25F	Standard full length radiographs	N/A	N/A	85.1 (males), 84.6 (females)	3.6 males, 3.1 females	−2.2 (males and females)	N/A
17	120 healthy Caucasian adult volunteers	range 25–60	60M, 60F	Standard full length radiographs	N/A	88.13°	86.85°	4.9 ± 0.7°	−1.2 ± 2.2°	N/A
20	100 healthy Iranian adult volunteers	range 15–32	50M, 50F	Standard full length radiographs	83.2 ± 3°	N/A	87.2	5.7 ± 1.2°	−1.5°(varus)	−1 ± 1.6°
21	118 healthy female Korean volunteers	range 20–39	118F	Standard full length radiographs	N/A	87.78 ± 1.68°	86.82 ± 1.61°	5.99 ± 0.7°	−1.35 ± 2.04°	N/A

criteria of "constitutional varus" defined as a hip-knee-ankle (HKA, equivalent to mTFA in this study) angle of 3° or greater varus. They further postulated that correcting such patients to a neutral mechanical axis through total knee replacement may lead to unfavorable outcomes. The authors noted one of the weaknesses of their study was the use of plain radiographs. They indicated that the rotational position of the extremities was controlled by positioning the subjects standing barefoot with the feet together and "standing at attention" with the patella oriented forward. Although this is a widely used technique, it is clear that all studies that use this methodology are at best estimating at the degree of rotation of the extremities. They considered the use of CT scans but were concerned about increased radiation. Our study addressed the issues discussed by Bellemans et al. By using CT scan generated models using preexisting scans, we avoided any additional radiation to patients. We also addressed the rotational variability of the positioning by placing the models on virtual planes and taking images in this position for the semiautomatic analysis. Song et al. explored the incident of constitutional varus in a controlled population of normal volunteers demonstrating a 20% incidence of constitutional varus in a group of Korean female volunteers [21]. Our data demonstrated a lower incidence of constitutional varus than both of these studies. This may reflect the different methodologies used (CT generated 3D models vs standard radiographs) as well as a different population (Belgian and Korean populations compared to a population from the USA).

A number of studies have evaluated the effect of rotation on lower extremity alignment parameters. Oswald et al. performed a cadaveric study on 38 lower extremity specimens using standard radiographs and analyzed the effect of rotation on the anatomic mechanical angle (AMA) [22]. At neutral, the AMA was 6.3°. They noted a change in this angle from 6.8° in 15° of internal rotation to 5.7° in 15° of external rotation for an average decrease in the AMA of 0.036° per degree of rotation. Radtke et al. performed a limited study on one lower extremity saw bone model in which a total knee replacement was implanted [23]. They then took five series of X-rays of that specimen measuring the AMA in various rotations from 20° of internal rotation (6.83°) to 20° of external rotation (4.63°) for an average decrease of 0.055° per degree of rotation. In our series, the AMA in the rotated studies was 5.33° at neutral and decreased from 5.43° to 5.08° between 12° of internal rotation and 12° of external rotation for an average decrease of 0.0146° per degree of rotation.

This study has a number of important weaknesses. The population included in this study was a random sample of patients undergoing CT angiography for vascular disease. As a result, the majority of the subjects were elderly with an average age of 66 years old. Furthermore, the characteristics of the population based on factors such as weight, height, or race could not be determined. In spite of our efforts to rule out patients with osteoarthritis of the knee, undoubtedly some degree of degeneration may have been present in this population. Second, we standardized the position of the femur relative to the coronal plane. However, there is some variability of the position of the tibia relative to that of the femur. We chose to standardize the femur since the methods for doing so are more reproducible based on the three points of contact of the femur on the coronal plane, namely the medial and lateral posterior condyles and the posterior greater trochanter. We operated under the assumption that the tibia would be relatively consistent in relation to the femur. Third, the software output was a three-dimensional reconstruction rather than a radiograph. These images do not demonstrate typical physical distortions such as parallax seen in standard radiographs, potentially limiting their comparisons to the traditional methods of alignment measurement used in previous publications. Fourth, in spite of our use of large monitor computer workstations, there is a possibility of some degree of inaccuracy of the measurements of the most distal aspect of each condyle and most proximal aspect of each tibial plateau due to the relatively low magnification of these regions relative to the entire image of the lower extremity. The number of patients included in the study was relatively low compared to some other population based studies. Another limitation of this study is that although there is a statistically significant error introduced with rotation of the leg for some of the parameters such as MPTA, the size of this error may not be clinically significant. It rests upon the reader to determine for themselves the clinically relevant range of error acceptable to them from a clinical perspective for the analysis or operation being considered. Some procedures may be more sensitive to variabilities in alignment than others.

In spite of these weaknesses, this study is one of the first to provide rotationally controlled values for commonly performed measurements of coronal alignment and one of the few studies that indicates the sensitivity of commonly performed measurements of coronal alignment to discreet small rotations of the entire lower extremity.

Conclusions

In conclusion, the current study validates the lower extremity alignment measurements that are commonly used in the fields of rheumatology and orthopedics with a more robust methodology that standardizes the rotational position of the lower extremity using three-dimensional models in a virtual environment. The study indicates that for some parameters, even a 3° rotational deviation can lead to a statistically significantly different value.

Abbreviations

aLDFA: Anatomical lateral distal femoral articular angle. The angle between the anatomical axis of the femur and the distal femoral articular axis; AMA: Anatomical-mechanical angle. The angle between the mechanical and anatomical axes of the femur; aTFA: Anatomic tibiofemoral angle. The angle between the anatomical axis of the femur and the mechanical/anatomical axis of the tibia; CT: Computerized tomography; HKA: Hip-knee-ankle angle. Equivalent to mTFA in this study; ICC: Intraclass correlation coefficients; JLCA: Joint line convergence angle. The angle between the proximal tibial and distal femoral articular axes; mLDFA: Mechanical lateral distal femoral articular angle. The lateral angle between the mechanical axis of the femur and the distal femoral articular axis; MPTA: Medial proximal tibial angle. The medial angle between the mechanical/anatomical axis of the tibia and the proximal tibial articular axis; mTFA: Mechanical tibiofemoral angle. The angle between the mechanical axis of the femur and the mechanical/anatomical axis of the tibia; PFSC: Proximal femoral shaft center. The geometric center of four points, two points on the lateral femoral surface and two points on the medial femoral surface in the subtrochanteric region of the femur; RMANOVA: Repeated measures analysis of variance

Acknowledgements

We would like to acknowledge the staff at the UC Davis Department of Radiology for their assistance with data acquisition protocols.

Funding

No external sources of funding were used for this study.

Authors' contributions

AAJ was the principal investigator and was involved in the study conception and manuscript preparation and submission. JPM was the co-principal investigator and was involved in the study conception and manuscript preparation and submission. NMM was the research resident and was involved in a large portion of the data acquisition and analysis as well as manuscript preparation. MJA was the research fellow and was involved in the remaining portion of the data acquisition and analysis as well as manuscript preparation. RL was the musculoskeletal radiologist and was involved in CT image acquisition, analysis, and data presentation. CP was the statistician and was involved in the presentation of the data and the statistical analysis and presentation of the results. All authors read and approved the final manuscript.

Competing interests

The authors declare that they have no competing interests.

Author details

[1]Joint Preservation Institute, 2825 J Street, Suite 440, Sacramento, CA 95816, USA. [2]UC Davis Medical Center, 4860 Y St., #4800, Sacramento, CA 95817, USA. [3]Department of Orthopaedic Surgery, University of California, Irvine, 101 The City Drive South, Pavillion III, Building 29A, Orange, CA 92868, USA. [4]UC Davis Department of Orthopaedics, 4635 2nd Ave, Research 1 Room 2000, Sacramento, CA 95817, USA. [5]UC Davis Department of Radiology, 4860 Y St., #3100, Sacramento, CA 95817, USA. [6]Sutter Institute for Medical Research, 2801 Capitol Ave Suite 400, Sacramento 95816, USA.

References

1. Cooke D, Scudamore A, Li J, Wyss U, Bryant T, Costigan P. Axial lower-limb alignment: comparison of knee geometry in normal volunteers and osteoarthritis patients. Osteoarthritis Cartilage. 1997;5:39–47.
2. Sharma L, Song J, Felson DT, Cahue S, Shamiyeh E, Dunlop DD. The role of knee alignment in disease progression and functional decline in knee osteoarthritis. JAMA. 2001;286:188–95.
3. Cooke TD, Harrison L, Khan B, Scudamore A, Chaudhary MA. Analysis of limb alignment in the pathogenesis of osteoarthritis: a comparison of Saudi Arabian and Canadian cases. Rheumatol Int. 2002;22:160–4.
4. Brouwer GM, van Tol AW, Bergink AP, Belo JN, Bernsen RM, Reijman M, Pols HA, Bierma-Zeinstra SM. Association between valgus and varus alignment and the development and progression of radiographic osteoarthritis of the knee. Arthritis Rheum. 2007;56:1204–11.
5. Paley D, Herzenberg JE, Tetsworth K, McKie J, Bhave A. Deformity planning for frontal and sagittal plane corrective osteotomies. Orthop Clin North Am. 1994;25:425–65.
6. Kettelkamp DB, Wenger DR, Chao EY, Thompson C. Results of proximal tibial osteotomy. The effects of tibiofemoral angle, stance-phase flexion-extension, and medial-plateau force. J Bone Joint Surg Am. 1976;58:952–60.
7. Rudan JF, Simurda MA. High tibial osteotomy. A prospective clinical and roentgenographic review. Clin Orthop Relat Res. 1990;255:251–6.
8. Terauchi M, Shirakura K, Kobuna Y, Fukasawa N. Axial parameters affecting lower limb alignment after hightibial osteotomy. Clin Orthop Relat Res. 1995;317:141–9.
9. Insall JN, Binazzi R, Soudry M, Mestriner LA. Total knee arthroplasty. Clin Orthop Relat Res. 1985;192:13–22.
10. Collier MB, Engh Jr CA, McAuley JP, Engh GA. Factors associated with the loss of thickness of polyethylene tibial bearings after knee arthroplasty. J Bone Joint Surg Am. 2007;89:1306–14.
11. Fang DM, Ritter MA, Davis KE. Coronal alignment in total knee arthroplasty: just how important is it? J Arthroplasty. 2009;24:39–43.
12. Howell SM, Howell SJ, Kuznik KT, Cohen J, Hull ML. Does a kinematically aligned total knee arthroplasty restore function without failure regardless of alignment category? Clin Orthop Relat Res. 2013;471:1000–7.
13. Parratte S, Pagnano MW, Trousdale RT, Berry DJ. Effect of postoperative mechanical axis alignment on the fifteen-year survival of modern, cemented total knee replacements. J Bone Joint Surg Am. 2010;92:2143–9.
14. Jamali AA, Deuel C, Perreira A, Salgado CJ, Hunter JC, Strong EB. Linear and angular measurements of computer-generated models: are they accurate, valid, and reliable? Comput Aided Surg. 2007;12:278–85.
15. Moreland JR, Bassett LW, Hanker GJ. Radiographic analysis of the axial alignment of the lower extremity. J Bone Joint Surg Am. 1987;69:745–9.
16. Paley D. Principles of deformity correction. 1st edn. New York: Spinger-Verlag; 2002.
17. Chao EY, Neluheni EV, Hsu RW, Paley D. Biomechanics of malalignment. Orthop Clin North Am. 1994;25:379–86.
18. Tang WM, Zhu YH, Chiu KY. Axial alignment of the lower extremity in Chinese adults. J Bone Joint Surg Am. 2000;82-A:1603–8.
19. Bellemans J, Colyn W, Vandenneucker H, Victor J. The Chitranjan Ranawat Award: is neutral mechanical alignment normal for all patients?: the concept of constitutional varus. Clin Orthop Relat Res. 2012;470(1):45–53.
20. Jabalameli M, Moghimi J, Yeganeh A, Nojomi M. Parameters of lower extremities alignment view in Iranian adult population. Acta Med Iran. 2015;53:293–6.
21. Song MH, Yoo SH, Kang SW, Kim YJ, Park GT, Pyeun YS. Coronal alignment of the lower limb and the incidence of constitutional varus knee in Korean females. Knee Surg Relat Res. 2015;27:49–55.
22. Oswald MH, Jakob RP, Schneider E, Hoogewoud HM. Radiological analysis of normal axial alignment of femur and tibia in view of total knee arthroplasty. J Arthroplasty. 1993;8:419–26.
23. Radtke K, Becher C, Noll Y, Ostermeier S. Effect of limb rotation on radiographic alignment in total knee arthroplasties. Arch Orthop Trauma Surg. 2010;130:451–7.

11

Local infiltration of analgesia and sciatic nerve block provide similar pain relief after total knee arthroplasty

Hidenori Tanikawa[1*], Kengo Harato[2], Ryo Ogawa[3], Tomoyuki Sato[4], Shu Kobayashi[2], So Nomoto[1], Yasuo Niki[2] and Kazunari Okuma[5]

Abstract

Background: Although femoral nerve block provides satisfactory analgesia after total knee arthroplasty (TKA), residual posterior knee pain may decrease patient satisfaction. We conducted a randomized controlled trial to clarify the efficacy of the sciatic nerve block (SNB) and local infiltration of analgesia with steroid (LIA) regarding postoperative analgesia after TKA, when administrated in addition to femoral nerve block (FNB).

Methods: Seventy-eight patients were randomly allocated to the two groups: concomitant administration of FNB and SNB or FNB and LIA. The outcome measures included post-operative pain, passive knee motion, C-reactive protein level, time to achieve rehabilitation goals, the Knee Society Score at the time of discharge, patient satisfaction level with anesthesia, length of hospital stay, surgical time, and complications related to local anesthesia.

Results: The patients in group SNB showed less pain than group LIA only on postoperative hours 0 and 3. Satisfactory postoperative analgesia after TKA was also achieved with LIA combined with FNB, while averting the risks associated with SNB. The influence on progress of rehabilitation and length of hospital stay was similar for both anesthesia techniques.

Conclusions: The LIA offers a potentially safer alternative to SNB as an adjunct to FNB, particularly for patients who have risk factors for sciatic nerve injury.

Keywords: Sciatic nerve block, Local infiltration of analgesia, Total knee arthroplasty

Background

Postoperative pain after total knee arthroplasty (TKA) is a major concern. In an effort to reduce postoperative pain and expedite recovery, femoral nerve block (FNB) shows higher quality of postoperative status after TKA [1, 2]. Although FNB has been found to provide effective analgesia, facilitate early ambulation, and reduce the length of hospitalization in patients undergoing TKA [3–5], previous research have shown that some patients experience significant postoperative pain despite the use of FNB [6–8].

Currently, anesthetic technique of sciatic nerve block (SNB) and local infiltration of analgesic agents (LIA) are two major options to supplement FNB. Many authors have shown that LIA provide improved pain relief compared

with no injection [9–12]. The analgesic effect of LIA varies due to the ingredients of the cocktail, and adding steroid in LIA has the effect of reducing inflammation, decreasing early pain relief, and improving recovery in TKA [13]. The addition of a SNB to a FNB also provides better pain relief than FNB alone [8, 14–16]. A previous study on the efficacy of SNB has shown that 67% of patients who had a preoperative FNB required the addition of a postoperative SNB [9].

The aim of this study was to compare the efficacy between SNB and LIA with steroid, when combined with the single-shot and continuous FNBs, in relieving postoperative pain, facilitating early rehabilitation, and reducing the length of hospital stay.

Methods

Study design

This was a double-blinded randomized controlled trial conducted in one centre. All patients received an explanation

* Correspondence: adriatic123sea@gmail.com
[1]Department of Orthopaedic Surgery, Saiseikai Yokohamashi Tobu Hospital, 3-6-1 Shimosueyoshi, Tsurumi, Yokohama, Kanagawa, Japan
Full list of author information is available at the end of the article

of the procedures and possible risks of the study, and gave written informed consent. This study was performed in conformity with the Declaration of Helsinki and was approved by the ethics review board at our institution. The inclusion criteria were primary TKA for osteoarthritis, American Society of Anesthesiologists (ASA) physical status classification 1–3, and full understanding of the informed consent. Exclusion criteria included patients with bilateral TKA, allergy to the drugs used in this study, neuromuscular disease, sensory disturbances of the legs, severe diabetes, heart failure, renal dysfunction, and liver dysfunction. Patients were randomized to one of two groups, combined FNB and SNB (SNB group) or combined FNB and LIA (LIA group) using sealed envelopes. Nurses and physiotherapists recording outcomes were blinded to the treatment.

Anesthetic and surgical techniques

Following general anesthesia, the anesthesiologist conducted one-shot FNB with 20 ml of 0.375% ropivacaine and then placed a catheter tip (Aesculap, B. Braun, Melsungen, Germany) for continuous FNB. For the patients in the SNB group, the anesthesiologist conducted one-shot SNB with 20 ml of 0.375% ropivacaine using an ultrasound-guided technique in combination with a nerve stimulus technique. For the patients in the LIA group, periarticular injection of local anesthetic was undertaken by the surgeons during surgery. A solution containing 200 mg of ropivacaine (100 ml of ropivacaine 0.2%), 6.6 mg of dexamethasone, and 0.5 ml of adrenaline (1 $mg \cdot ml^{-1}$) was administered as follows: 20 ml administered subcutaneously around the skin incision at the beginning of surgery; 50 ml administered into the posterior capsule, collateral ligaments, and quadriceps muscles before implant fixation; 30 ml was administered into the joint space at the end of surgery. All surgeries were performed by the same team of orthopedists using three types of TKA implant model.

Postoperative care

After surgery, 0.2% ropivacaine infusion at 5 $ml \cdot h^{-1}$ was initiated via the femoral nerve catheter and was continued for 48 h after surgery. Self-reported pain at rest was assessed by nurses using NRS (0 = no pain; 10 = worst pain). When a patient reported a NRS score >3 at rest, 25 mg diclofenac was administered by suppository. Nurses recorded the time when the patients were able to move his or her toes, and the following complications: nausea and vomiting, bleeding from the catheter, and toxic symptoms of local anesthesia including dizziness, tinnitus, tongue numbness, and spasm. All the patients were questioned on post-operative day (POD) 3 about the satisfaction level of the anesthesia received, which was evaluated with a categorical scale from 1 to 5 (1 = very dissatisfied, 2 = dissatisfied, 3 = neither, 4 = satisfied,

5 = very satisfied). Postoperative physiotherapy was started from the day after surgery. Maximum knee flexion angle was recorded by physiotherapists on PODs 7, 14, and 21. Physiotherapists also measured the number of days taken to achieve the following exercises: ambulation using a walker (10 m), ambulation using a cane (10 m), and climbing up and down the stairs (5 steps). Our hospital integrates acute-phase postoperative management and late-phase rehabilitation treatment, therefore the discharge criteria in our hospital includes stable 300 m ambulation using a cane, climbing up and down the stairs using a rail, and passive knee flexion of 120°.

Outcome measures

The primary outcome measure was post-operative pain, measured on a NRS on post-operative hours 0, 3, 6, 12, 24, 48, and PODs 3 to 21. Secondary outcome measures included passive knee motion, C-reactive protein (CRP) level, time to achieve rehabilitation goals, the Knee Society Score (KSS) at the time of discharge, patient satisfaction level, length of hospital stay, induction time, surgical time, and complications related to local anesthesia. We defined the induction time and surgical time as duration from oxygen administration to initial skin incision, and duration from initial skin incision to application of surgical dressings, respectively.

Statistics

Statistical analysis was performed using statistical software (SPSS 16.0 for Windows; SPSS Inc, Chicago, IL). The Mann–Whitney U test was used to analyze the nonparametric data, and the Student's t test was used to analyze the parametric data. Statistical significance was defined as $P < 0.05$.

Results

One hundred and thirty-two patients consented for the study. Fifty patients were excluded before randomization because they did not match the criteria. Two patients were lost to follow-up, and one patient was excluded because she removed the tube for continuous femoral nerve block by herself. Therefore, 79 patients were analyzed in this study (Fig. 1). No significant differences were observed in patient characteristics or intraoperative data between the two groups (Table 1).

The patients in group SNB showed less pain than group LIA on postoperative hours 0 and 3, and showed greater pain than group LIA on postoperative hours 24. After that, there was no significant difference between the SNB group and the LIA group concerning postoperative pain in the first 21 days (Fig. 2). The SNB group and the LIA group achieved similar passive knee flexion angle on POD 7, 14, and 21. The postoperative CRP level on POD 1 was significantly lower in LIA group compared with SNB

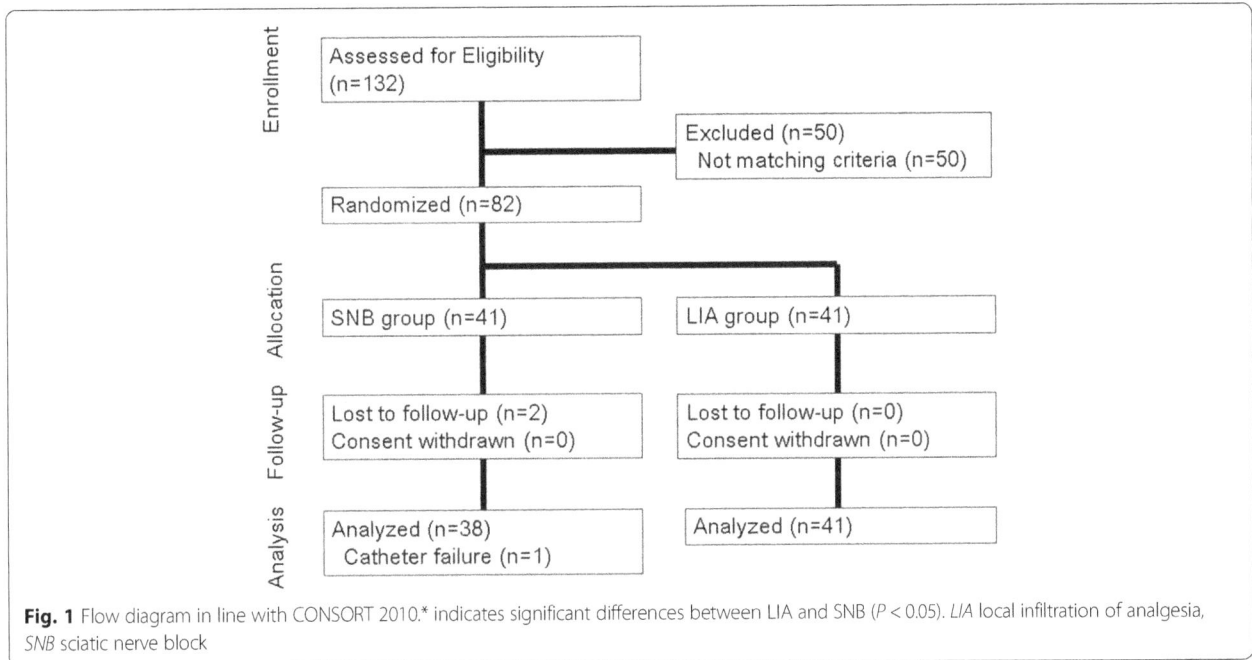

Fig. 1 Flow diagram in line with CONSORT 2010.* indicates significant differences between LIA and SNB (*P* < 0.05). *LIA* local infiltration of analgesia, *SNB* sciatic nerve block

group. The surgical time was similar between LIA group and SNB group, whereas the induction time was significantly smaller in LIA group (Table 2). There was no significant difference between the two groups in the rehabilitation progress, the length of stay, the KSS score, and the adverse effects of local anesthesia (Table 2).

Discussion

The main findings of our study show that SNB was more effective than LIA in reducing pain immediately after the surgery (within 3 h), however, SNB was less effective than LIA at 24 h after the surgery. Furthermore, 14.6% patients (six patients) in group LIA expressed severe pain (NRS > 7), whereas none of the patients in group SNB expressed severe pain. There are two possible reasons for the lower analgesic effect of LIA immediately after the surgery. First, the anesthesiologist used an ultrasound guidance technique and nerve stimulation equipment to carry out SNB, therefore accurate injection of the anesthetic agent to the sciatic nerve was achieved. In comparison, the surgeons blindly injected the anesthetic agent to the sensory nerve at the rear of knee joint in the LIA group, which may result in

variability among the analgesic effect of LIA. The second reason is the timing of the procedure. The anesthesiologist performed SNB before the surgery, whereas LIA was carried out during the surgery (at the beginning of the surgery, before implant fixation, after closing the capsule), therefore the analgesic effect in LIA group might not have taken effect at the end of the surgery and at 3 h after surgery. Since the patients in LIA group expressed less pain than SNB group at 24 h after the surgery, LIA may have a longer acting time than SNB. Considering that a previous report found that 3 or less NRS score meant successful analgesia [17], our results showed that both patients in group LIA and SNB would experience enough reduction in pain after surgery. The maximum difference of NRS between the two groups was 0.98 on POD 12, which was considered to be of subclinical difference, since a change of 1.3 points on a 10 cm VAS has been reported as clinically significant [18, 19]. Our result is supported by a study comparing SNB and periarticular infiltration as an adjunct to FNB, reporting that morphine consumption, VAS scores, and knee flexion angle in the first 48 h were comparable between the two groups [16]. Although a statistically significant difference

Table 1 Patient characteristics

Variables	LIA group (*n* = 41)	SNB group (*n* = 38)	*P* value
Age (years)	74 (68–80)	76 (71–80.5)	0.356
Body mass index (kg · m^{-2})	25.0 ± 3.84	24.6 ± 3.46	0.475
Sex, F/M	30/11	29/9	0.750
ASA I/II/III	5/35/1	1/37/0	0.265

Data are presented as absolute number or median (interquartile range) as appropriate for the variables and compared by Mann-Whitney *U* test. LIA = local infiltration of analgesia; *SNB* sciatic nerve block, *ASA* American Society of Anesthesiologists

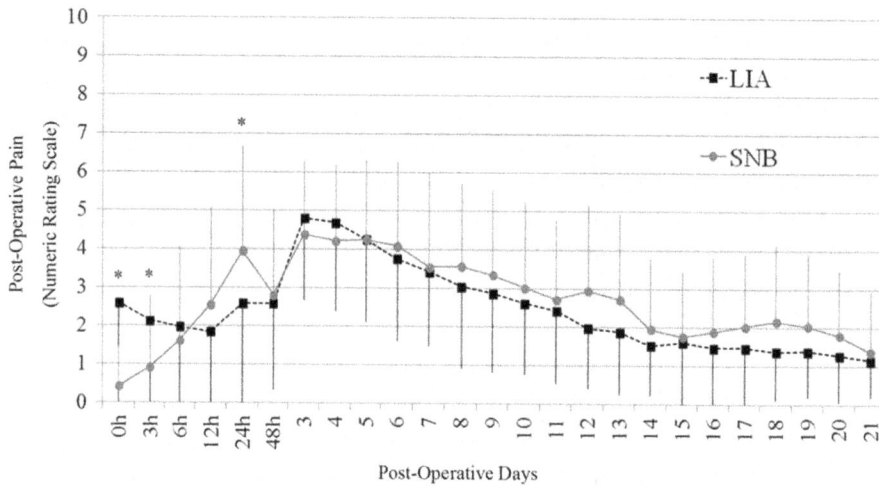

Fig. 2 Post-operative pain (numeric rating scale) after total knee arthroplasty. Data are expressed as mean ± SD and are analyzed using the independent Student's t test. * indicates significant differences between LIA and SNB ($P < 0.05$). *LIA* local infiltration of analgesia, *SNB* sciatic nerve block

was not seen, our results show that postoperative NRS remained at a low level in both groups, and sufficient postoperative analgesia was achieved with either SNB or LIA technique combined with one-shot and continuous FNBs.

Dexamethasone is a long-acting glucocorticoid with potent anti-inflammatory properties. Its anti-inflammatory effects, both locally and systemically, were confirmed in the past study by evaluating Interleukin-6 in drain and serum CRP [13]. The postoperative CRP levels were lower in LIA group compared with SNB group, and significant difference was found in CRP levels on POD 1, possibly due to the addition of steroid to local anesthetics in the LIA group. Ikeuchi et al. evaluated the efficacy of the addition of steroid to local anesthetics in LIA and concluded that adding steroid to local anesthetics reduced inflammation, resulting in early pain relief and rapid recovery in TKA [13]. The most important possible risks with steroid in the postoperative period include gastric ulcers, impaired wound healing, and wound infections [20, 21]. These risks are mostly associated with chronic glucocorticoid use, however, careful consideration to use steroids for post-operative analgesia should be given in patients with a high-risk comorbidity prior.

The current study did not find any significant difference in progress of rehabilitation, knee mobilization, and length of hospital stay between the SNB group and the LIA group. The result makes sense given that the duration of activity of the analgesic agents were essentially limited to the first 24 to 36 h [4]. Furthermore, our result is consistent with past reports that concluded SNB or LIA were of no benefit concerning knee functional recovery or length of hospital stay [16, 22–24].

The time needed to perform SNB or LIA is also important to shorten the anesthetic time and to improve the efficiency of the operating room. The induction time

was 6.9 min longer in the SNB group, while there was no significant difference in the surgical time between the two groups. LIA is an easy and fast technique, and surgeons can eliminate wasting time by injecting the drugs into the posterior of knee joint capsule while preparing the cement for implant fixation. Also, an accurate and fast SNB procedure was achieved using an ultrasound-aided peripheral nerve stimulated technique, which offers the potential benefit of accelerating the procedure, reducing the dose of local anesthetics, and resulting in higher block success rates [25–28].

SNB has similar complication rates as with any other nerve blocks, with permanent injury being exceptionally rare. Even in the absence of a SNB, TKA can place significant stress on the sciatic nerve, and sciatic nerve injury is a generally known complication after TKA with an incidence of 1.3 to 2.2% [29, 30]. Several risk factors for sciatic nerve injury after TKA have been reported, such as valgus deformity > 10°, total tourniquet time > 120 min, preexisting neuropathy, and uncontrollable postoperative bleeding [30]. Although none of the patients in SNB group sustained nerve injury in this study, it took approximately 6 h until we could confirm the toe motion. We should take account that performing a SNB could cloud the diagnosis of sciatic nerve injury and delay treatment.

There are several limitations to be noted regarding this study. Firstly, randomization by sealed envelope is open to selection bias, and a better method would have been computer generated off-site randomization to reduce this bias. Secondly, the orthopaedic surgeons who analyzed the data were not blinded to the treatment. Thirdly, the results of this study using dexamethasone cannot be applied to other types of steroid because of the variety of the pharmacological characteristics. Fourthly, combining various implant

Table 2 Post-surgical clinical data and rehabilitation milestones in LIA and SNB patients

Variables	LIA group (n = 41)	SNB group (n = 38)	P value
Passive knee flexion angle (degrees)			
POD 7	108 ± 13	104 ± 14	0.150
POD 14	119 ± 12	116 ± 12	0.337
POD 21	123 ± 12	123 ± 8	0.978
C-reactive protein level (mg/dl)			
POD 1	1.39 ± 0.71	3.77 ± 1.78	<0.001*
POD 3	12.14 ± 5.22	15.47 ± 4.20	0.006*
POD 7	5.53 ± 7.02	6.13 ± 8.68	0.762
POD 14	1.19 ± 1.42	1.26 ± 0.99	0.841
Time to achieve rehabilitation milestones (days)			
Ambulation with a walker	2.0 (2.0-3.0)	2.0 (1.25–3.0)	0.648
Straight leg raise	3.0 (3.0–4.0)	3.0 (3.0–4.0)	0.821
Ambulation with a cane	9.0 (7.0–11.5)	8.0 (7.0–10.0)	0.818
Stairs with a rail	11.0 (9.0–17.0)	12.0 (9.0–16.25)	0.886
Length of hospital stay (days)	24.0 (20.0–32.0)	24.0 (22.0–30.0)	0.738
Knee Society Score (function)			
Before surgery	39.2 ± 25.2	41.9 ± 28.2	0.624
At discharge	49.3 ± 16.2	51.6 ± 14.1	0.791
Knee Society Score (knee)			
Before surgery	44.9 ± 13.7	47.5 ± 17.5	0.661
At discharge	83.9 ± 10.0	84.9 ± 11.8	0.325
Induction time (min)	54.1 ± 6.4	61.0 ± 8.5	<0.001*
Surgical time (min)	73.5 ± 15.6	69.5 ± 13.1	0.215
Time of motor block in toe motion (h)	1.5 ± 4.4	6.7 ± 4.8	<0.001*
Requirement of diclofenac (mg)	0 (0–25)	0 (0–50)	0.159
Adverse effects			
Nausea or vomiting (%)	5 (12.2)	7 (18.4)	0.444
Symptoms of local anesthetic poisoning (%)	0 (0)	0 (0)	1.00

Data are presented as absolute number (percentage), median (interquartile range), or mean (SD) as appropriate for the variables and compared by Mann-Whitney U test or chi-square test. * Statistically significant P < 0.05. *LIA* local infiltration of analgesia, *SNB* sciatic nerve block, *POD* post-operative day

models may have an unknown effect on postoperative pain and knee function. Lastly, our hospital integrates acute-phase postoperative management and late-phase rehabilitation treatment, so the discharge criteria are different from international standard. This discrepancy may be a major restriction to expanding this study into international practice.

Conclusions

In conclusion, satisfactory postoperative analgesia after TKA was achieved with LIA combined with FNB, while averting the risks associated with SNB, and the influence on progress of rehabilitation and length of hospital stay was similar in both anesthesia techniques. Therefore, the combination of LIA and FNB may be a safer way of anesthesia for TKA, particularly for patients who have risk factors for sciatic nerve injury after TKA.

Abbreviations
ASA: American society of anesthesiologists; CRP: C-reactive protein; FNB: Femoral nerve block; KSS: Knee society score; LIA: Local infiltration of analgesia; NRS: Numeric rating scale; NSAIDs: Non-steroidal anti-inflammatory drugs; POD: Post-operative day; SNB: Sciatic nerve block; TKA: Total knee arthroplasty; VAS: Visual analogue scale

Acknowledgements
We would like to thank Ms. Sumi Yamashita, Ms. Mari Nagafuchi, and Ms. Akemi Uematsu for their valuable collaboration for the care of study patients and data collection. Additionally, we also thank Hiroko Tanikawa for technical assistance.

Funding
The study was not funded.

Authors' contributions

HT and TS designed the study. YN and SK helped in the data acquisition. HT and KH carried out the formal analysis. HT and KO performed the investigation. HT and TS provided the methodology. SN and YN helped in the project administration. KH and SN are responsible for the software. SN supervised the study. HT and RO wrote, reviewed, and edited the paper. All authors read and approved the final manuscript.

Competing interests

The authors declare that they have no competing interests.

Author details

[1]Department of Orthopaedic Surgery, Saiseikai Yokohamashi Tobu Hospital, 3-6-1 Shimosueyoshi, Tsurumi, Yokohama, Kanagawa, Japan. [2]Department of Orthopaedic Surgery, Keio University School of Medicine, Shinjyuku, Tokyo, Japan. [3]Department of Orthopaedic Surgery, Kitasato University Kitasato Institute Hospital, Minato-ku, Tokyo, Japan. [4]Department of Anesthesiology, Saiseikai Yokohamashi Tobu Hospital, Yokohama, Kanagawa, Japan. [5]Department of Orthopaedic Surgery, Saitama City Hospital, Saitama-shi, Saitama, Japan.

References

1. Allen HW, Liu SS, Ware PD, Naim CS, Owens BD. Peripheral nerve blocks improve analgesia after total knee replacement surgery. Anesth Analg. 1998;87:93–7.
2. Hirst GC, Lang SA, Dust WN, Cassidy JD, Yip RW. Femoral nerve block. Single injection versus continuous infusion for total knee arthroplasty. RegAnesth. 1996;21:292–7.
3. Capdevila X, Barthelet Y, Biboulet P, Ryckwaert Y, Rubenovitch J, d'Athis F. Effects of perioperative analgesic technique on the surgical outcome and duration of rehabilitation after major knee surgery. Anesthesiology. 1999;91:8–15.
4. Wang H, Boctor B, Verner J. The effect of single-injection femoral nerve block on rehabilitation and length of hospital stay after total knee replacement. RegAnesth Pain Med. 2002;27:139–44.
5. Fischer HB, Simanski CJ, Sharp C, Bonnet F, Camu F, Neugebauer EA, Rawal N, Joshi GP, Schug SA, Kehlet H, Working Group PROSPECT. A procedure-specific systematic review and consensus recommendations for postoperative analgesia following total knee arthroplasty. Anaesthesia. 2008;63:1105–23.
6. Davies AF, Segar EP, Murdoch J, Wright DE, Wilson IH. Epidural infusion or combined femoral and sciatic nerve blocks as perioperative analgesia for knee arthroplasty. Br J Anaesth. 2004;93:368–74.
7. Tierney E, Lewis G, Hurtig JB, Johnson D. Femoral nerve block with bupivacaine 0.25 per cent for postoperative analgesia after open knee surgery. Can J Anaesth. 1987;34:455–8.
8. Weber A, Fournier R, Van Gessel E, Gamulin Z. Sciatic nerve block and the improvement of femoral nerve block analgesia after total knee replacement. Eur J Anaesthesiol. 2002;19:834–6.
9. Vendittoli PA, Makinen P, Drolet P, Lavigne M, Fallaha M, Guertin MC, Varin F. A multimodal analgesia protocol for total knee arthroplasty. A randomized, controlled study. J Bone Joint Surg Am. 2006;88:282–9.
10. Koh IJ, Kang YG, Chang CB, Kwon SK, Seo ES, Seong SC, Kim TK. Additional pain relieving effect of intraoperative periarticular injections after simultaneous bilateral TKA: a randomized, controlled study. Knee Surg Sports Traumatol Arthrosc. 2010;18:916–22.
11. Gómez-Cardero P, Rodríguez-Merchán EC. Postoperative analgesia in TKA: ropivacaine continuous intraarticular infusion. Clin Orthop Relat Res. 2010; 468:1242–7.
12. Andersen KV, Bak M, Christensen BV, Harazuk J, Pedersen NA, Søballe K. A randomized, controlled trial comparing local infiltration analgesia with epidural infusion for total knee arthroplasty. Acta Orthop. 2010;81:606–10.
13. Ikeuchi M, Kamimoto Y, Izumi M, Fukunaga K, Aso K, Sugimura N, Yokoyama M, Tani T. Effects of dexamethasone on local infiltration analgesia in total knee arthroplasty: a randomized controlled trial. Knee Surg Sports Traumatol Arthrosc. 2014;22:1638–43.
14. McNamee DA, Parks L, Milligan KR. Post-operative analgesia following total knee replacement: an evaluation of the addition of an obturator nerve block to combined femoral and sciatic nerve block. Acta Anaesthesiol Scand. 2002;46:95–9.
15. Ben-David B, Schmalenberger K, Chelly JE. Analgesia after total knee arthroplasty: is continuous sciatic blockade needed in addition to continuous femoral blockade? Anesth Analg. 2004;98:747–9.
16. Mahadevan D, Walter RP, Minto G, Gale TC, McAllen CJ, Oldman M. Combined femoral and sciatic nerve block vs combined femoral and periarticular infiltration in total knee arthroplasty: a randomized controlled trial. J Arthroplasty. 2012;27:1806–11.
17. Farrar JT, Young Jr JP, LaMoreaux L, Werth JL, Poole RM. Clinical importance of changes in chronic pain intensity measured on an 11-point numerical pain rating scale. Pain. 2001;94:149–58.
18. Affas F, Nygårds EB, Stiller CO, Wretenberg P, Olofsson C. Pain control after total knee arthroplasty: a randomized trial comparing local infiltration anesthesia and continuous femoral block. Acta Orthop. 2011;82:441–7.
19. Gallagher EJ, Liebman M, Bijur PE. Prospective validation of clinically important changes in pain severity measured on a visual analog scale. Ann Emerg Med. 2001;38:633–8.
20. Cutolo M, Seriolo B, Pizzorni C, Secchi ME, Soldano S, Paolino S, Montagna P, Sulli A. Use of glucocorticoids and risk of infections. Autoimmun Rev. 2008;8:153–5.
21. Wicke C, Halliday B, Allen D, Roche NS, Scheuenstuhl H, Spencer MM, Roberts AB, Hunt TK. Effects of steroids and retinoids on wound healing. Arch Surg. 2000;135:1265–70.
22. Carli F, Clemente A, Asenjo JF, Kim DJ, Mistraletti G, Gomarasca M, Morabito A, Tanzer M. Analgesia and functional outcome after total knee arthroplasty: periarticular infiltration vs continuous femoral nerve block. Br J Anaesth. 2010;105:185–95.
23. Toftdahl K, Nikolajsen L, Haraldsted V, Madsen F, Tønnesen EK, Søballe K. Comparison of peri- and intraarticular analgesia with femoral nerve block after total knee arthroplasty: a randomized clinical trial. Acta Orthop. 2007; 78:172–9.
24. Wegener JT, van Ooij B, van Dijk CN, Hollmann MW, Preckel B, Stevens MF. Value of single-injection or continuous sciatic nerve block in addition to a continuous femoral nerve block in patients undergoing total knee arthroplasty: a prospective, randomized, controlled trial. Reg Anesth Pain Med. 2011;36:481–8.
25. Mariano ER, Loland VJ, Sandhu NS, Bishop ML, Lee DK, Schwartz AK, Girard PJ, Ferguson EJ, Ilfeld BM. Comparative efficacy of ultrasound-guided and stimulating popliteal-sciatic perineural catheters for postoperative analgesia. Can J Anaesth. 2010;57:919–26.
26. Casati A, Baciarello M, Di Cianni S, Danelli G, De Marco G, Leone S, Rossi M, Fanelli G. Effects of ultrasound guidance on the minimum effective anaesthetic volume required to block the femoral nerve. Br J Anaesth. 2007; 98:823–7.
27. Perlas A, Brull R, Chan VW, McCartney CJ, Nuica A, Abbas S. Ultrasound guidance improves the success of sciatic nerve block at the popliteal fossa. Reg Anesth Pain Med. 2008;33:259–65.
28. Orebaugh SL, Williams BA, Kentor ML. Ultrasound guidance with nerve stimulation reduces the time necessary for resident peripheral nerve blockade. Reg Anesth Pain Med. 2007;32:448–54.
29. Schinsky MF, Macaulay W, Parks ML, Kiernan H, Nercessian OA. Nerve injury after primary total knee arthroplasty. J Arthroplasty. 2001;16:1048–54.
30. Horlocker TT, Cabanela ME, Wedel DJ. Does postoperative epidural analgesia increase the risk of peroneal nerve palsy after total knee arthroplasty? Anesth Analg. 1994;79:495–500.

12

Subscapularis- and deltoid-sparing vs traditional deltopectoral approach in reverse shoulder arthroplasty: a prospective case-control study

Alexandre Lädermann[1,2,3]* ⓘ, Patrick Joel Denard[4,5], Jérome Tirefort[3], Philippe Collin[6], Alexandra Nowak[1] and Adrien Jean-Pierre Schwitzguebel[1]

Abstract

Background: With the growth of reverse shoulder arthroplasty (RSA), it is becoming increasingly necessary to establish the most cost-effective methods for the procedure. The surgical approach is one factor that may influence the cost and outcome of RSA. The purpose of this study was to compare the clinical results of a subscapularis- and deltoid-sparing (SSCS) approach to a traditional deltopectoral (TDP) approach for RSA. The hypothesis was that the SSCS approach would be associated with decreased length of stay (LOS), equal complication rate, and better short-term outcomes compared to the TDP approach.

Methods: A prospective evaluation was performed on patients undergoing RSA over a 2-year period. A deltopectoral incision was used followed by either an SSCS approach or a traditional tenotomy of the subscapularis (TDP). LOS, adverse events, physical therapy utilization, and patient satisfaction were collected in the 12 months following RSA.

Results: LOS was shorter with the SSCS approach compared to the TDP approach (from 8.2 ± 6.4 days to 15.2 ± 11.9 days; $P = 0.04$). At 3 months postoperative, the single assessment numeric evaluation score ($80 \pm 11\%$ vs $70 \pm 6\%$; $P = 0.04$) and active elevation ($130 \pm 22°$ vs $109 \pm 24°$; $P = 0.01$) were higher in the SSCS group. The SSCS approach resulted in a net cost savings of $5900 per patient. Postoperative physical therapy, pain levels, and patient satisfaction were comparable in both groups. No immediate intraoperative complications were noted.

Conclusion: Using a SSCS approach is an option for patients requiring RSA. Overall LOS is minimized compared to a TDP approach with subscapularis tenotomy. The SSCS approach may provide substantial healthcare cost savings, without increasing complication rate or decreasing patient satisfaction.

Keywords: Shoulder, Reverse shoulder arthroplasty, Length of stay, Deltopectoral approach, Subscapularis sparing, Approach, Cost-effectiveness, Results

Background

The use of reverse shoulder arthroplasty (RSA) has increased substantially in recent years [1]. While the introduction of RSA has provided a solution for several previously untreatable conditions, as with most technological advancements, this has led to increased healthcare utilization and cost. Concurrently, from a macroscopic perspective, there has been growing interest within health systems to identify the most valuable or cost-effective treatments.

The bundled payment initiative has brought attention to examining multiple aspects of cost in the entire phase of care. In addition to implant cost, potential areas of cost savings include length of stay (LOS), complication and readmission rate, and postoperative rehabilitation center or physical therapy utilization. The impact of surgical approach for RSA on the aforementioned factors

* Correspondence: alexandre.laedermann@gmail.com
[1]Division of Orthopaedics and Trauma Surgery, La Tour Hospital, Rue J.-D. Maillard 3, 1217 Meyrin, Switzerland
[2]Faculty of Medicine, University of Geneva, Rue Michel-Servet 1, 1211 Geneva 4, Switzerland
Full list of author information is available at the end of the article

has not been previously studied. The most common surgical approach for RSA is a deltopectoral incision that includes a tenotomy or peel of the subscapularis to gain access to the glenohumeral joint. Recently, an approach which uses a deltopectoral incision but spares the subscapularis has been reported with good short-term clinical results [2]. Since this approach is subscapularis and deltoid sparing (SSCS), immediate active range of motion (ROM) without immobilization is allowed [2]. This fast-track rehabilitation protocol may therefore lead to cost savings.

The purpose of this study was to compare the clinical results of the SSCS and the TDP for RSA. The hypothesis was that the SSCS approach would be associated with decreased LOS, equal complication rate, and better short-term outcomes compared to a traditional deltopectoral (TDP) approach.

Methods
Patient selection
Between May 2013 and June 2015, all patients who had a primary RSA performed by one author (A.L.) with minimum follow-up of 3 months were considered potentially eligible for inclusion in this prospective case-control study that estimated the cost savings of a TDP approach compared to the SSCS approach. Patients with fractures, previous infection, shoulder malignancy, and

revision surgery were excluded. Forty-three patients were considered potentially eligible for the study. Among them, five were excluded for revision shoulder arthroplasty, one for shoulder malignancy, and two for previous glenohumeral septic arthritis. Thus, there were 35 patients (35 RSAs) that met the study criteria. There were 18 patients in the TDP group and 17 patients in the SSCS group (Fig. 1). The study protocol was approved by the hospital ethics committee (AMG: 12–26), and all patients gave informed written consent.

Surgical technique
All patients had general anesthesia with muscle relaxants used to facilitate glenoid exposure. Prior to skin incision, prophylactic intravenous antibiotics (cefazolin) were administered. In all cases, a deltopectoral incision was used [3]. The two approaches vary at the point of addressing the subscapularis tendon. If the subscapularis was torn, the remaining subscapularis and/or capsular tissue was tenotomized to gain access to the glenohumeral joint [4]. Conversely, if the subscapularis was intact, a SSCS approach was utilized as previously described [2]. For both approaches, the humeral head was cut with 20° of retroversion [5–7]. A circular baseplate (Aequalis Reversed; Tornier, Montbonnot, France) was implanted at the inferior edge of the glenoid. The glenosphere was usually eccentric to limit friction-type impingement in

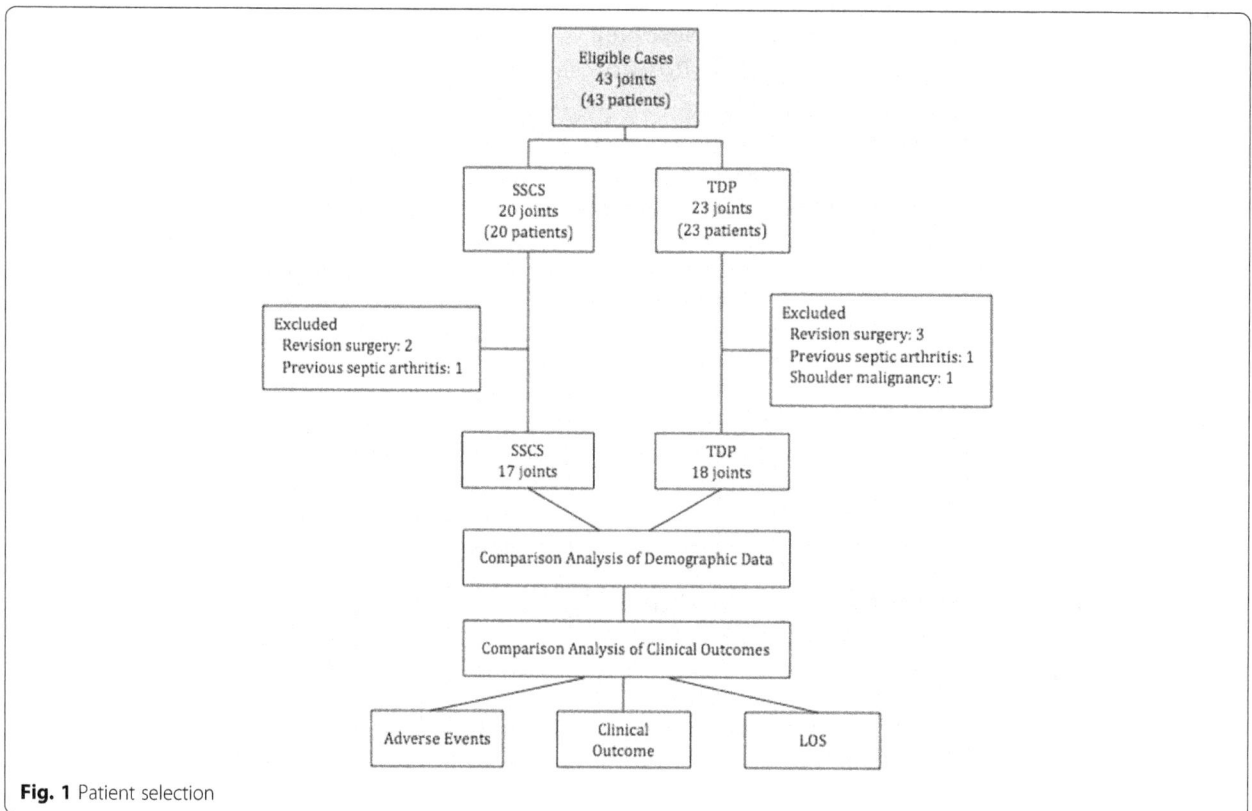

Fig. 1 Patient selection

adduction, extension, and external rotation [8]. An onlay humeral stem with a final humeral inclination of 145° and an eccentric humeral plate was implanted. The eccentric infero-medial position was always used to limit arm lengthening and to maximize lateralization [9]. After closure of the incision, 160 mg of gentamicin mixed in 20 mL of saline was injected into the glenohumeral joint [10].

Postoperative rehabilitation

In the case of a TDP approach, a standardized rehabilitation protocol was followed [11]. Patients were placed in a sling for 4 weeks. Passive ROM was initiated immediately, and active motion was allowed at 4 weeks. Strengthening was allowed at 8 weeks. With the SSCS approach, immediate active ROM was allowed with a sling for comfort only during the first few postoperative days [2] and strengthening was allowed at 6 weeks.

Baseline characteristics and study variables

Baseline clinical characteristics extracted from the prospective database included age, sex, dominant hand, initial diagnosis (Hamada 1 to 2, Hamada 3 to 5, dislocation arthropathy, post-traumatic), previous shoulder surgeries, prior deltoid or subscapularis insufficiency, and baseline functional outcome and ROM. Baseline characteristics are summarized in Table 1.

The primary outcome was LOS, including hospitalization and rehabilitation or post acute care. LOS during hospitalization was determined by the ability of the patient to return home. If unable, rehabilitation or post acute care was prescribed until the patient was able to independently return home. All costs were expressed in US dollars and estimated by adding the costs of the immediate postoperative hospital stay and rehabilitation stay. At our institution, the average cost of a hospital stay per night is approximately $1500 and the cost of a rehabilitation stay per night is approximately $647. Implant costs were excluded since

we used the same implant in all cases and were not evaluating implant costs.

Secondary outcomes were adverse events (readmission and complication), number of postoperative physical therapy sessions, and clinical outcome at 3 months in terms of pain (visual analogue scale (VAS)), functional outcome (single assessment numeric evaluation (SANE)), and ROM in elevation, external rotation, and internal rotation) and at 12 months with Constant score [12]. Preoperative outcomes are summarized in Table 2.

Statistical analysis

Statistical analysis was performed with R v3.1.2 Portable (Free Software Foundation Inc, Vienna, Austria). Basic descriptive statistics (mean and percentages) were used for baseline clinical parameters and functional evaluation (VAS, SANE, and ROM). Clinical parameters of interest were compared between SSCS and TDS approach with two-tailed Student's t or chi-squared test, when appropriate. Level of significance was set at $P < 0.05$.

Results

There were no statistically significant differences between the two groups at baseline (Tables 1 and 2).

With the SSCS approach, the total length of stay was significantly shorter compared to the TDP approach. Hospitalization and rehabilitation stay costs were lower in the SSCS approach compared to the TDP approach (Table 3). There were no statistically significant differences between groups with respect to the number of physical therapy sessions. The SSCS approach was associated with a better functional outcome at 3 months in regard to SANE score and arm elevation. There was no statistically significant difference between the two groups in postoperative pain or range of internal and external rotation at 3 months postoperative (Table 4) and in Constant score at 1 year (68.1 ± 15.6 with SSCS approach vs 77.3 ± 12.9 with TDP approach; $P = 0.07$, respectively).

Table 1 Baseline patient characteristics

	All prosthesis (N = 35)	SSCS approach (N = 17)	TDP approach (N = 18)	P
DRG insurance coverage	14	9	5	0.13
Failed cuff repair	3	0	3	0.08
Cuff tear arthropathy Hamada 1–2	14	10	4	0.03
Cuff tear arthropathy Hamada 3–5	10	5	5	0.91
Malunion	8	2	6	0.13
Age	78 ± 7	78 ± 7	78 ± 8	0.82
Sex (male)	8 (23%)	4 (24%)	4 (22%)	1
Dominant arm	18 (51%)	7 (41%)	11 (61%)	0.4
Previous surgeries	20 (61%)	5 (29%)	15 (94%)	0.23

DRG diagnosis-related group, *TDP* traditional deltopectoral, *SSCS* subscapularis and deltoid sparing

Table 2 Preoperative outcomes

	All prosthesis (N = 35)	SSCS approach (N = 17)	TDP approach (N = 18)	P
Pain VAS	6.9 ± 2.3	6.9 ± 1.9	6.8 ± 2.7	0.84
SANE	32 ± 19	37 ± 14	27 ± 22	0.12
Forward elevation	95 ± 50	111 ± 58	75 ± 31	0.04
ER	19 ± 20	20 ± 21	19 ± 18	0.9
IR (median spinal height)	L4	L1	Sacrum	0.27

ER external rotation, *IR* internal rotation, *TDP* traditional deltopectoral, *SANE* single shoulder numeric assessment, *SSCS* subscapularis and deltoid sparing, *VAS* visual analogue scale

Table 4 Clinical outcome evaluated at 3 months post-surgery

	All prosthesis (N = 35)	SSCS (N = 17)	TDP (N = 18)	P value
Pain VAS	1.2 ± 1.4	1.2 ± 1.5	1.2 ± 1.4	0.89
SANE	75 ± 15	80 ± 11	70 ± 16	0.04
Forward elevation	119 ± 25	130 ± 22	109 ± 24	0.01
ER	20 ± 24	25 ± 27	15 ± 21	0.29
IR (median spinal level)	L4	L1	L4	0.27

ER external rotation, *IR* internal rotation, *TDP* traditional deltopectoral, *SANE* Single shoulder numeric assessment, *SSCS* subscapularis and deltoid sparing, *VAS* visual analogue scale

During the follow-up period of 18 ± 11 months (range, 12 to 46 months), only one patient had a complication. This patient had a TDP approach and suffered a prosthetic dislocation 6 weeks postoperatively, which has been successfully managed with closed reduction. The same patient also experienced an acromial stress fracture that was managed conservatively. No subscapularis avulsion or iatrogenic tuberosity fracture was observed due to retraction during the SSCS approach.

Discussion

The results of the current study support the hypothesis that the SSCS approach is associated with lower cost and equal complication compared to a TDP approach.

It is notable that the population is aging and older patients are the most likely to benefit from RSA [13]. However, the average hospital cost for shoulder arthroplasty is estimated to be $17,000 [14]. Consequently, it is important to find a solution to reduce the overall costs to provide continued access to RSA. LOS has recently been analyzed after shoulder arthroplasty in women, seniors, and comorbidity patients, with insurance coverage and diagnosis significantly contributing to increase in LOS [13, 15, 16]. In addition, hospital volume and surgeon experience have been associated with a lower LOS and cost compared to lower volume facilities and surgeons [17]. The current study examines an additional variable—that of surgical approach—which may affect cost. After controlling for preoperative and surgical variables, utilization of a SSCS approach compared to the current standard of a TDP approach for RSA resulted in an economic savings of $5881, corresponding to an average

LOS of 7 days. By decreasing LOS and allowing earlier mobilization, such an approach may also help lower hospital-acquired infection rates [18], decrease risk factors for readmission [19], and improve patient satisfaction [20].

In addition to cost savings, the SSCS approach group was also significantly associated with a better functional outcome at 3 months compared to the TDP approach. At least four reasons could explain these differences. First, the subscapularis plays a crucial role in anterior elevation. Collin et al. previously demonstrated that the subscapularis is the most important rotator cuff muscle for elevation in native shoulders [21]. Although the RSA design partially changes the role of the subscapularis, an intact inferior subscapularis assures the joint protection necessary for ROM [22] and the superior subscapularis provides a positive vector force and function as an abductor [23]. Second, preservation of the subscapularis may improve internal rotation. A deficit in internal rotation is common after RSA, and while not well-studied, lack of healing of the subscapularis may partially account for this deficit. Third, if tenotomized or preoperatively torn, the subscapularis should be repaired whenever possible and protected in order to obtain healing as it plays a role in postoperative stability [24] at least in Medial Glenoid/Medial Humerus designs. Fourth, and finally, the SSCS approach allows immediate ROM. Immobilization has been shown to be associated with increased shoulder stiffness [25]. Postoperative immobilization following shoulder arthroplasty has been designed to balance the optimization of healing and prevention of stiffness. A 6-week period of immobilization is typically used to allow the tendon bone interface to

Table 3 Cost by surgical approach evaluated at 3 months post-surgery

	All prosthesis (N = 35)	SSCS approach (N = 17)	TDP approach (N = 18)	P value
Hospitalization stay	11.9 ± 10.2	8.2 ± 6.4	15.2 ± 11.9	0.04
Hospitalization costs (dollars)	13,600 ± 7900	10,500 ± 5200	16,400 ± 8700	0.02
Complication rate	1 (3%)	0 (0%)	1 (6%)	1
Number of outpatient care physical therapy sessions	14.1 ± 13.7	15.9 ± 17.9	12.4 ± 8.7	0.48

TDP traditional deltopectoral, *SSCS* subscapularis and deltoid sparing

progress through the normal healing phases of inflammation, proliferation, and remodeling [26]. After subscapularis repair in anatomic total shoulder arthroplasty, 4 weeks of immobilization lead to higher healing rates [27]. However, with a SSCS approach, immobilization may be avoided since there is no need to obtain subscapularis healing. Such early mobilization likely explains our superior clinical results in the SSCS group at short term. Nevertheless, the results were no different at 1 year.

Complications after RSA are related to etiology [28], prosthetic design [9, 29], arm lengthening [30, 31], and experience of the surgeon [32]. Traditionally, the rate of short-term complications after RSA is around 20% [28, 33, 34]. In this case-control series of 35 patients, the rate of short-term complications (3%) was lower than previously reported. In particular, we did not observe any technical problems with the SSCS approach. While further study with a larger cohort is needed, the early results with deltopectoral approach (with or without subscapularis sparing) are encouraging.

Strengths and limitations

This prospective case-control study was the first to analyze the impact of a SSCS approach for RSA on cost. We observed substantial economic savings to the system, improved short-term results, and a minimal complication rate that may have the potential to change the standard for approach during RSA. However, there are several limitations that warrant discussion. First, different insurance coverages have been included in the study. The calculation was based on private division fees. Therefore, formal cost analysis was not possible for DRG patients [35] (i.e., patients without a private insurance coverage). Indeed, the cost of RSA for patients with DRG is not dependent of the length of the hospitalization stay. We consequently extrapolated the price regarding the loss of earnings for the hospital. Second, this study represents the learning curve and experience of one surgeon. Results could vary by learning curve and different geographical regions or health care systems. Concern has been expressed about cost savings from small changes in systems and techniques [36]. To date, no study has examined the economic effect of more widespread use of such approach, as it may not deliver significant savings at the macro scale. Effectively, it has not been proven that an anterosuperior approach [37], which involves the splitting of the deltoid muscle to avoid cutting the subscapularis tendon, is associated with lower cost or better functional results [38]. Third, we also recognize that SSCS approach might be challenging in certain cases (i.e., stiff shoulders) and may not be practical or possible in all circumstances. Fourth, our LOS was long. The latter is dependent of many factors, including patient factors (i.e., pain and ability to do ADLs) and health system factors. For example, in our

country, our insurance system often imposes a minimum stay which artificially prolongs the LOS. In a recent study, Padegimas et al. demonstrated that LOS at orthopedic specialty hospitals is significantly shorter than at tertiary referral centers [39]. Their findings may be the result not only of fast-track rehabilitation and strict disposition protocols but also of less invasive surgical techniques. The cost-effectiveness of the SSCS approach is now even more apparent in our practice as patients are routinely discharging after only one to two nights in the hospital and no longer require an acute care stay and do not have therapy in the first 6 weeks postoperative. Fifth, due to the limited sample size, some of the comparisons performed might lack statistical power (type II error). Multicenter and prospective investigation will be necessary to determine the role of independent variables such as surgical approach, fast-track surgery, rehabilitation protocols, or health care systems.

Conclusion

Using a SSCS approach is an option for patients requiring RSA. Overall, LOS is minimized compared to a TDP approach with subscapularis tenotomy. The SSCS approach may provide substantial healthcare cost savings, without increasing complication rate or decreasing patient satisfaction.

Abbreviations

DRG: Diagnosis-related group; LOS: Length of stay; ROM: Range of motion; RSA: Reverse shoulder arthroplasty; SANE: Single assessment numeric evaluation; SSCS: Subscapularis and deltoid sparing; TDP: Traditional deltopectoral; VAS: Visual analogue scale

Acknowledgements

Not applicable.

Funding

No funding was received for this study.

Authors' contributions

AL conceived of the study, operated the patients, participated in its design and coordination, and helped to draft the manuscript. JT and AN who were not involved in the surgical procedures analyzed the medical records, operative reports, and radiographs for each patient. PJD and PC helped to draft and to write the manuscript. AS participated in the design of the study and performed the statistical analysis. All authors read and approved the final manuscript.

Competing interests

PJD received royalties and is a paid consultant for Arthrex. PC is a paid consultant from Wright and Smith and Nephew and received royalties from Wright, Storz, and Advanced Medical Application. The other authors certify that they or any members of their immediate families have no non-financial or financial disclosures (e.g., consultancies, stock ownership, equity interest, patent/licensing arrangements) that might pose a conflict of interest in connection with the submitted article.

Author details

[1]Division of Orthopaedics and Trauma Surgery, La Tour Hospital, Rue J.-D. Maillard 3, 1217 Meyrin, Switzerland. [2]Faculty of Medicine, University of Geneva, Rue Michel-Servet 1, 1211 Geneva 4, Switzerland. [3]Division of Orthopaedics and Trauma Surgery, Department of Surgery, Geneva University Hospitals, Rue Gabrielle-Perret-Gentil 4, CH-1211 Geneva 14, Switzerland. [4]Southern Oregon Orthopedics, Medford, Oregon, USA. [5]Department of Orthopaedics and Rehabilitation, Oregon Health & Science University, Portland, Oregon, USA. [6]Saint-Grégoire Private Hospital Center, Boulevard Boutière 6, 35768 Saint-Grégoire cedex, France.

References

1. Schairer WW, Nwachukwu BU, Lyman S, Craig EV, Gulotta LV. National utilization of reverse total shoulder arthroplasty in the United States. J Shoulder Elbow Surg. 2015;24:91-7.

2. Lädermann A, Lo EY, Schwitzguebel AJ, Yates E. Subscapularis and deltoid preserving anterior approach for reverse shoulder arthroplasty. Orthop Traumatol Surg Res. 2016;102:905-8.

3. Walch G, Wall B. Indication and techniques of revision arthroplasty with a reverse prosthesis. In: Walch G, Boileau P, Mole D, Favard L, Lévigne C, Sirveaux F, editors. Reverse shoulder arthroplasty. Montpellier: Sauramps Medical; 2006. p. 243-6.

4. Boileau P, Walch G. The surgical anatomy and osteotomy technique for the humeral head. In: Walch GBP, editor. Shoulder arthroplasty. Berlin: Springer-Verlag; 1999. p. 107-55.

5. Berhouet J, Garaud P, Favard L. Evaluation of the role of glenosphere design and humeral component retroversion in avoiding scapular notching during reverse shoulder arthroplasty. J Shoulder Elbow Surg. 2014;23:151-8.

6. Gulotta LV, Choi D, Marinello P, Knutson Z, Lipman J, Wright T, Cordasco FA, Craig EV, Warren RF. Humeral component retroversion in reverse total shoulder arthroplasty: a biomechanical study. J Shoulder Elbow Surg. 2012; 21:1121-7.

7. Stephenson DR, Oh JH, McGarry MH, Rick Hatch 3rd GF, Lee TQ. Effect of humeral component version on impingement in reverse total shoulder arthroplasty. J Shoulder Elbow Surg. 2011;20:652-8.

8. Lädermann A, Gueorguiev B, Charbonnier C, Stimec BV, Fasel JH, Zderic I, Hagen J, Walch G. Scapular notching on kinematic simulated range of motion after reverse shoulder arthroplasty is not the result of impingement in adduction. Medicine (Baltimore). 2015;94:e1615.

9. Lädermann A, Denard PJ, Boileau P, Farron A, Deransart P, Terrier A, Ston J, Walch G. Effect of humeral stem design on humeral position and range of motion in reverse shoulder arthroplasty. Int Orthop. 2015;39:2205-13.

10. Lovallo J, Helming J, Jafari SM, Owusu-Forfie A, Donovan S, Minnock C, Adib F. Intraoperative intra-articular injection of gentamicin: will it decrease the risk of infection in total shoulder arthroplasty? J Shoulder Elbow Surg. 2014; 23:1272-6.

11. Liotard J. Painful shoulder rehabilitation: how to do it simple. Revue du rhumatisme monographies. 2010;77(3):239-45.

12. Constant CR, Murley AH. A clinical method of functional assessment of the shoulder. Clin Orthop Relat Res. 1987;214:160-4.

13. Menendez ME, Baker DK, Fryberger CT, Ponce BA. Predictors of extended length of stay after elective shoulder arthroplasty. J Shoulder Elbow Surg. 2015;24:1527-33.

14. Bachman D, Nyland J, Krupp R. Reverse-total shoulder arthroplasty cost-effectiveness: a quality-adjusted life years comparison with total hip arthroplasty. World J Orthop. 2016;7:123-7.

15. Garcia GH, Fu MC, Dines DM, Craig EV, Gulotta LV. Malnutrition: a marker for increased complications, mortality, and length of stay after total shoulder arthroplasty. J Shoulder Elbow Surg. 2016;25:193-200.

16. Sivasundaram L, Heckmann N, Pannell WC, Alluri RK, Omid R, Hatch 3rd GF. Preoperative risk factors for discharge to a postacute care facility after shoulder arthroplasty. J Shoulder Elbow Surg. 2016;25:201-6.

17. Hammond JW, Queale WS, Kim TK, McFarland EG. Surgeon experience and clinical and economic outcomes for shoulder arthroplasty. J Bone Joint Surg Am. 2003;85-A:2318-24.

18. Hassan M, Tuckman HP, Patrick RH, Kountz DS, Kohn JL. Cost of hospital-acquired infection. Hosp Top. 2010;88:82-9.

19. Xu S, Baker DK, Woods JC, Brabston 3rd EW, Ponce BA. Risk factors for early readmission after anatomical or reverse total shoulder arthroplasty. Am J Orthop (Belle Mead NJ). 2016;45:E386-92.

20. Husted H, Holm G, Jacobsen S. Predictors of length of stay and patient satisfaction after hip and knee replacement surgery: fast-track experience in 712 patients. Acta Orthop. 2008;79:168-73.

21. Collin P, Matsumura N, Lädermann A, Denard PJ, Walch G. Relationship between massive chronic rotator cuff tear pattern and loss of active shoulder range of motion. J Shoulder Elbow Surg. 2014;23:1195-202.

22. Collin P, Lädermann A, Le Bourg M, Walch G. Subscapularis minor—an analogue of the Teres minor? Orthop Traumatol Surg Res. 2013;99:S255-8.

23. Gulotta LV, Choi D, Marinello P, Wright T, Cordasco FA, Craig EV, Warren RF. Anterior deltoid deficiency in reverse total shoulder replacement: a biomechanical study with cadavers. J Bone Joint Surg (Br). 2012;94:1666-9.

24. Edwards TB, Williams MD, Labriola JE, Elkousy HA, Gartsman GM, O'Connor DP. Subscapularis insufficiency and the risk of shoulder dislocation after reverse shoulder arthroplasty. J Shoulder Elbow Surg. 2009;18:892-6.

25. Sarver JJ, Peltz CD, Dourte L, Reddy S, Williams GR, Soslowsky LJ. After rotator cuff repair, stiffness—but not the loss in range of motion—increased transiently for immobilized shoulders in a rat model. J Shoulder Elbow Surg. 2008;17:108S-13.

26. Millett PJ, Wilcox 3rd RB, O'Holleran JD, Warner JJ. Rehabilitation of the rotator cuff: an evaluation-based approach. J Am Acad Orthop Surg. 2006; 14:599-609.

27. Denard PJ, Lädermann A. Immediate versus delayed passive range of motion following total shoulder arthroplasty. J Shoulder Elbow Surg. 2016; 25:1918-24.

28. Wall B, Nove-Josserand L, O'Connor DP, Edwards TB, Walch G. Reverse total shoulder arthroplasty: a review of results according to etiology. J Bone Joint Surg Am. 2007;89:1476-85.

29. Farshad M, Gerber C. Reverse total shoulder arthroplasty—from the most to the least common complication. Int Orthop. 2010;34:1075-82.

30. Lädermann A, Edwards TB, Walch G. Arm lengthening after reverse shoulder arthroplasty: a review. Int Orthop. 2014;38:991-1000.

31. Lädermann A, Lubbeke A, Melis B, Stern R, Christofilopoulos P, Bacle G, Walch G. Prevalence of neurologic lesions after total shoulder arthroplasty. J Bone Joint Surg Am. 2011;93:1288-93.

32. Walch G, Bacle G, Lädermann A, Nove-Josserand L, Smithers CJ. Do the indications, results, and complications of reverse shoulder arthroplasty change with surgeon's experience? J Shoulder Elbow Surg. 2012;21:1470-7.

33. Clark JC, Ritchie J, Song FS, Kissenberth MJ, Tolan SJ, Hart ND, Hawkins RJ. Complication rates, dislocation, pain, and postoperative range of motion after reverse shoulder arthroplasty in patients with and without repair of the subscapularis. J Shoulder Elbow Surg. 2012;21:36-41.

34. Mulieri P, Dunning P, Klein S, Pupello D, Frankle M. Reverse shoulder arthroplasty for the treatment of irreparable rotator cuff tear without glenohumeral arthritis. J Bone Joint Surg Am. 2010;92:2544-56.

35. Busse R, Geissler A, Aaviksoo A, Cots F, Hakkinen U, Kobel C, Mateus C, Or Z, O'Reilly J, Serden L, et al. Diagnosis related groups in Europe: moving towards transparency, efficiency, and quality in hospitals? BMJ. 2013;346: f3197.

36. Marshall M, Ovretveit J. Can we save money by improving quality? BMJ Qual Saf. 2011;20:293-6.

37. Mole D, Wein F, Dezaly C, Valenti P, Sirveaux F. Surgical technique: the anterosuperior approach for reverse shoulder arthroplasty. Clin Orthop Relat Res. 2011;469:2461-8.

38. Lädermann A, Lubbeke A, Collin P, Edwards TB, Sirveaux F, Walch G. Influence of surgical approach on functional outcome in reverse shoulder arthroplasty. Orthop Traumatol Surg Res. 2011;97:579-82.

39. Padegimas EM, Zmistowski BM, Clyde CT, Restrepo C, Abboud JA, Lazarus MD, Ramsey ML, Williams GR, Namdari S. Length of stay after shoulder arthroplasty-the effect of an orthopedic specialty hospital. J Shoulder Elbow Surg. 2016;25:1404-11.

13

Intrathecal morphine versus femoral nerve block for pain control after total knee arthroplasty

Yi Tang, Xu Tang, Qinghua Wei and Hui Zhang[*]

Abstract

Background: This meta-analysis aims to illustrate the efficacy and safety of intrathecal morphine (ITM) versus femoral nerve block (FNB) for pain control after total knee arthroplasty (TKA).

Methods: In April 2017, a systematic computer-based search was conducted in PubMed, EMBASE, Web of Science, Cochrane Database of Systematic Reviews, Cami Info. Inc., Casalini databases, EBSCO databases, Verlag database and Google database. Data on patients prepared for TKA surgery in studies that compared ITM versus FNB for pain control after TKA were collected. The main outcomes were the visual analogue scale (VAS) at 6, 12, 24, 48 and 72 and total morphine consumption at 12, 24 and 48 h. The secondary outcomes were complications that included postoperative nausea and vomiting (PONV) and itching. Stata 12.0 was used for pooling the data.

Results: Five clinical studies with a total of 225 patients (ITM group = 114, FNB group = 111) were ultimately included in the meta-analysis. The results revealed that the ITM group was associated with a reduction of VAS at 6, 12, 24, 48 and 72 h and total morphine consumption at 12, 24 and 48 h. There was no significant difference between the occurrences of PONV. However, the ITM group was associated with an increased occurrence of itching after TKA.

Conclusions: Some immediate analgesic efficacy and opioid-sparing effects were obtained with the administration of ITM when compared with FNB. The complications of itching in the ITM group were greater than in the FNB group. The sample size and the quality of the included studies were limited. A multi-centre RCT is needed to identify the optimal method for reaching maximum pain control after TKA.

Keywords: Intrathecal morphine, Total knee arthroplasty, Femoral nerve block, Meta-analysis

Background

Total knee arthroplasty (TKA) leads to considerable post-operative pain [1, 2]. Ineffective pain control after TKA can cause many side effects [3]. Optimal pain control can not only decrease complications but also facilitate fast recovery during the immediate postoperative period [4]. Currently, a multimodal technique, a new concept, is accepted by most surgeons. Multimodal analgesia includes regional techniques, systemic opioids and preoperative administration gabapentin. Thus, femoral nerve block (FNB) and intrathecal morphine (ITM) are seldom used alone for the management of postoperative pain, though they are known to provide excellent analgesia [5]. Since the

recommendation by the PROSPECT working group [6], FNB and ITM have become two common methods for postoperative analgesia management following TKA.

Regarding the efficacy and safety of ITM and FNB for pain control after TKA, there has yet to be a consensus. Recently, Li et al. [7] conducted a meta-analysis for this topic. However, several disadvantages existed in that meta-analysis. First it ignored important randomized controlled trials (RCTs), which may have had an important influence on the final results [8]. Furthermore, continuous FNB and single-shot FNB were not compared in a subgroup analysis. Thus, the purpose of this meta-analysis is to compare the efficacy and safety of ITM and FNB for pain control after TKA (Table 1).

* Correspondence: zhanghui201707@qq.com
Department of Orthopedics, People's Hospital of JianYang, No. 180, Yiyuan Road, Jiancheng zhen, Jianyang, Sichuan Province, China

Table 1 The general characteristic of the included studies.

Study	Country	FNB Group			Surgery	ITM Group			Outcomes	Follow-up
		No. of patients	Method	Drug		No. of patients	Dose	Concomitant pain management		
Frassanito 2010	Italy	26	SFNB	Ropivacaine 0.75% 25 ml	TKA	26	Hyperbaric bupivacaine 15 mg plus 0.1 mg of morphine sulphate	Paracetamol 1 g i.v. four times daily and intravenous. Ketorolac 30 mg 2 times every 24 h	1, 2, 3, 4	48 h
Mohamed 2016	Egypt	20	SFNB	Hyperbaric bupivacaine 15 mg	TKA	20	0.2 mg morphine	PCA with morphine	1, 2, 3, 4	3 month
Olive 2015	Australia	27	CFNB	20 ml bottle of 0.5% bupivacaine	TKA	28	0.5% bupivacaine 3.5 ml plus 0.175 mg morphine	0.5% bupivacaine 3.5 mL	1, 2, 3, 4	1 year
Sites 2004	USA	20	SFNB	40 mL of 0.5% ropivacaine with 75 mg of clonidine and 5 mg/mL of epinephrine	TKA	20	0.25 mg morphine and 15 mg hyperbaric bupivacaine	30 mg ketorolac IV every 6 h	1, 2, 3, 4	48 h
Tarkkila 1998	India	18	CFNB	0.25% bupivacaine at a rate of 0.1 mL kg 1 h 1	TKA	20	0.3 mg morphine mixed with bupivacaine	Oxycodone 0.1–0.14 mg/kg	1, 2, 3, 4	48 h

FNB femoral nerve block, *ITM* intrathecal morphine, *TKA* total knee arthroplasty

Methods

This systematic review was reported according to the preferred reporting items for systematic reviews and meta-analyses (PRISMA) guidelines [9].

Search strategies

The following databases were searched in September 2016 without restrictions on location or publication types: PubMed (1950–April 2017), EMBASE (1974–April 2017), the Cochrane Library (April 2017, Issue 4), Cami info. Lnc (1950–April 2017), Casalini databases (1950–April 2017), EBSCO databases (1950–April 2017), Verlag database (1950–April 2017) and Google database (1950–April 2017). The Mesh terms and their combinations used in the search were as follows: "analgesia" OR "pain management" OR "anaesthetic agents" OR "total knee arthroplasty" OR "total knee replacement" OR "TKA" OR "TKR" OR ""Arthroplasty, Replacement, Knee"[Mesh]" AND "intrathecal morphine" OR "femoral nerve block". The reference lists of related reviews and original articles were searched for any relevant studies, including RCTs involving adult humans. There was no language restriction for this meta-analysis. When multiple reports describing the same sample were published, the most recent or complete report was used. This meta-analysis gathered data from published articles, and thus, no ethics approval was necessary for this article.

Inclusion criteria and study selection

Patients: patients prepared for primary unilateral TKA; Intervention: use ITM as an intervention group; Comparison: use FNB as a comparison group; Outcomes: VAS at 6, 12, 24, 48 and 72 h, total morphine consumption at 12, 24 and 48, and related complications (postoperative nausea and vomiting (PONV) and itching); Study design: RCTs (Fig. 1).

Two independent reviewers screened the title and abstracts of the identified studies after removing the duplicates from the search results. Any disagreements about the inclusion or exclusion of a study were solved through discussion or consultation with an expert (skilled in pain control and TKA). The reliability of the study selection was determined by Cohen's kappa test, and the acceptable threshold value was set at 0.61 [6, 7].

Data abstraction and quality assessment

A specific extraction was conducted to collect data in a pre-generated standard Microsoft® Excel (Microsoft Corporation, Redmond, Washington, USA) file. The items extracted from relevant studies were as follows: first author and publication year, country, sample size of the intervention and control groups, preoperative and postoperative doses, timing and frequency and the total dose of gabapentin per number of days and follow-ups. Abstracted and recorded in the spreadsheet were outcomes such as the

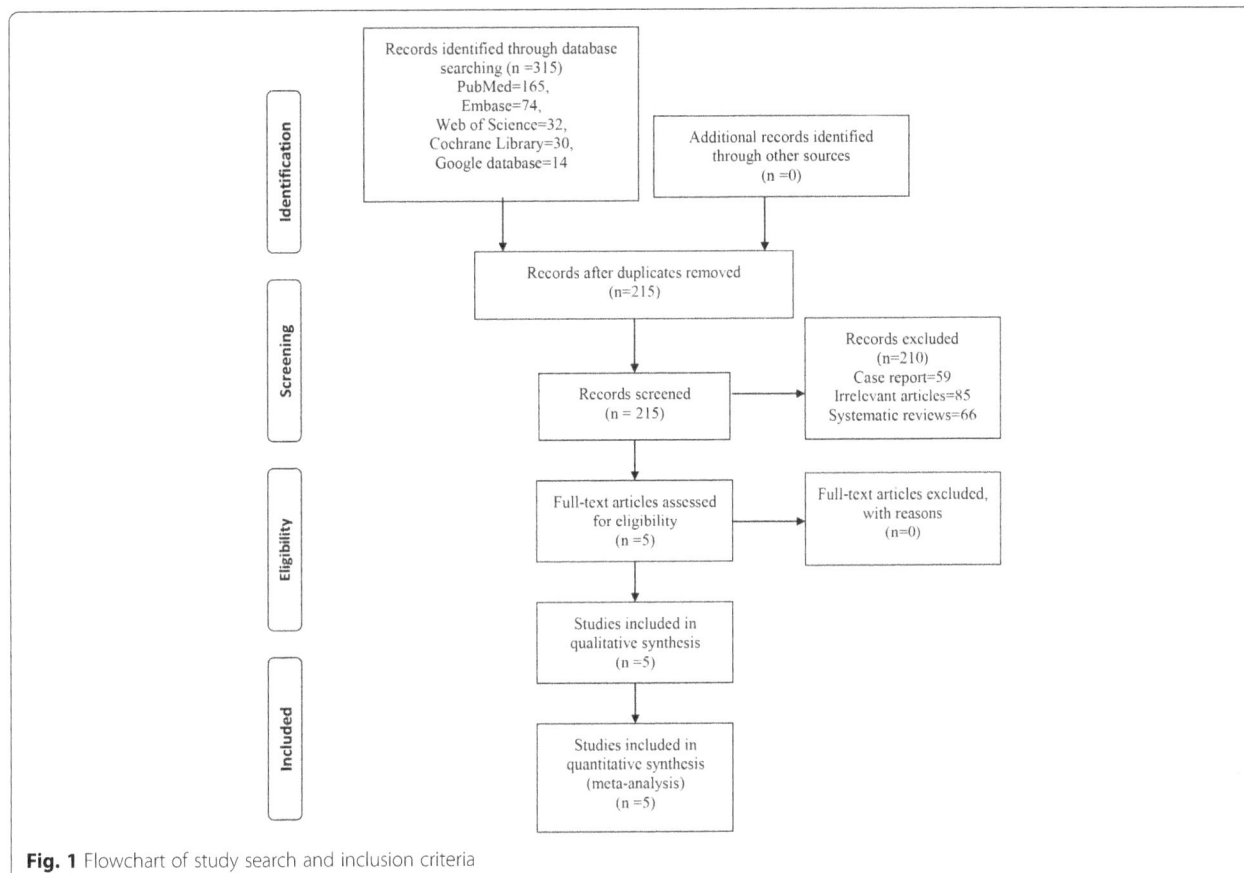

Fig. 1 Flowchart of study search and inclusion criteria

VAS at 6, 12, 24, 48 and 72 h; total morphine consumption at 12, 24 and 48 h; and related complications (PONV and itching). Postoperative pain intensity was measured using a 110-point VAS (0 = no pain and 100 = extreme pain). When the numerical rating scale (NRS) was reported, it was converted to a VAS. Additionally, a 10-point VAS was converted to a 100-point VAS [10]. Data in other forms (i.e. median, interquartile range, and mean ± 95% confidence interval (CI)) were converted to the mean ± standard deviation (SD) according to the Cochrane Handbook [11]. If the data were not reported numerically, we extracted these data using the "GetData Graph Digitizer" software from the published figures. All the data were extracted by two independent reviewers, and disagreements were resolved through discussion.

The quality of all included trials was independently assessed by two reviewers on the basis of the Cochrane Handbook for Systematic Reviews of Interventions, version 5.1.0 (http://training.cochrane.org/handbook/) [11]. A total of seven domains were used to assess the overall quality: random sequence generation, allocation concealment, blinding of participant and personnel, blinding of outcome assessment, incomplete outcome data, selective reporting and other bias. Each domain was measured as low bias, unclear bias or high bias.

Outcome measures and statistical analysis

Continuous outcomes (VAS at 6, 12, 24, 48 and 72 h and total morphine consumption at 12, 24 and 48 h) were expressed as weighted mean differences (WMD) with 95% CI. Dichotomous outcomes (the occurrence of PONV and itching) were expressed as a risk ratio (RR) with 95% CI. Statistical significance was set at $P < 0.05$ to summarize the findings across the trials. Variables in the meta-analysis were calculated using Stata software, version 12.0 (Stata Corp., College Station, TX). Statistical heterogeneity was evaluated using the chi-square test and the I^2 statistic. When there was no statistical evidence of heterogeneity ($I^2 < 50\%$, $P > 0.1$), a fixed-effects model was adopted; otherwise, a random-effects model was chosen. Publication bias was tested using funnel plots. Publication bias was visually assessed using funnel plots and was quantitatively assessed using Begg's test. Subgroup analysis was conducted according to the type of continuous FNB (CFNB) or single shot FNB (SFNB). We did not perform the publication bias since the numbers were less than ten.

Results

Search results and quality assessment

In the initial search, a total of 386 studies were identified from the electronic databases (PubMed = 165, EMBASE = 74,

Web of Science = 32, Cochrane Database of Systematic Reviews = 30, Google database = 14). Then, all papers were input into Endnote X7 (Thomson Reuters Corp., USA) software for the removal of duplicate papers. A total of 308 papers were reviewed, and 209 papers were removed according to the inclusion criteria at abstract and title levels. Ultimately, five clinical studies with 225 patients (ITM group = 114, FNB group = 111) were included in this meta-analysis [8, 12–15].

The quality assessment of the included studies is summarized in Figs. 2 and 3. All studies describe the random sequence generation procedure. Two studies did not describe allocation concealment and the blinding of participants and personnel and thus had an unclear risk of bias. The rest of the items all had a low risk of bias. The overall kappa value for the evaluation of the risk of bias of included RCTs was 0.763, indicating that the agreement between the two reviewers was acceptable.

VAS at 6, 12, 24, 48 and 72 h
Postoperative VAS scores at 6 h were reported in three studies, and the pooled results indicated that ITM can decrease VAS scores at 6 h (WMD = −3.04, 95% CI −5.19,

−0.89, P = 0.006, Fig. 4) when compared with the FNB group. Postoperative VAS scores at 6 h in the included studies had a large heterogeneity (I^2 = 88.8%, P = 0.000), which required a random-effects model that was performed to analyse the data.

The meta-analysis results indicated that ITM can decrease VAS scores at 12 h (WMD = −9.90, 95% CI −15.05, −4.74, P = 0.000, Fig. 4) when compared with the FNB group. Postoperative VAS scores at 12 h in the included studies had a large heterogeneity (I^2 = 74.9%, P = 0.003), which required a random-effects model that was performed to analyse the relevant data.

The results of the meta-analysis indicated that ITM can decrease VAS scores at 24 h (WMD = −10.27, 95% CI −12.16, −8.39, P = 0.001, Fig. 4) when compared with the FNB group. Postoperative VAS scores at 24 h in the included studies had a large heterogeneity (I^2 = 84.7%, P = 0.000), which required a random-effects model that was performed to analyse the relevant data.

The results of the meta-analysis indicated that ITM can decrease VAS scores at 48 h (WMD = −10.27, 95% CI −12.16, −8.39, P = 0.000, Fig. 4) compared with the FNB group. Postoperative VAS scores at 48 h in the included studies had little heterogeneity (I^2 = 24.7%, P = 0.249).

The results of the meta-analysis indicated that ITM can decrease VAS scores at 72 h (WMD = −9.00, 95% CI −10.39, −7.61, P = 0.000, Fig. 4) when compared with the FNB group.

Total morphine consumption at 12, 24 and 48 h
Total morphine consumption was presented in six studies. The pooled results indicated that ITM can reduce total morphine consumption at 12 h (WMD = −1.17, 95% CI −1.61, −0.73, P = 0.000, Fig. 5), 24 h (WMD = −3.96, 95% CI −4.43, −3.48, P = 0.000, Fig. 5) and 48 h (WMD = −2.76, 95% CI −3.72, −1.80, P = 0.000, Fig. 5).

The occurrence of PONV
There were no significant differences between the groups in the occurrence of PONV (RR = 1.10, 95% CI 0.57, 2.12, P = 0.769, Fig. 6). There was high heterogeneity between the included studies (I^2 = 76.5%, P = 0.005), and thus, a random-effect model was performed.

The occurrence of itching
The occurrence of itching was presented in three studies. Compared with the FNB group, ITM was associated with an increase of the occurrence of itching (RR = 2.50, 95% CI 1.05, 5.93, P = 0.038, Fig. 7). There was a high heterogeneity (I^2 = 61.8%, P = 0.073) among the included studies, and thus, a random-effects model was performed.

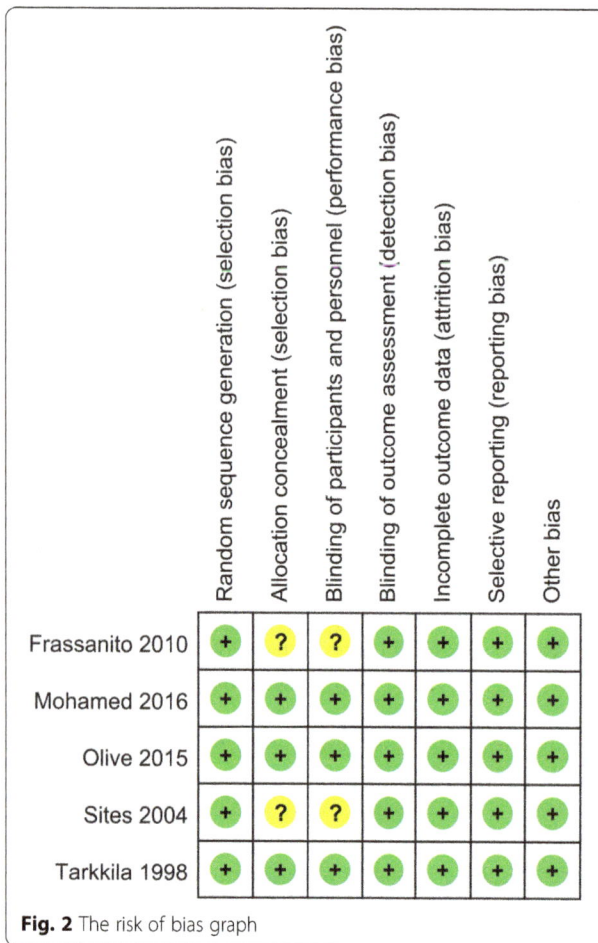

Fig. 2 The risk of bias graph

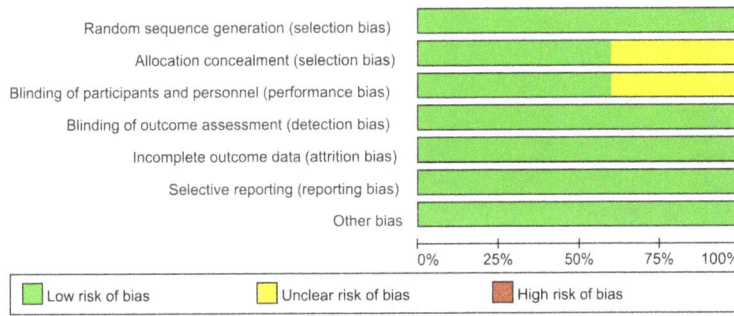

Fig. 3 Risk of bias summary of included randomized controlled trials. +, no bias; −, bias;?, bias unknown

Subgroup analysis and dose-response relationship

Subgroup analysis was conducted according to the type of FNB (CFNB or SFNB). The results are shown in Additional file 1 and indicate that there was no significant difference between the CFNB and SFNB in terms of VAS at 6, 12 and 24 h.

Discussion

This meta-analysis aimed to illustrate the optimal method of pain control in TKA patients using ITM and FNB. Pooled results indicated that the ITM group had lower pain scores at 6, 12, 24, 48 and 72 h after TKA.

Furthermore, ITM was associated with less total morphine consumption at 12, 24 and 48 h after TKA. However, ITM was associated with an increase of the occurrence of itching. There was no significant difference in the occurrence of PONV after TKA. A major strength of this meta-analysis was that we comprehensively searched the electronic databases and used a rigorous statistical calculation. A total of five relevant studies were included, and the risk of bias was relatively high.

TKA is characterized by severe postoperative pain and morphine-related complications. A meta-analysis has identified that the administration of FNB was associated

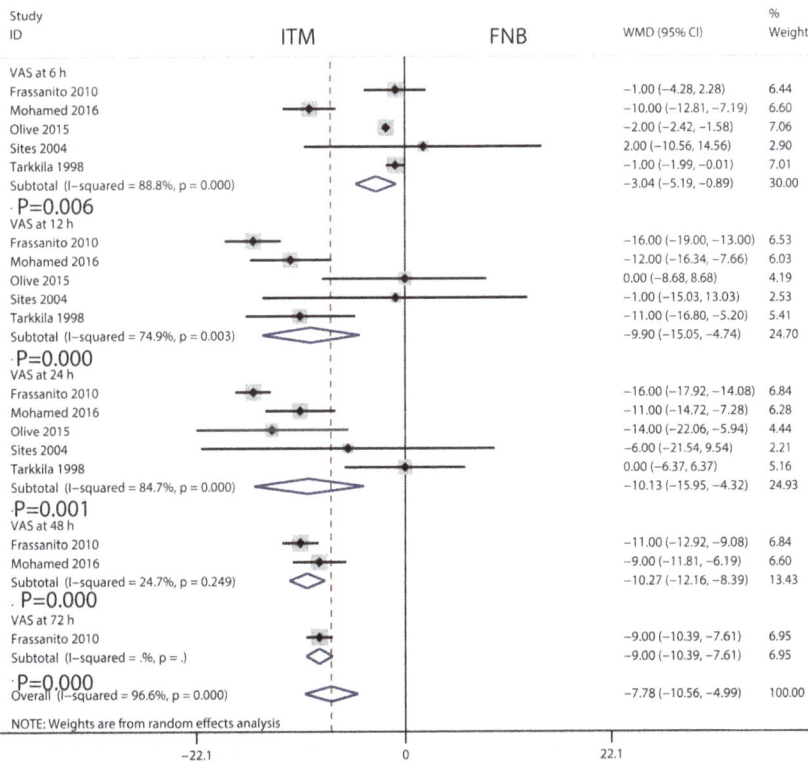

Fig. 4 Forest plots of the included studies comparing the VAS at 6, 12, 24, 48 and 72 h

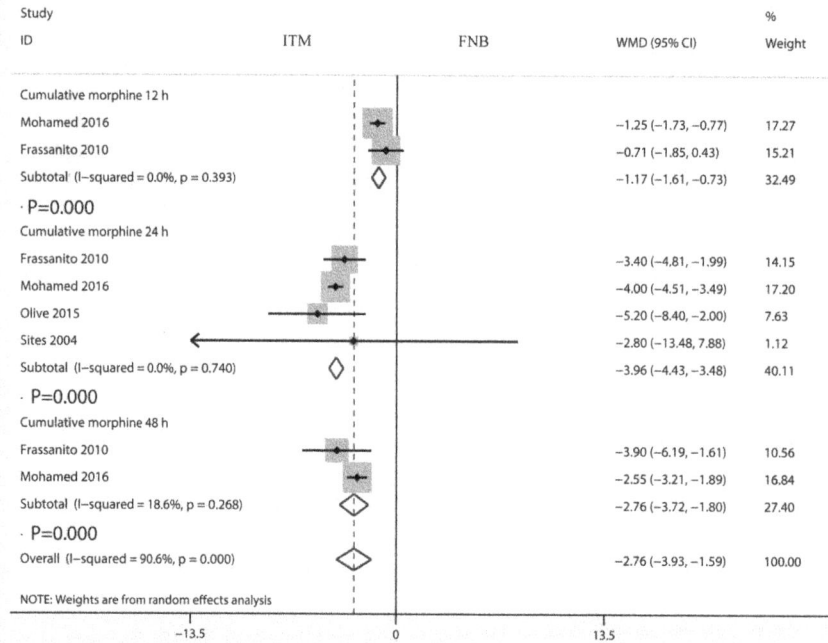

Fig. 5 Forest plots of the included studies comparing the total morphine consumption at 12, 24 and 48h

with a reduction in pain intensity after TKA [5]. FNB has been identified as an effective method for decreasing postoperative pain and morphine consumption after TKA. Alternatively, there is solid evidence supporting the use of ITM [16, 17]. Currently, there is no consensus regarding which methods are more effective after TKA surgery. Thus, we performed this meta-analysis to provide summary evidence for surgeons for a better choice of pain control following TKA. The current meta-analysis indicated that ITM was more effective than FNB at 6, 12, 24, 48 and 72 h after TKA. The doses of ITM ranged from 0.1 to 0.5 mg [18]. A meta-analysis showed that the rate of episodes of respiratory depression (doses <0.3 mg) was equal to that of the systemic opioids group [19]. The dose of morphine in the ITM group in the meta-analysis ranged from 0.1 to 0.3 mg, and this may be due to heterogeneity

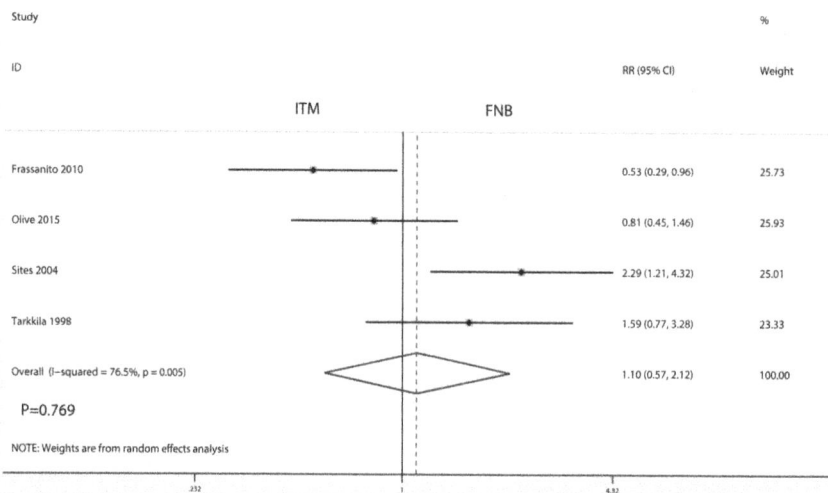

Fig. 6 Forest plots of the included studies comparing the occurrence of PONV

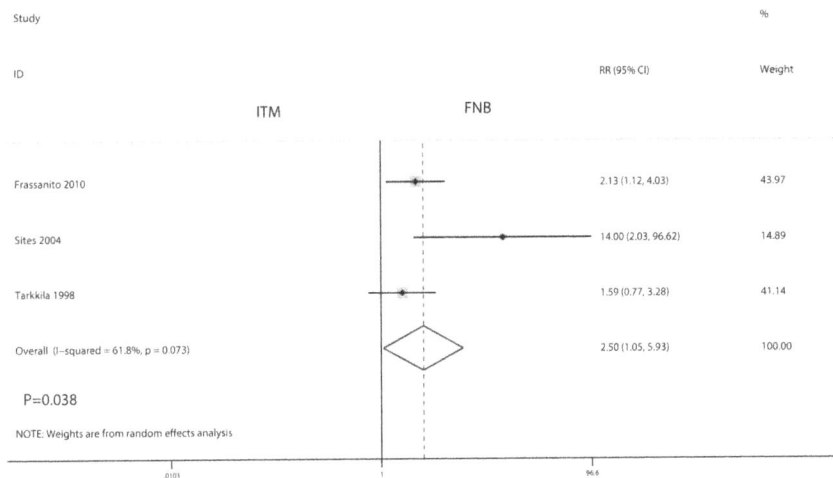

Fig. 7 Forest plots of the included studies comparing the occurrence of itching

in the sources of different studies. Meanwhile, two studies performed the CFNB, and the remaining three studies performed the SFNB.

Since pain intensity was decreased in the ITM group, morphine consumption as a supplement for pain control was decreased correspondingly. Pooled results indicated that the ITM group was associated with a reduction of total morphine consumption at 12 h by 1.17 mg (WMD = −1.17, 95% CI −1.61, −0.73, P = 0.000) and 3.96 mg at 24 h (WMD = −3.96, 95% CI −4.43, −3.48, P = 0.000) and 48 h (WMD = −2.76, 95% CI −3.72, −1.80, P = 0.000). Li et al. [7] found that total morphine consumption in the ITM group was less than in the FNB group, at appropriately 0.84 mg. Chang et al. [20] reported that the addition of IT morphine 0.1 mg to continuous femoral 3-in-1 nerve block improves postoperative analgesia and morphine consumption after TKA.

Another issue that must be addressed is that FNB requires the use of an ultrasound machine and a special needle, which add to the cost. Additionally, another anaesthetist is needed to perform FNB, and thus, it may add to the total operation time. In this regard, ITM is very cost effective, time-saving and a relatively simple technique.

There were a total of six limitations in this meta-analysis: (1) only five RCTs were included, which may have affected the precision of the effect size estimations; (2) follow-up in the included studies ranged from 24 h to 6 months, and the relatively short-term follow-up may underestimate the complication rate; (3) the dosage of ITM differed between the studies, and although a subgroup analysis was conducted to decrease heterogeneity, that could affect the precision of the results; (4) the

dosage, drugs and type of FNB differed between the studies, which could affect the precision of the results; (5) multiple analgesic approaches differed from one another, and consistent multiple analgesic approaches are needed to identify the most effective pain control method; and (6) publication bias was not performed due to the limited number of included studies, and there was potential publication bias.

Conclusion

In conclusion, some immediate analgesic efficacy and opioid-sparing effects were obtained with the administration of ITM when compared with FNB. Complications of itching in the ITM group were greater than in the FNB group. Because the sample size and the number of included studies were limited, a multi-centre RCT is needed to identify the effects of ITM in reducing acute pain following TKA surgery.

Abbreviations
CFNB: Continuous femoral nerve block; CI: Confidence interval; DVT: Deep venous thrombosis; FNB: Femoral nerve block; ITM: Intrathecal morphine; NRS: Numerical rating scale; PONV: Postoperative nausea and vomiting; PRISMA: Preferred Reporting Items for Systematic Reviews and Meta-analyses; RCTs: Randomized controlled trials; RR: Relative risk; SD: Standard deviation; SFNB: Single shot femoral nerve block; TKA: Total knee arthroplasty; VAS: Visual analogue scale; WMD: Weight mean difference

Acknowledgements
We thank Aaberish, Dong Lin and Yong-long Liu for searching the French, German, Spanish and Italian literatures.

Funding
There is no funding for this article.

Authors' contributions

TY and XT conceived the study design. QHW and HZ performed the study, collected the data and contributed to the study design. TY and QHW prepared the manuscript. HZ and TY edited the manuscript. All authors read and approved the final manuscript.

Competing interests

The authors declare that they have no competing interests.

References

1. Keijsers R, van den Bekerom M, van Delft R, van Lotten M, Rademakers M, Nolte PA. Continuous local infiltration analgesia after TKA: a meta-analysis. J Knee Surg. 2016;29(4):310–21.
2. Sun XL, Zhao ZH, Ma JX, et al. Continuous local infiltration analgesia for pain control after total knee arthroplasty: a meta-analysis of randomized controlled trials. Medicine (Baltimore). 2015;94(45):e2005.
3. Dong J, Li W, Wang Y. The effect of pregabalin on acute postoperative pain in patients undergoing total knee arthroplasty: a meta-analysis. Int J Surg. 2016;34:148–60.
4. Kehlet H, Holte K. Effect of postoperative analgesia on surgical outcome. Br J Anaesth. 2001;87(1):62–72.
5. Chan EY, Fransen M, Parker DA, Assam PN, Chua N. Femoral nerve blocks for acute postoperative pain after knee replacement surgery. Cochrane Database Syst Rev. 2014;13(5):Cd009941.
6. Fischer HB, Simanski CJ, Sharp C, et al. A procedure-specific systematic review and consensus recommendations for postoperative analgesia following total knee arthroplasty. Anaesthesia. 2008;63(10):1105–23.
7. Li XM, Huang CM, Zhong CF. Intrathecal morphine verse femoral nerve block for pain control in total knee arthroplasty: a meta-analysis from randomized control trials. Int J Surg. 2016;32:89–98.
8. Mohamed, A. A., Maghraby, H. H., Abdelghaffar, H. S. Comparison of combined intrathecal morphine and sonar-guided single shot femoral nerve block vs. either technique alone for postoperative analgesia in patients undergoing total knee replacement surgery. (2016).
9. Liberati A, Altman DG, Tetzlaff J, et al. The PRISMA statement for reporting systematic reviews and meta-analyses of studies that evaluate healthcare interventions: explanation and elaboration. BMJ. 2009;339:b2700.
10. Wang C, Cai X-Z, Yan S-G. Comparison of periarticular multimodal drug injection and femoral nerve block for postoperative pain management in total knee arthroplasty: a systematic review and meta-analysis. The Journal of arthroplasty. 2015;30(7):1281–6.
11. GS, H. J. Cochrane handbook for systematic reviews of interventions version 5.1.0. [http://handbook.cochrane.org/]. Accessed 2011.
12. Frassanito L, Vergari A, Zanghi F, Messina A, Bitondo M, Antonelli M. Post-operative analgesia following total knee arthroplasty: comparison of low-dose intrathecal morphine and single-shot ultrasound-guided femoral nerve block: a randomized, single blinded, controlled study. Eur Rev Med Pharmacol Sci. 2010;14(7):589–96.
13. Olive DJ, Barrington MJ, Simone SA, Kluger R. A randomised controlled trial comparing three analgesia regimens following total knee joint replacement: continuous femoral nerve block, intrathecal morphine or both. Anaesth Intensive Care. 2015;43(4):454–60.
14. Sites BD, Beach M, Gallagher JD, Jarrett RA, Sparks MB, Lundberg CJ. A single injection ultrasound-assisted femoral nerve block provides side effect-sparing analgesia when compared with intrathecal morphine in patients undergoing total knee arthroplasty. Anesth Analg. 2004;99(5):1539–43. table of contents
15. Tarkkila P, Tuominen M, Huhtala J, Lindgren L. Comparison of intrathecal morphine and continuous femoral 3-in-1 block for pain after major knee surgery under spinal anaesthesia. Eur J Anaesthesiol. 1998;15(1):6–9.
16. Karlsen AP, Wetterslev M, Hansen SE, Hansen MS, Mathiesen O, Dahl JB. Postoperative pain treatment after total knee arthroplasty: a systematic review. PLoS One. 2017;12(3):e0173107.
17. Kilickaya R, Orak Y, Balci MA, Balci F, Unal I. Comparison of the effects of intrathecal fentanyl and intrathecal morphine on pain in elective total knee replacement surgery. Pain Res Manag. 2016;2016:3256583.
18. Mugabure Bujedo B. A clinical approach to neuraxial morphine for the treatment of postoperative pain. Pain Res Treat. 2012;2012:612145.
19. Gehling M, Tryba M. Risks and side-effects of intrathecal morphine combined with spinal anaesthesia: a meta-analysis. Anaesthesia. 2009;64(6):643–51.
20. Chang KP, Cho CK, Shin HH, Cho JH. The effect of intrathecal morphine added to continuous femoral 3-in-1 nerve block for analgesia after total knee replacement. Korean Journal of Anesthesiology. 2008;54(5):544–51.

14

Comparison of arthroplasty vs. osteosynthesis for displaced femoral neck fractures

Feng-Jen Tseng[1,2], Wei-Tso Chia[3], Ru-Yu Pan[4], Leou-Chyr Lin[4], Hsian-Chung Shen[4], Chih-Hung Wang[5], Jia-Fwu Shyu[6] and Ching-Feng Weng[1*]

Abstract

Background: This meta-analysis compared clinical outcomes of arthroplasty vs. osteosynthesis for displaced femoral neck fractures.

Methods: Meta-analysis was performed on the difference in revision rate and overall mortality between participants undergoing osteosynthesis vs. total hip arthroplasty (THA), osteosynthesis vs. hemiarthroplasty (HA), or THA vs. HA.

Results: Pooled direct and indirect results indicated no significant difference in mortality between THA and HA (pooled OR = 0.87, 95% CI 0.55 to 1.38; P = 0.556), between THA and osteosynthesis (pooled OR = 1.17, 95% CI 0.69 to 1.99; P = 0.553), and between HA and osteosynthesis (pooled OR = 1.21, 95% CI 0.84 to 1.74; P = 0.304). Pooled direct and indirect results indicated no significant difference in revision rates between THA and HA (pooled OR = 0.90, 95% CI 0.26 to 3.19; P = 0.874). But, fewer revisions (OR = 0.19, 95% CI 0.10 to 0.34; P = 0.000) were seen in patients treated with THA than osteosynthesis and also in those treated with HA than osteosynthesis (OR = 0.12, 95% CI 0.07 to 0.20; P = 0.000). After excluding studies without showing normal cognition in inclusion criteria, pooled direct and indirect results also indicated no significant difference in mortality between THA, HA, and osteosynthesis. Similarly, there was no significant difference in revision rates between THA and HA, but HA and THA had significantly lower revision rates compared with osteosynthesis.

Conclusions: There was no significant difference in overall mortality among osteosynthesis, HA, and THA. However, HA and THA had significantly lower revision rates compared with osteosynthesis. Results of the present study provide support for the use of hip arthroplasty to treat displaced fractures of the femoral neck.

Keywords: Meta-analysis, Displaced femoral neck fractures, Arthroplasty, Osteosynthesis, Elderly, Open reduction internal fixation

Background

Approximately 250,000 proximal femoral fractures occur in the USA each year, and 90% of these fractures occur in patients older than 50 years of age [1, 2]. Fractures of the femoral neck can be categorized into either non-displaced or displaced fractures in order to facilitate appropriate management, particularly in the elderly [3, 4]. Displaced femoral neck fractures are defined as unstable fractures that can impair blood supply to the femoral head, resulting in avascular necrosis [5, 6]. These fractures are associated with substantial fracture-related mortality and morbidity [6, 7]. An additional contributor to femoral head osteonecrosis involves the quality of the reduction or fracture fixation [8].

Osteosynthesis refers to the percutaneous placement of several parallel cannulated lag screws, and in the younger patient, such internal fixation is the standard treatment for displaced fractures [8]. Hip arthroplasty, on the other hand, refers to replacement of all or part of the hip joint with a prosthetic implant [6, 9] and can be divided into either total hip arthroplasty (THA) or

* Correspondence: cfweng@mail.ndhu.edu.tw
[1]Department of Life Science and the Institute of Biotechnology, National Dong Hwa University, Hualien 974, Taiwan, Republic of China
Full list of author information is available at the end of the article

hemiarthroplasty (HA). THA involves replacement of both the femoral head and the acetabular articular surface, whereas in HA, only the femoral head is replaced with an artificial implant, while the patient's own acetabulum is retained [5, 6, 9].

Although internal fixation is recommended for most non-displaced fractures of the femoral neck, the optimal treatment for displaced fractures of the femoral neck is still controversial [10–12]. HA was once considered the procedure of choice for elderly patients with displaced (Garden stage III or IV) femoral neck fractures [13], but a Swedish study concluded that THA should be performed for displaced femoral neck fractures in older patients with normal mental function and high function [14], a conclusion that has been echoed in several more recent publications [15, 16]. Davison et al., on the other hand, recommended either reduction with internal fixation or cemented HA as alternative treatments for a displaced intracapsular fracture in a mobile and mentally competent patient under 80 years of age [10].

The literature also contains conflicting evidence regarding rates of mortality, major postoperative complications, and function in elderly patients with displaced femoral neck fractures treated either by internal fixation or arthroplasty [17]. In fact, the choice of surgical treatment for a displaced intracapsular fracture of the proximal femur in the elderly remains as controversial now as it was over 50 years ago when it was designated as "the unsolved fracture" [10, 12, 18]. This meta-analysis was designed, therefore, to address this controversy by comparing outcomes after internal fixation, hemiarthroplasty, and THA, with particular reference to mortality and revision rates because until now, few studies have compared these three alternative treatments [10]. In addition, due to the limited number of studies with head-to-head comparison of HA and total hip replacement, a statistical analysis (comprised of both direct and indirect comparisons) was utilized to achieve this study's objective.

Methods

Selection criteria

Only English language publications of randomized controlled trials (RCTs) or prospective comparative studies of patients with displaced femoral neck fractures were included. Patient subjects had to be elderly (60 years of age or older) and capable of walking independently (without relying on another person), with or without aids prior to the injury. In addition, only studies that involved one or more comparisons of at least two types of intervention: (1) osteosynthesis vs. THA, (2) osteosynthesis vs. HA, or (3) THA vs. HA were included in the analysis.

Retrospective studies, letters, comments, editorials, case reports, technical reports, and non-English publications were excluded. In addition, any retrospective comparative

study or single-arm study was excluded. Any study design that contained no numerical information about the outcomes of interest was also excluded.

Search strategy

This meta-analysis was conducted in accordance with the PRISMA guidelines [19]. Medline, Cochrane, and Embase databases were searched until August 31, 2014. In addition, the reference lists of relevant studies were manually searched. Keywords used for the search included femoral neck, fracture, total hip replacement, internal fixation, open reduction internal fixation, ORIF, osteosynthesis, HA, and arthroplasty.

Study selection and data extraction

Studies were identified by two independent reviewers using the designated search strategy. Where there was uncertainty regarding eligibility, a third reviewer was consulted. Data extraction was also performed by two independent reviewers, and a third reviewer was consulted for any uncertainties. The following data were extracted from studies that met the inclusion criteria: the name of the first author; year of publication; study design; number of participants in each treatment group; demographic data of participants, such as age and gender; diagnostic criteria; treatment methods; and duration of follow-up.

Quality assessment

The Cochrane Risk of Bias Tool was utilized to assess the included studies [20]. The quality assessment was performed by the independent reviewers, and a third reviewer was consulted for any uncertainties.

Outcome measures

The primary endpoint in the meta-analysis was the overall mortality, and the secondary endpoint was the revision rate. Economic outcomes, quality of life (QoL), and functional outcomes were not assessed. However, additional analysis was performed on a subgroup of studies involving only elderly subjects with no significant or severe cognitive impairment. This approach was used to determine if any differences existed regarding mortality and revision rates within this subgroup, who underwent either HA, THA, or osteosynthesis.

Statistical analysis

The odds ratio (OR) and 95% confidence interval (CI) were calculated for binary outcomes and then compared between two different interventions. A chi-square-based test of homogeneity was performed, and the inconsistency index (I^2) statistic was determined. When heterogeneity existed between studies ($I^2 > 50\%$), a random-effects model was used. Otherwise, fixed-effects models were applied. Pooled summary statistics for ORs of the individual studies were reported. Sensitivity analysis was performed by using the leave-one-out cross-validation approach [21]. In addition, publication bias was not assessed in groups of fewer than five studies because more than ten studies are required to detect funnel plot asymmetry [22]. Direct pairwise meta-analyses were performed using Comprehensive Meta-Analysis, version 2 (Biostat, Englewood, NJ). Adjusted indirect comparisons of pooled estimates using inverse variance weighting were then performed according to the methods of Bucher and colleagues using the indirect treatment comparison computer program, version 1.0 [23]. We calculated an indirect result between THA and HA groups.

Results

Literature search
After initially identifying 274 articles, 223 articles were excluded and 51 studies were assessed for eligibility. After full-text review, 17 additional articles were excluded, as shown in Fig. 1. The remaining 34 articles [10, 15, 24–55] were included in the qualitative and quantitative analyses.

Study characteristics
Twenty-six studies (reported in the 34 articles) were included in the systematic review. All studies compared arthroplasty with osteosynthesis (Table 1); five studies (encompassing references [15, 24–29]) compared THA ($n = 218$) with osteosynthesis ($n = 235$), 14 studies (encompassing references [10, 30–44]) compared HA ($n = 1518$) with osteosynthesis ($n = 1178$), and only seven studies (encompassing references [45–55]) compared THA ($n = 432$) and HA ($n = 462$). Postoperative follow-up ranged from 14.5 months [26] to 17 years [15].

As shown in Table 1, ages of participants were similar among studies and between groups of different interventions, and the majority of participants were female.

Primary outcome measure: overall mortality
Total hip arthroplasty vs. hemiarthroplasty
Direct pairwise comparison All seven studies reported mortality [45, 48, 49, 51–53, 55]. A random-effects model of analysis was used due to heterogeneity among the studies ($Q = 14.044$, $P = 0.029$; $I^2 = 57.28\%$). Meta-analysis revealed no significant difference in mortality between THA and HA (pooled OR = 0.85, 95% CI 0.52 to 1.41; $P = 0.537$) (Fig. 2a).

Indirect comparison Results of the adjusted indirect comparison for mortality between THA and HA are shown in Fig. 2a (OR = 0.97, 95% CI 0.51 to 1.83; $P = 0.918$). The pooled results from direct and indirect

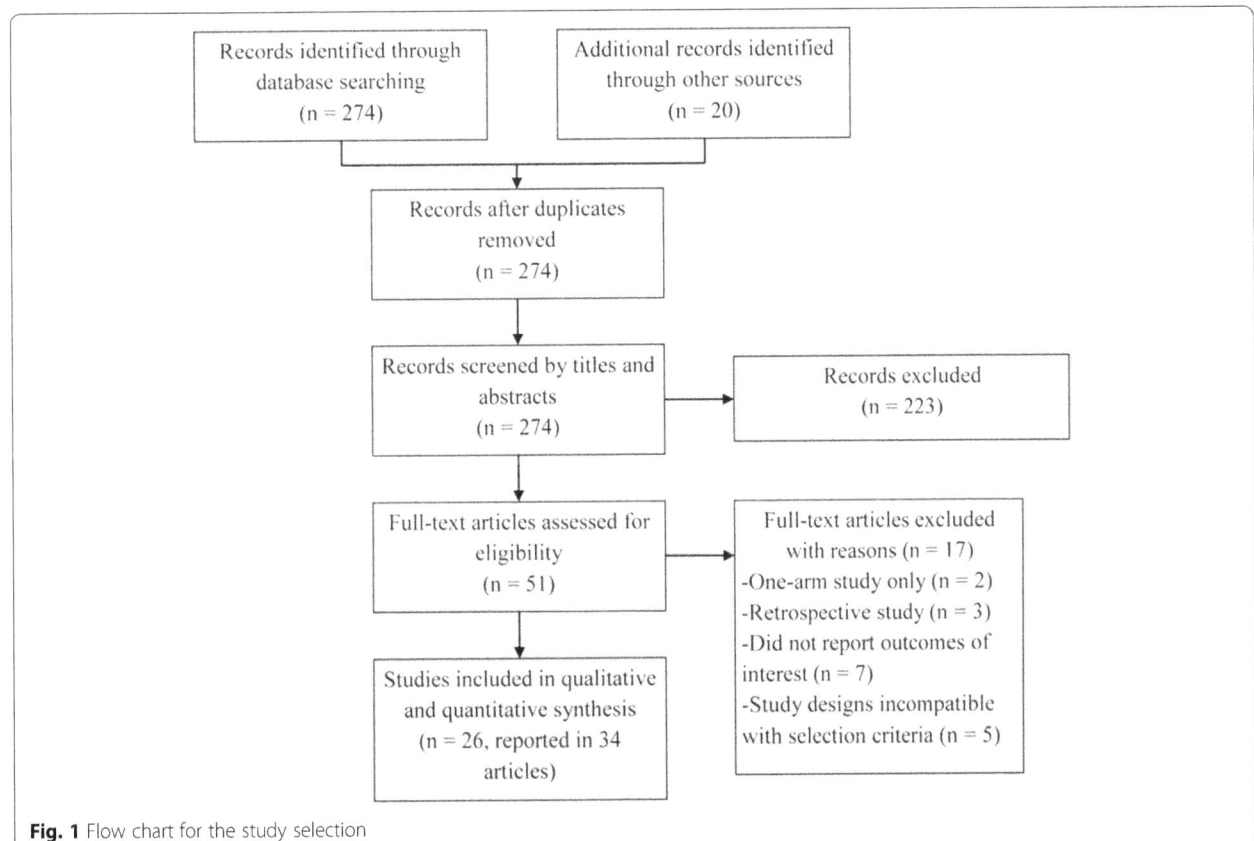

Fig. 1 Flow chart for the study selection

Table 1 A list of included studies and demography of the study subjects

First author	Normal cognition	Interventions	No. of patients	Age (years)	Male (%)	Duration of follow-up	Tools for functional measurement
Total hip arthroplasty vs. hemiarthroplasty							
Avery (2011) [45] and Baker (2006) [46]	Yes	Total hip arthroplasty	40	74	20	8.83 (7.2 to 10.3) years	Oxford Hip Score
		Hemiarthroplasty	41	76	22	8.6 (7.2 to 10) years	
Cadossi (2013) [49]	Yes	Total hip arthroplasty	42	82	19	28.6 (22 to 52) months	Harris Hip Score
		Hemiarthroplasty	41	84	32	30.1 (23 to 50) months	
Hedbeck (2011) [48] and Blomfeldt (2007) [47]	Yes	Total hip arthroplasty	60	81	22	4 years	Harris Hip Score
		Hemiarthroplasty	60	81	10		
Keating (2006) [51] and Keating (2005) [50]	Yes	Total hip arthroplasty	69	75	25	2 years	Hip rating questionnaire
		Hemiarthroplasty	69	75	22		
Macaulay (2008) [52]	Yes	Total hip arthroplasty	17	82	59	34 (29 to 42) months	Harris Hip Score
		Hemiarthroplasty	23	77	39		
Ravikumar (2000) [53] and Skinner (1989) [54]	No	Total hip arthroplasty	89	81	10	13 years	Harris Hip Score
		Hemiarthroplasty	91	82			
van den Bekerom (2010) [55]	Yes	Total hip arthroplasty	115	82	22	5 years	Harris Hip Score
		Hemiarthroplasty	137	80	16		
Total hip arthroplasty vs. osteosynthesis							
Bachrach-Lindström (2000) [24]	No	Total hip arthroplasty	50	84	20	1 year	NA
		Closed reduction and internal fixation	50	84	24		
Blomfeldt (2005a) [27], Tidermark (2003) [28], and Tidermark (2003) [29]	Yes	Total hip replacement	49	79	18	4 years	Charnley's numerical classification
		Closed reduction and internal fixation	53	81	21		
Chammout (2012) [15]	Yes	Total hip replacement	43	78	12	17 years	Harris Hip Score
		Open reduction and internal fixation	57	79	28		
Jónsson (1996) [25]	NA	Total hip replacement	23	80[a]	22	2 years	Walking ability, pain or social function
		Closed reduction and internal fixation	24	79[a]	25		
Söreide (1979) [26]	NA	Total hip replacement	53	78	13	14.5 (12–23) months	Stinchfield's classification system
		Reduction and internal fixation	51	78	26	14.7 (12–24) months	
Hemiarthroplasty vs. osteosynthesis							
Bjorgul (2006) [30]	NA	Hemiarthroplasty	455	82	20	6 years	NA
		Internal fixation	228	82	31		
Blomfeldt (2005b) [31]	No	Hemiarthroplasty	30	84	7	2 years	Charnley's numerical classification
		Internal fixation	30	84	13		
Davison (2001) [10]	Yes	Thompson unipolar hemiarthroplasty	90	76[a]	21	5 years	Harris Hip Score
		Monk bipolar hemiarthroplasty	97	75[a]	26		
			93	73[a]	25		

Table 1 A list of included studies and demography of the study subjects *(Continued)*

		Reduction and internal fixation					
El-Abed (2005) [32]	Yes	Hemiarthroplasty	62	74	35	3 (3 to 4.5) years	Matta Scoring System
		Dynamic screw fixation	60	72	30		
Frihagen (2007) [41] and Støen (2014) [42]	No	Hemiarthroplasty	110	83	29	6 (5 to 7) years	Harris Hip Score
		Internal fixation	112	83	22		
Hedbeck (2013) [33]	No	Hemiarthroplasty	29	85	17	2 years	Charnley's numerical classification
		Internal fixation	30	84	17		
Heetveld (2007) [34]	No	Hemiarthroplasty	109	83	17	2 years	Harris Hip Score
		Internal fixation	115	77	34		
Parker (2002) [44] and Parker (2010) [43]	No	Hemiarthroplasty	229	82	20	11 years	Charnley's numerical classification
		Internal fixation	226	82	20		
Puolakka (2001) [35]	NA	Hemiarthroplasty	15	82	7	2 years	NA
		Internal fixation	17	81	24		
Rödén (2003) [36]	Yes	Prosthesis	47	81	28	5 years	NA
		Internal fixation	53	81	30		
Sikorski (1981) [37]	NA	Posterior Thompson	57	80	16	2 years	Pain and mobility
		Anterior Thompson	57		9		
		Internal fixation	76		21		
van Dortmont (2000) [38]	No	Hemiarthroplasty	29	84	24	16.5 (0.167 to 69.5) months	NA
		Internal fixation	31	84	3		
van Vugt (1993) [39]	Yes	Hemiarthroplasty	22	76	36	3 years	Sheperd's pain and the hip mobility score
		Osteosynthesis	21	75	48		
Waaler Bjornelv (2012) [40]	No	Hemiarthroplasty	80	82	29	2 years	Harris Hip Score
		Internal fixation	86		22		

NA not available
[a]Data are shown as median numbers

results showed no significant difference in mortality between THA and HA (pooled OR = 0.87, 95% CI 0.55 to 1.38; P = 0.556) (Fig. 2a). A random-effects model was used because of heterogeneity existed (Q = 14.074, P = 0.05; I^2 = 50.26%).

Total hip arthroplasty vs. osteosynthesis
Of the five studies, four reported patient mortality [24–27]. A fixed-effect model of analysis was used because no heterogeneity existed among the studies (Q = 0.333, P = 0.954; I^2 = 0%). The results indicated no significant difference in mortality between THA and osteosynthesis (pooled OR = 1.17, 95% CI 0.69 to 1.99; P = 0.553) (Fig. 2b).

Hemiarthroplasty vs. osteosynthesis
Of the 14 studies, 12 studies reported mortality [10, 30–32, 34–39, 41–44]. A random-effects model was used due to heterogeneity among the studies (Q = 34.206, P < 0.001; I^2 = 67.84%). There was no significant difference in

mortality between HA and osteosynthesis (pooled OR = 1.21, 95% CI 0.84 to 1.74; P = 0.304) (Fig. 2c).

Secondary outcome measure: revision rate
Total hip arthroplasty vs. hemiarthroplasty
Direct pairwise comparison Of the seven studies evaluated, five reported revision rates [45, 48, 49, 53, 55]. A random-effects model of analysis was used to evaluate heterogeneity among the studies (Q = 11.128, P = 0.025; I^2 = 64.05%). The meta-analysis showed no significant difference in revision rates between THA and HA (pooled OR = 0.76, 95% CI 0.18 to 3.21; P = 0.710) (Fig. 3a).

Indirect comparison Results of the adjusted indirect comparison of revision rates between THA and HA are shown in Fig. 3a (OR = 1.58, 95% CI 0.70 to 3.58; P = 0.271). The pool of the direct and indirect results showed no significant difference in revision rates between THA and HA (pooled OR = 0.90, 95% CI 0.26 to 3.19; P = 0.874) (Fig. 3a). A random-effects model was used due

Fig. 2 Meta-analysis forest plot for odds ratio of mortality for **a** total hip arthroplasty vs. hemiarthroplasty, **b** total hip arthroplasty vs. osteosynthesis, and **c** hemiarthroplasty vs. osteosynthesis

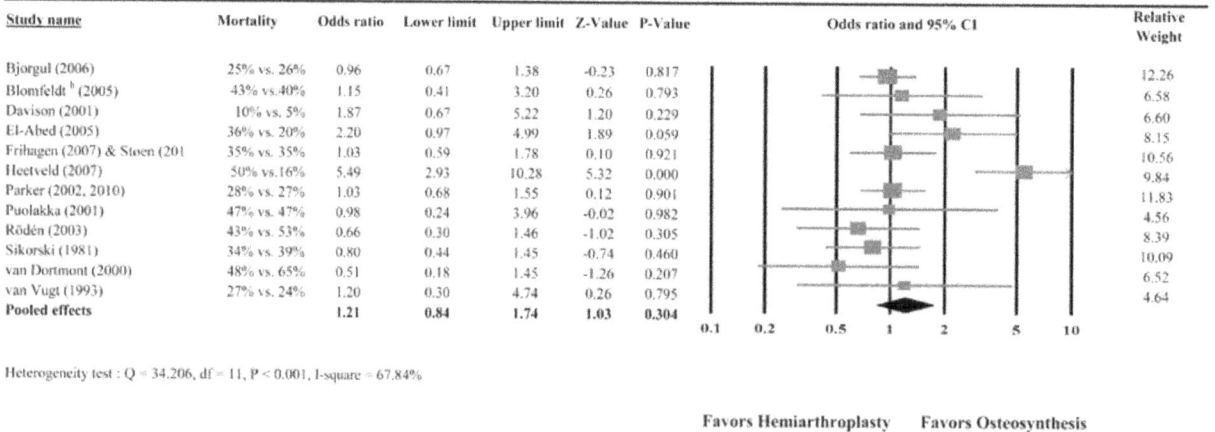

to heterogeneity among the studies (Q = 17.141, P = 0.004; I^2 = 70.83%).

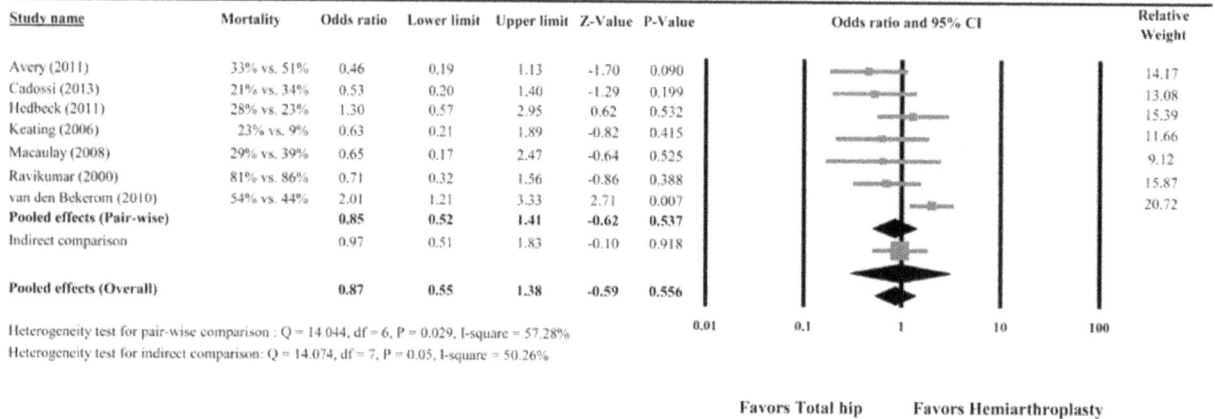

Total hip arthroplasty vs. osteosynthesis

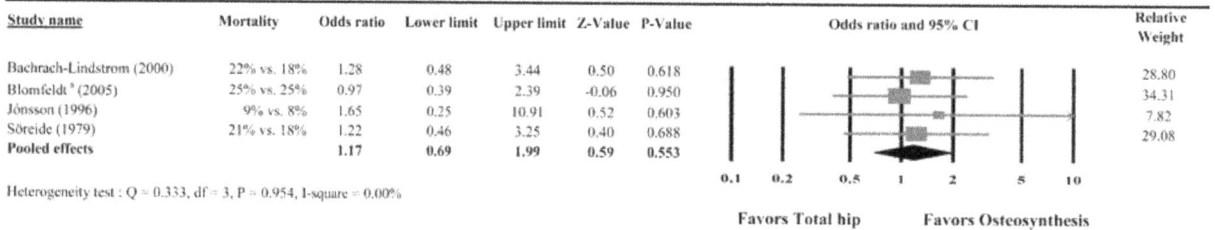

Of the five studies, four reported revision rates [15, 25–27]. A fixed-effect model of analysis was used due to homogeneity among the studies (Q = 4.396, P = 0.222; I^2 = 31.76%). The pooled results showed fewer (OR = 0.19, 95% CI 0.10

to 0.35; P = 0.000) revisions in patients treated by THA than by osteosynthesis (Fig. 3b).

Hemiarthroplasty vs. osteosynthesis

Of the 14 studies, 11 studies reported revision rates [10, 30–36, 38, 41–44]. A random-effects model was used, due to heterogeneity among the studies (Q = 23.06, P = 0.011; I^2 = 56.63%). The pooled results showed fewer (OR = 0.12,

Fig. 3 Meta-analysis forest plot for odds ratio of revision for (**a**) total hip arthroplasty vs. hemiarthroplasty, (**b**) total hip arthroplasty vs. osteosynthesis, and (**c**) hemiarthroplasty vs. osteosynthesis

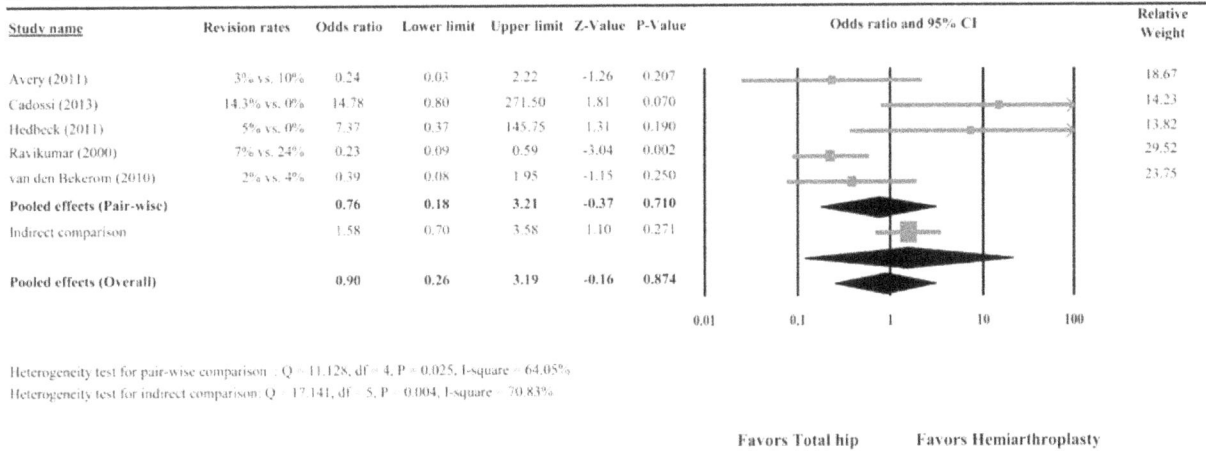

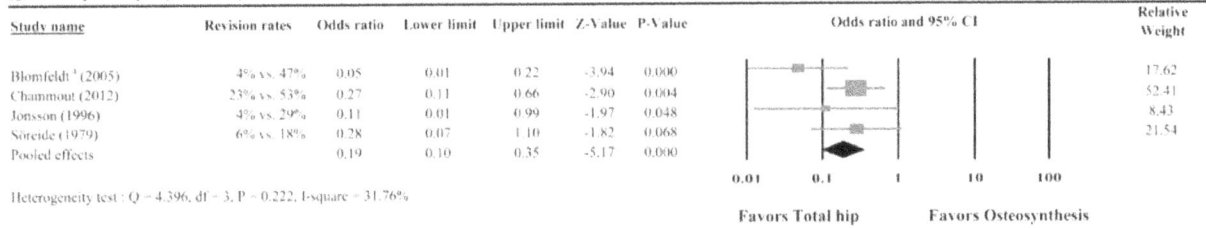

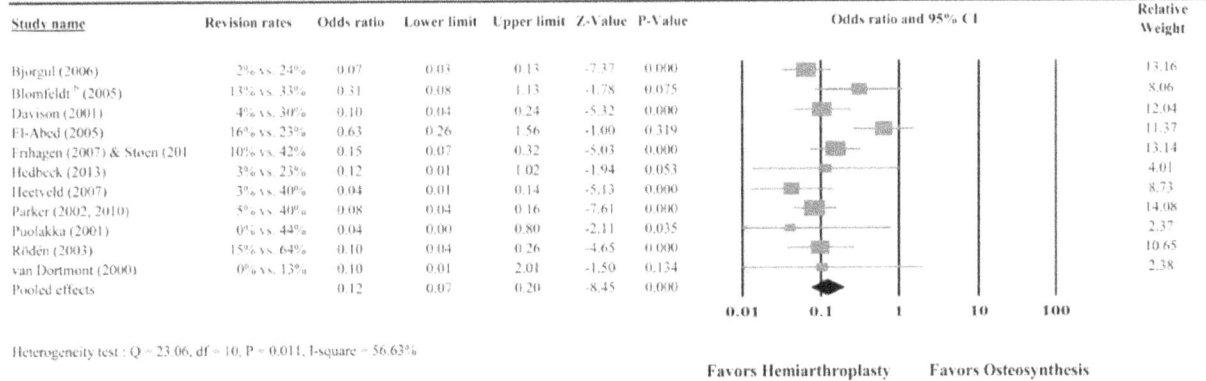

95% CI 0.07 to 0.20; $P = 0.000$) revisions for HA compared with osteosynthesis (Fig. 3c). That is to say, patients who underwent osteosynthesis were approximately eight times more likely to need a second operation.

Sensitivity analyses and publication bias

The sensitivity tests showed no obvious influence of any individual study on the pooled estimates (Table 2). In addition, it was not possible to assess publication bias

for mortality and revision rates due to the small number of studies used in the meta-analysis.

Outcome measures involving a subgroup of patients with normal cognition

After excluding studies without showing normal cognition in inclusion criteria, six studies were included in the meta-analysis for the odds ratio of mortality rate for THA vs. HA. A random-effects model was used due to large heterogeneity among studies ($Q = 13.008$, $P = 0.023$; $I^2 = 61.56\%$).

Table 2 Sensitivity analyses: a leave-one-out cross-validation approach

Study name	Odds ratio	Lower limit	Upper limit	Z value	P value
Mortality					
(A) Total hip arthroplasty vs. hemiarthroplasty					
Avery (2011) [45]	0.98	0.65	1.49	− 0.08	0.938
Cadossi (2013) [49]	0.95	0.61	1.46	− 0.25	0.805
Hedbeck (2011) [48]	0.83	0.52	1.33	− 0.79	0.432
Keating (2006) [51]	0.91	0.58	1.43	− 0.40	0.693
Macaulay (2008) [52]	0.90	0.58	1.41	− 0.45	0.655
Ravikumar (2000) [53]	0.91	0.57	1.45	− 0.39	0.694
van den Bekerom (2010) [55]	0.76	0.55	1.06	− 1.62	0.106
(B) Total hip arthroplasty vs. osteosynthesis					
Bachrach-Lindstrom (2000) [24]	1.13	0.60	2.11	0.39	0.700
Blomfeldt (2005) [27]	1.29	0.67	2.48	0.78	0.437
Jónsson (1996) [25]	1.14	0.66	1.98	0.47	0.641
Söreide (1979) [26]	1.15	0.62	2.16	0.45	0.655
(C) Hemiarthroplasty vs. osteosynthesis					
Bjorgul (2006) [30]	1.25	0.82	1.90	1.02	0.310
Blomfeldt (2005) [31]	1.21	0.83	1.78	0.98	0.325
Davison (2001) [10]	1.17	0.80	1.71	0.82	0.415
El-Abed (2005) [32]	1.15	0.79	1.67	0.71	0.479
Frihagen (2007) [41] and Støen (2014) [42]	1.23	0.82	1.85	1.00	0.315
Heetveld (2007) [34]	1.00	0.82	1.21	0.00	0.999
Parker (2002, 2010) [43, 44]	1.23	0.81	1.88	0.98	0.329
Puolakka (2001) [35]	1.22	0.84	1.78	1.03	0.301
Rödén (2003) [36]	1.28	0.87	1.87	1.26	0.208
Sikorski (1981) [37]	1.27	0.85	1.88	1.17	0.241
van Dortmont (2000) [38]	1.28	0.88	1.86	1.31	0.189
van Vugt (1993) [39]	1.21	0.83	1.77	0.98	0.326
Revision rates					
(A) Total hip arthroplasty vs. hemiarthroplasty					
Avery (2011) [45]	1.12	0.29	4.26	0.16	0.871
Cadossi (2013) [49]	0.63	0.20	2.00	− 0.78	0.433
Hedbeck (2011) [48]	0.69	0.20	2.38	− 0.58	0.560
Ravikumar (2000) [53]	1.29	0.38	4.39	0.41	0.684
van den Bekerom (2010) [55]	1.11	0.26	4.68	0.14	0.888
(B) Total hip arthroplasty vs. osteosynthesis					
Blomfeldt (2005) [27]	0.25	0.12	0.50	− 3.88	< 0.001
Chammout (2012) [15]	0.12	0.05	0.31	− 4.45	< 0.001
Jónsson (1996) [25]	0.20	0.10	0.38	− 4.81	< 0.001
Söreide (1979) [26]	0.17	0.08	0.34	− 4.88	< 0.001
(C) Hemiarthroplasty vs. osteosynthesis					
Bjorgul (2006) [30]	0.13	0.08	0.23	− 7.45	< 0.001
Blomfeldt (2005) [31]	0.11	0.07	0.18	− 8.49	< 0.001
Davison (2001) [10]	0.12	0.07	0.22	− 7.33	< 0.001
El-Abed (2005) [32]	0.10	0.07	0.13	− 14.80	< 0.001

Table 2 Sensitivity analyses: a leave-one-out cross-validation approach *(Continued)*

Study name	Odds ratio	Lower limit	Upper limit	Z value	P value
Frihagen (2007) [41] and Støen (2014) [42]	0.12	0.07	0.20	−7.48	<0.001
Hedbeck (2013) [33]	0.12	0.07	0.20	−8.02	<0.001
Heetveld (2007) [34]	0.13	0.08	0.22	−7.88	<0.001
Parker (2002, 2010) [43, 44]	0.13	0.07	0.22	−7.14	<0.001
Puolakka (2001) [35]	0.12	0.07	0.21	−8.11	<0.001
Rödén (2003) [36]	0.12	0.07	0.21	−7.47	<0.001
van Dortmont (2000) [38]	0.12	0.07	0.20	−8.11	<0.001

The pooled odds ratio was 0.87 (95% CI 0.49 to 1.56; $P = 0.648$; Fig. 4a), suggesting that there was no significant difference in the odds ratio of mortality between patients treated with THA and HA. For the comparison between HA and osteosynthesis, four studies designed for patients with normal cognition were analyzed. A fixed-effects model was used since there was no evidence of heterogeneity among the four studies ($Q = 4.895$, $P = 0.180$; $I^2 = 38.71\%$; Fig. 4b). No significant difference in the odds ratio of mortality was found between patients treated with HA and osteosynthesis (OR = 1.30, 95% CI 0.82 to 2.08; $P = 0.267$).

Four studies of patients with normal cognition were included to examine the odds ratio of revision rate for THA vs. HA. A random-effects model was used ($Q = 7.8665$, $P = 0.049$; $I^2 = 61.86\%$). There was no difference in the odds ratio of revision between the THA and HA groups (OR = 1.35, 95% CI 0.20 to 9.11; $P = 0.761$; Fig. 5a). To compare differences in revision

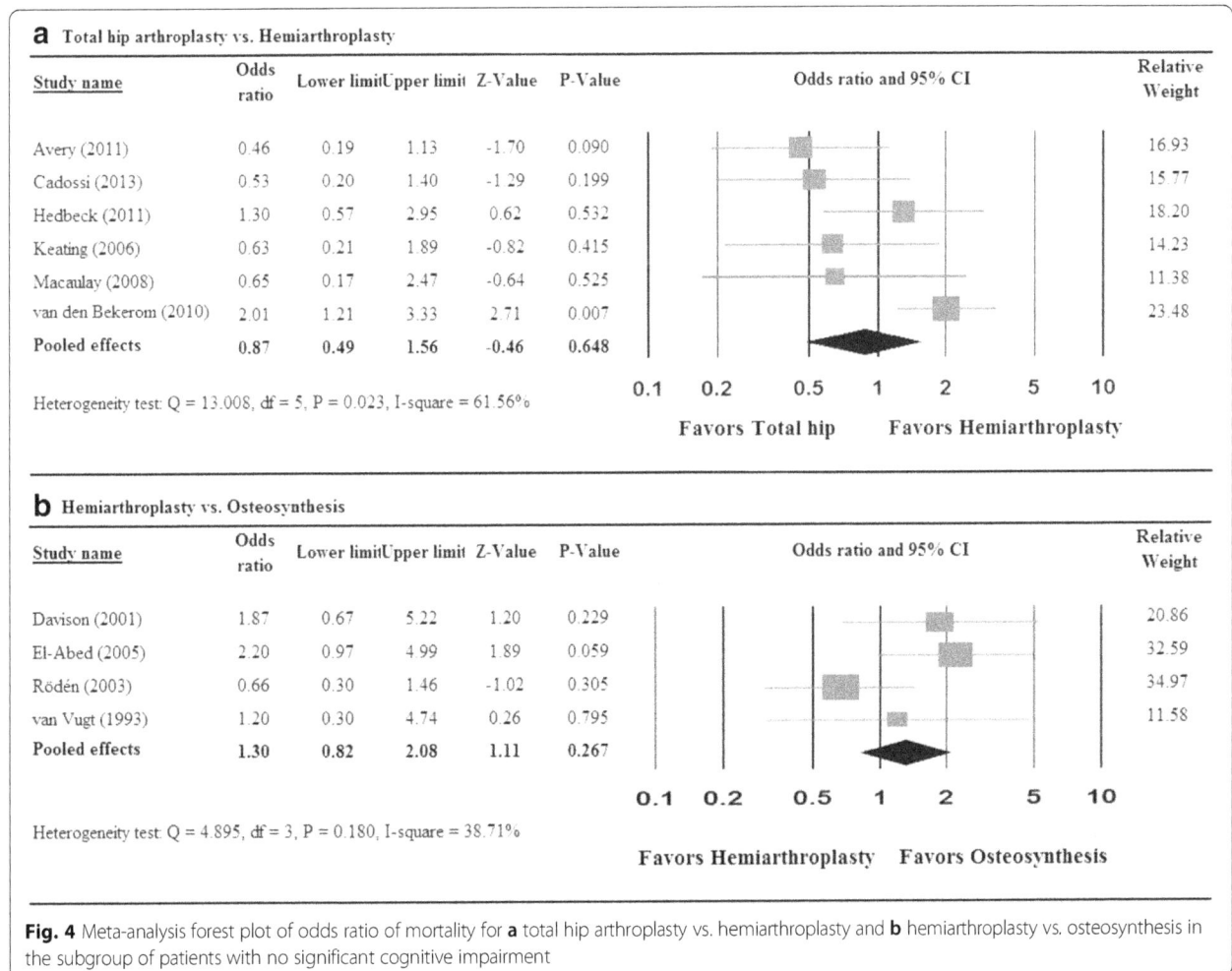

Fig. 4 Meta-analysis forest plot of odds ratio of mortality for **a** total hip arthroplasty vs. hemiarthroplasty and **b** hemiarthroplasty vs. osteosynthesis in the subgroup of patients with no significant cognitive impairment

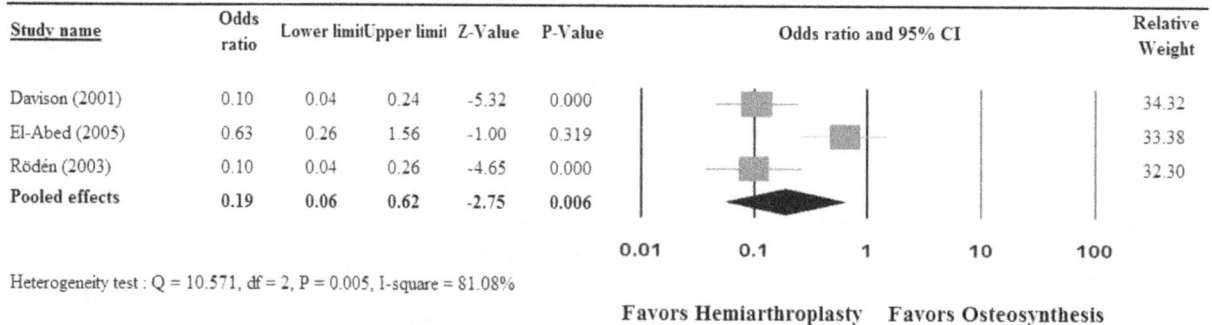

Fig. 5 Meta-analysis forest plot of odds ratio of revision for **a** total hip arthroplasty vs. hemiarthroplasty, **b** total hip arthroplasty vs. osteosynthesis, and **c** hemiarthroplasty vs. osteosynthesis, in the subgroup of patients with no significant cognitive impairment

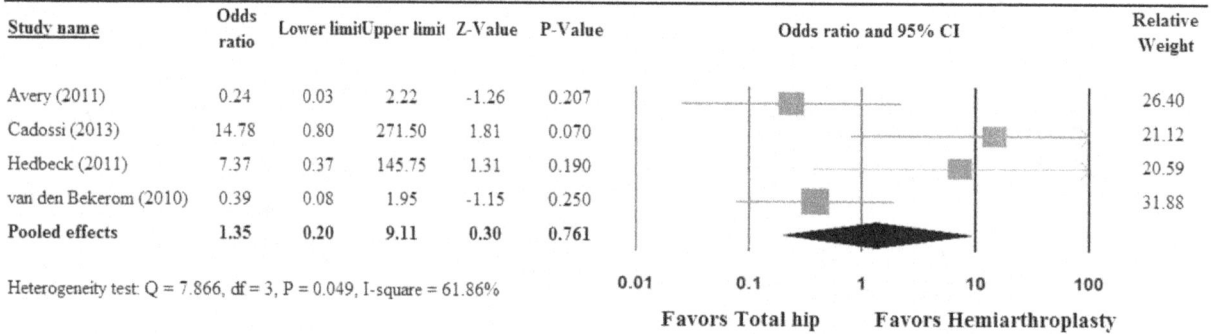

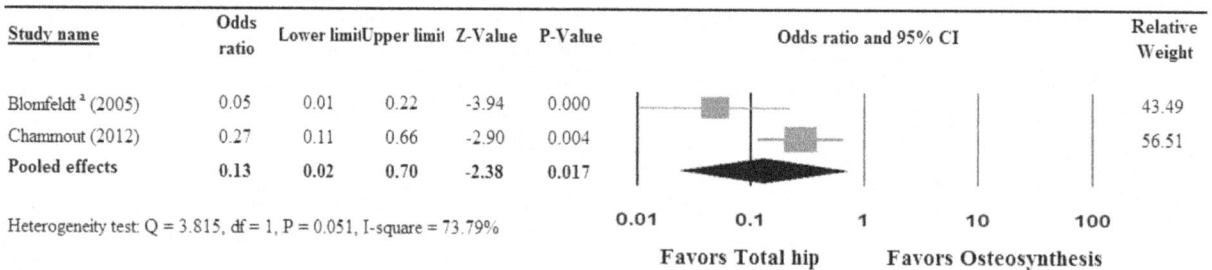

rate between THA and osteosynthesis groups, two studies of patients with normal cognition were included with large heterogeneity ($Q = 3.815$, $P = 0.051$; $I^2 = 73.79\%$). Patients treated with THA had significantly lower revision rates than did those with osteosynthesis (OR = 0.13, 95% CI 0.02 to 0.70; $P = 0.017$; Fig. 5b). For the comparison between HA and osteosynthesis, three studies designed for patients with normal cognition were analyzed. A random-effects model was used due to large heterogeneity among studies ($Q = 10.571$, $P = 0.005$; $I^2 = 81.08\%$). The pooled results showed that patients treated with HA had lower revision rates than those treated with osteosynthesis (OR = 0.19, 95% CI 0.06 to 0.62; $P = 0.006$; Fig. 5c).

Quality assessment

The results of quality assessment are shown in Fig. 6. In this figure, Fig. 6a shows the potential risk of bias in an individual study, and Fig. 6b shows the summary of bias for included studies. The most potential risk of bias came from performance bias and detection bias because of inadequate blinding of participants and outcome assessors.

Discussion

This meta-analysis compared the overall mortality and revision rates between arthroplasty (HA and THA) vs. osteosynthesis for displaced femoral neck fractures in the elderly. Advanced statistical analysis (indirect comparison)

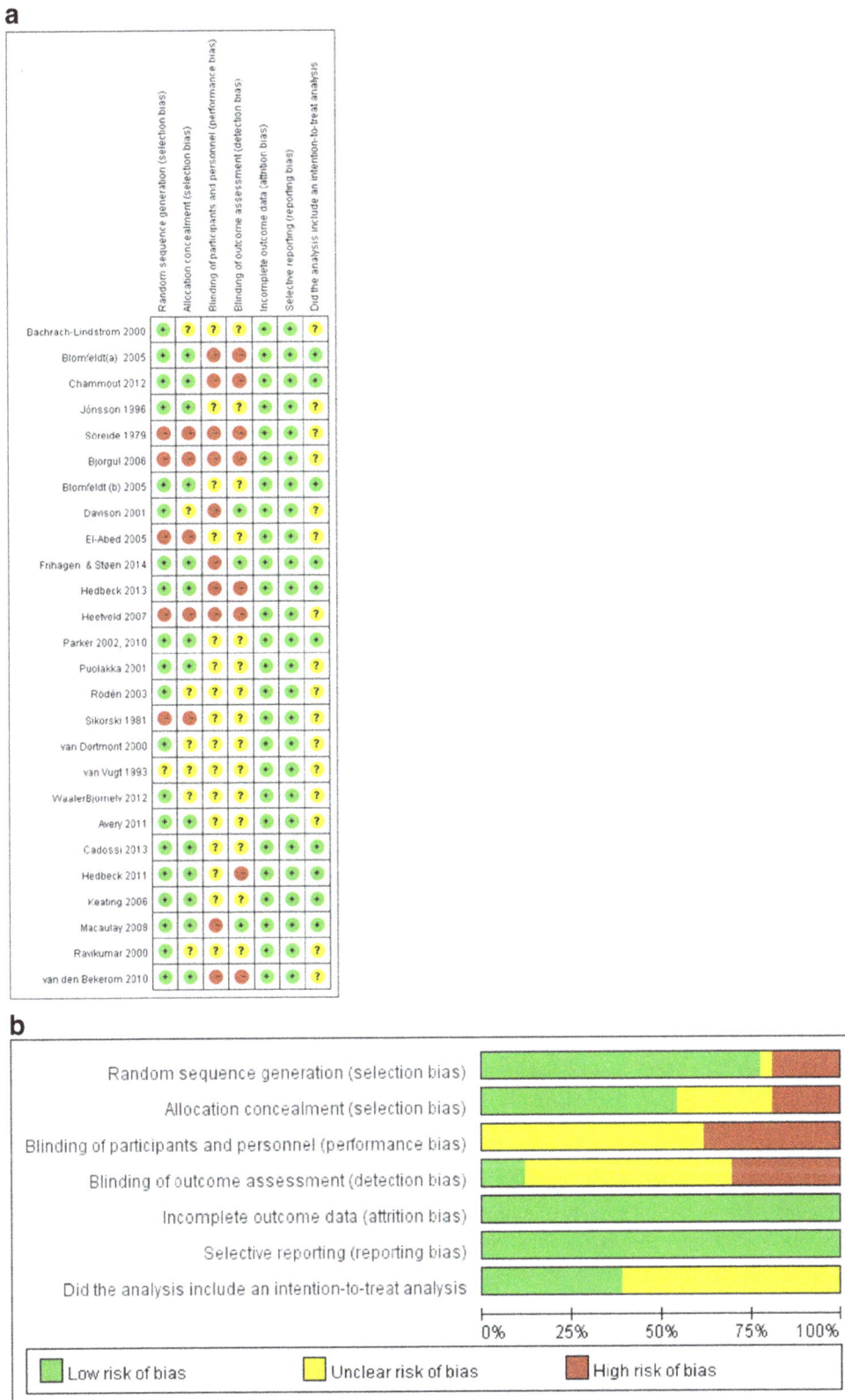

Fig. 6 The results of quality assessment for **a** individual studies. **b** The summary of bias for all included studies

was used simultaneously to compare THA and HA in order to resolve the lack of studies with head-to-head comparison between THA and HA. We also compared clinical outcomes of arthroplasty (THA and HA) vs. osteosynthesis (internal fixation) for displaced femoral neck fractures.

This meta-analysis found no significant difference in mortality rates between THA, HA, and OS. In addition, no significant difference in revision rates was found between THA and HA, but osteosynthesis had higher revision rates than either THA or HA. The additional subgroup analysis, using only studies involving elderly subjects without significant cognitive impairment, provided similar results for mortality (i.e., no difference between HA and osteosynthesis) and revision rates (no difference between THA and HA), but OS had higher revision rates than either THA or HA.

One study (two articles) showed the mean survival time of persons who died for both THA (5.3 years, range 1.3 to 9.1 years) and HA (3.8 years, range 0.003 to 7.5 years) [45, 46]. Two studies (three articles) assessed the mean survival time after intervention. Davison et al. [10] found that patients who received Thompson unipolar HA, Monk (hard-top) bipolar HA, and reduction/internal fixation had mean survival times of 61, 68, and 79 months, respectively. There was a significant difference in mean survival time between groups (P = 0.008). Parker et al. [43, 44] found that the patients who received HA and internal fixation had mean survival times of 2.7 years (95% CI 2.2–3.1) and 3.2 years (95% CI 2.5–3.9), respectively. No significant difference was found between groups. Due to the limitation in the number of available studies, the survival time after interventions (osteosynthesis, HA, and THA) was not included in the meta-analysis.

No meta-analysis was conducted for the functional outcome after interventions since the methods or scales for evaluating hip function were heterogeneous among the included articles (Table 1), including the Oxford Hip Score [45, 46], Harris Hip Score [10, 15, 34, 40–42, 47–49, 52–55], hip rating questionnaire [50, 51], Charnley's numerical classification [27–29, 31, 33, 43, 44], Matta Scoring System [32], Stinchfield's classification system [26], and Sheperd's pain and hip mobility score [39]. In addition, no data for baseline measurement were shown in most of the studies. Therefore, it was impossible to estimate the difference in mean change before and after the intervention between the two groups.

To the best of our knowledge, this is the first meta-analysis to compare three types of interventions for displaced femoral neck fractures in one meta-analysis. Although a meta-analysis comparing THA, HA, and osteosynthesis was reported in 2012 by Gao et al. [17], the need to revisit this issue (by conducting another meta-analysis) remained because the meta-analysis by Gao et al. compared the outcomes between arthroplasty and internal fixation and thus pooled together the outcomes of HA and total hip replacement [17]. Fisher et al. [56], in their review of 3423 cases of ORIF, THA, and HA, found no differences in the 30-day mortality rates among the ORIF, HA, and THA groups, similar to our findings. ORIF and HA also resulted in a lower likelihood of developing respiratory complications than did THA [56]. A meta-analysis comparing THA and HA was reported by Burgers et al. [57]. Given the heterogeneity in surgical technique and experience over time, we felt an update of the evidence was necessary. We have updated the search, but our results were consistent with this meta-analysis that no significant difference was found in mortality and revision rates between THA and HA, but they demonstrated that THA may lead to higher dislocation rates compared with HA [57]. Therefore, it was felt that the optimal choice of arthroplasty (THA or HA) for treating femoral neck fractures had not yet been established.

It appears that the choice between arthroplasty and internal fixation in some studies was based primarily on the survival time of the implant. For example, in Davison et al. [10], HA was not recommended due to the shorter mean survival time of the implant compared with internal fixation despite the fact that internal fixation was associated with a 30% risk of failure [10]. They reported a mean patient survival which was significantly higher in the group undergoing reduction and internal fixation (79 months) compared with that with a cemented Thompson HA or a cemented Monk bipolar HA (61 and 68 months, respectively). We also found that the revision rates were lower in arthroplasty compared with internal fixation, but survival was the same among all three types of intervention (HA, THA, and osteosynthesis). These differences are likely related to the type of arthroplasty used. As in our evaluation, there was significant heterogeneity both in the implant used and the technique applied (for example, cementless HA [31, 32] vs. cemented HA [10, 30], articulation of metal on ultra-high-molecular-weight polyethylene in THR vs. metal on articular cartilage following HA [45]).

Nikitovic [6], on the basis of two systematic reviews evaluating the effectiveness of THA in comparison with HA for treatment of displaced femoral neck fractures, found a significant reduction in revision rates among patients receiving THA in comparison with HA. In addition, his recent study showed a significant improvement in functional outcome among patients receiving THA in comparison with HA, using the Harris Hip Score for the assessment. THA was favored over HA based on improvements in QoL using mobility and pain measures [6].

No meta-analysis was conducted for the QoL after interventions since the methods or scales for evaluating QoL were heterogeneous among the included articles. SF-36 was used in three studies (four articles), including three articles for THA vs. HA [45, 46, 52] and one article for HA vs. osteosynthesis [32]. EQ-5D was used in six studies (ten articles), including four articles for THA vs. HA [47, 48, 50, 51], three articles for THA vs. osteosynthesis [27–29], and three articles for HA vs. osteosynthesis [31, 33, 40]. Although we did not evaluate QoL, some studies have placed emphasis on social functioning after intervention. Jónsson et al. evaluated 50 patients with Garden stage 3 and 4 femoral neck fractures randomized for treatment using either osteosynthesis with the Hansson hook pins or THA with the Charnley prosthesis [25]. The patients were followed for up to 2 years, and their social function was evaluated using a standardized questionnaire. The authors concluded that a patient over 70 years of age who was relatively healthy, mobile, and socially independent should be considered for a primary hip prosthesis even if late complications, such as mechanical loosening, were taken into account. This conclusion was based on the fact that the majority of patients over 70 years of age are less likely to live long enough to develop implant loosening. For very old, frail, or immobile patients, however, osteosynthesis was the preferred treatment [25]. And, these findings were echoed in a more recent study from Sweden [24]. Bachrach-Lindström et al. found that a primary THA group performed better than an osteosynthesis group in weight change over time, locomotion, and pain. They also showed that primary THA could be performed safely in the elderly without increasing postoperative mortality [24].

As part of our study, we performed a sensitivity analysis and tested for homogeneity and quality. Since our analysis showed heterogeneity among the majority of studies, a random-effects model was primarily applied. We also tested for reliability based on sensitivity analysis. The direction and magnitude of the combined estimates did not change markedly with the exclusion of individual studies, indicating that our meta-analysis had good reliability. The results of quality assessment showed that the most potential risk of bias came from performance bias and detection bias because of inadequate blinding of participants and outcome assessors.

We also tested for publication bias. Although significant evidence of publication bias was found regarding differences in survival between THA and HA, we adjusted the effect of publication bias, and the adjusted point estimates of OR on mortality increased to 1.13 (95% CI 0.77 to 1.67, Fig. 2c).

In the 26 studies evaluated as part of our meta-analysis, almost all subjects had freedom of mobility or were capable of independent walking before their injury, and there was a female predominance. This is not surprising, as the incidence of proximal femoral fractures among females is two to three times greater than the incidence of such fractures in males [1]. Other risk factors for proximal femoral fractures include osteoporosis [1], a maternal history of hip fractures [58], excessive alcohol consumption and high caffeine intake [59], and physical inactivity [60], to name a few. Owing to our aging population, the risk of sustaining a proximal femoral fracture doubles every 10 years after the age of 50 [1]. Therefore, this study has clinical relevance in that it is an attempt to identify the best treatment option for these elderly patients.

Our study had several limitations. Potential performance and detection biases might exist in most of the included studies. We also did not assess functional status of the patients after the reconstructive procedures, and this was an inevitable shortcoming of this study. Notably for a patient with severe cognitive dysfunction, the lack of a surgical revision might correlate with a limited capacity for independent ambulation and with an inability to verbally express the features of a potentially symptomatic hip. We did perform an analysis on a subgroup of elderly patients without severe cognitive impairment and found no significant difference in the results regarding mortality and revision rates. But, the ways in which cognitive impairment was defined as significant or severe differed among studies. In addition, several studies only included patients with acute displaced femoral neck fractures with different time periods between fracture occurrence and admission; this ranged from 12 to 96 h. In addition, the studies included different types of femoral neck fractures, and not all studies specified the Garden stages of fractures. For all these reasons, more future studies comparing these three types of interventions are still needed to confirm our findings. Furthermore, there was significant heterogeneity among studies, especially with respect to the types of implants used for HA and THA and the types of screws used for osteosynthesis. The optimal choice of screw or reduction method (open or closed) for osteosynthesis remains unclear. Among included studies, only a few [15, 25, 45–48] chose independent living as a selection criterion, and it is arguable whether living independently or in a nursing home could have an impact on the results. Furthermore, the surgeons' experiences and the different numbers and types of procedures performed at the various medical centers were possible confounding factors that may have affected the results and influenced the heterogeneity among studies.

Conclusion

In conclusion, HA and THA provided similar overall mortality and revision rates, but both HA and THA had significantly lower revision rates compared with osteosynthesis. The results were not affected by excluding studies without showing normal cognition in inclusion criteria. Results of the present study provide evidence to support using hip arthroplasty for the treatment of femoral neck displaced fractures. To compare the clinical outcomes, functional outcomes, and health-related QoL between hip arthroplasty and osteosynthesis, a well-designed randomized control trial is warranted.

Abbreviations

CI: Confidence interval; HA: Hemiarthroplasty; I^2: Inconsistency index; OR: Odds ratio; QoL: Quality of life; RCT: Randomized controlled trial; THA: Total hip arthroplasty

Acknowledgements

Not applicable.

Funding

Not applicable.

Authors' contributions

F-JT: guarantor of integrity of the entire study, study concepts, study design, definition of intellectual content, literature research, data acquisition, statistical analysis, manuscript preparation; W-TC: study concepts, definition of intellectual content, literature research, data acquisition, statistical analysis, manuscript preparation; R-YP: study concepts, study design, definition of intellectual content, literature research, data acquisition, statistical analysis, manuscript preparation, manuscript editing, manuscript review; L-CL: study concepts, manuscript editing; H-CS: study concepts, manuscript editing; C-HW: manuscript editing; J-FS: manuscript review; C-FW: guarantor of integrity of the entire study, study design, manuscript editing, manuscript review. All authors read and approved the study.

Competing interests

The authors declare that they have no competing interests.

Author details

[1]Department of Life Science and the Institute of Biotechnology, National Dong Hwa University, Hualien 974, Taiwan, Republic of China. [2]Department of Orthopedics, Hualien Armed Force General Hospital, Hualien 971, Taiwan, Republic of China. [3]Department of Health, Hsin Chu General Hospital, Hsinchu 300, Taiwan, Republic of China. [4]Department of Orthopaedics, Tri-Service General Hospital, National Defense Medical Center, Neihu 114, Taipei, Taiwan, Republic of China. [5]Graduate Institute of Medical Science, National Defense Medical Center, Neihu 114, Taipei, Taiwan, Republic of China. [6]Department of Biology and Anatomy, National Defense Medical Center, Neihu 114, Taipei, Taiwan, Republic of China.

References

1. Zuckerman JD. Hip fracture. N Engl J Med. 1996;334:1519–25.
2. Fox KM, Magaziner J, Hebel JR, Kenzora JE, Kashner TM. Intertrochanteric versus femoral neck fractures: differential characteristics, treatment, and sequelae. J Gerontol A Biol Sci Med Sci. 1999;54:M635–M40.
3. Garden RS. Low-angle fixation in fractures of the femoral neck. J Bone Joint Surg Br. 1961;43:647–63.
4. Pauyo T, Drager J, Albers A, Harvey EJ. Management of femoral neck fractures in the young patient: a critical analysis review. World J Orthop. 2014;5:204–17.
5. Butler M, Forte M, Kane RL, Joglekar S, Duval SJ, Swiontkowski M, et al. Treatment of common hip fractures. Evid Rep Tech Assess. 2009;184:1–85.
6. Nikitovic M. Total hip arthroplasty versus hemiarthroplasty for displaced femoral neck fractures: a rapid review. 2013. 22p. Available from: http://www.hqontario.ca/Portals/0/Documents/evidence/rapid-reviews/hip-anthroplasty-130423-en.pdf.
7. Parker MJ. The management of intracapsular fractures of the proximal femur. J Bone Joint Surg Br. 2010;82:937–41.
8. Upadhyay A, Jain P, Mishra P, Maini L, Gautum VK, Dhaon BK. Delayed internal fixation of fractures of the neck of the femur in young adults. A prospective, randomised study comparing closed and open reduction. J Bone Joint Surg Br. 2004;86:1035–40.
9. Parker MJ, Gurusamy KS, Azegami S. Arthroplasties (with and without bone cement) for proximal femoral fractures in adults. Cochrane Database Syst Rev. 2010;6:CD001706.
10. Davison JN, Calder SJ, Anderson GH, Ward G, Jagger C, Harper WM, et al. Treatment for displaced intracapsular fracture of the proximal femur. A prospective, randomised trial in patients aged 65 to 79 years. J Bone Joint Surg Br. 2001;83:206–12.
11. Healy WL, Iorio R. Total hip arthroplasty: optimal treatment for displaced femoral neck fractures in elderly patients. Clin Orthop Relat Res. 2004;429:43–8.
12. Bhandari M, Devereaux PJ, Tornetta P 3rd, Swiontkowski MF, Berry DJ, Haidukewych G, et al. Operative management of displaced femoral neck fractures in elderly patients. An international survey. J Bone Joint Surg Am. 2005;87:2122–30.
13. Guyton JL. Fractures of hip, acetabulum, and pelvis. In: Canale ST, editor. Campbell's operative orthopedics. 9th ed. St. Louis: Mosby; 1998. p. 2181–276.
14. Johansson T, Jacobsson SA, Ivarsson I, Knutsson A, Wahlström O. Internal fixation versus total hip arthroplasty in the treatment of displaced femoral neck fractures: a prospective randomized study of 100 hips. Acta Orthop Scand. 2000;71:597–602.
15. Chammout GK, Mukka SS, Carlsson T, Neander GF, Stark AW, Skoldenberg OG. Total hip replacement versus open reduction and internal fixation of displaced femoral neck fractures: a randomized long-term follow-up study. J Bone Joint Surg Am. 2012;94:1921–8.
16. Rogmark C, Johnell O. Primary arthroplasty is better than internal fixation of displaced femoral neck fractures: a meta-analysis of 14 randomized studies with 2,289 patients. Acta Orthop. 2006;77:359–67.
17. Gao H, Liu Z, Xing D, Gong M. Which is the best alternative for displaced femoral neck fractures in the elderly?: a meta-analysis. Clin Orthop Relat Res. 2012;470:1782–91.
18. Speed K. Fractures; a fifty year review of teaching and treatment. Illinois Med J. 1952;102:114–7.
19. Liberati A, Altman DG, Tetzlaff J, Mulrow C, Gøtzsche PC, Ioannidis JP, et al. The PRISMA statement for reporting systematic reviews and meta-analyses of studies that evaluate health care interventions: explanation and elaboration. Ann Intern Med. 2009;151:W65–94.
20. Cochrane Handbook for Systematic. Reviews of Interventions. Version 5.1.0. (updated March, 2011). The Cochrane Collaboration Available at: http://handbook-5-1.cochrane.org/ (Accessed date: 1 Dec 2014).
21. Sutton AJ, Song F, Gilbody SM, Abrams KR. Modelling publication bias in meta-analysis: a review. Stat Methods Med Res. 2000;9:421–45.
22. Sterne JA, Sutton AJ, Ioannidis JP, Terrin N, Jones DR, Lau J, et al. Recommendations for examining and interpreting funnel plot asymmetry in meta-analyses of randomised controlled trials. BMJ. 2011; d4002:343.
23. Wells GA, Sultran SA, Chen L, Khan M, Coyle D. Indirect treatment comparison [computer program]. Version 1.0. Canadian Agency for Drugs and Technologies in Health: Ottawa; 2009.
24. Bachrach-Lindström M, Johansson T, Unosson M, Ek AC, Wahlström O. Nutritional status and functional capacity after femoral neck fractures: a prospective randomized one-year follow-up study. Aging (Milano). 2000;12:366–74.
25. Jónsson B, Sernbo I, Carlsson A, Fredin H, Johnell O. Social function after cervical hip fracture. A comparison of hook-pins and total hip replacement in 47 patients. Acta Orthop Scand. 1996;67:431–4.
26. Söreide O, Molster A, Raugstad TS. Internal fixation versus primary prosthetic replacement in acute femoral neck fractures: a prospective, randomized clinical study. Br J Surg. 1979;66:56–60.
27. Blomfeldt R, Törnkvist H, Ponzer S, Söderqvist A, Tidermark J. Comparison of internal fixation with total hip replacement for displaced femoral neck fractures. Randomized, controlled trial performed at four years. J Bone Joint Surg Am. 2005; 87:1680–8.
28. Tidermark J, Bergström G, Svensson O, Törnkvist H, Ponzer S. Responsiveness of the EuroQol (EQ 5-D) and the SF-36 in elderly patients with displaced femoral neck fractures. Qual Life Res. 2003;12:1069–79.
29. Tidermark J, Ponzer S, Svensson O, Söderqvist A, Törnkvist H. Internal fixation compared with total hip replacement for displaced femoral neck fractures in the elderly. A randomised, controlled trial. J Bone Joint Surg Br. 2003;85:380–8.
30. Bjorgul K, Reikeras O. Hemiarthroplasty in worst cases is better than internal

fixation in best cases of displaced femoral neck fractures: a prospective study of 683 patients treated with hemiarthroplasty or internal fixation. Acta Orthop. 2006;77:368–74.

31. Blomfeldt R, Törnkvist H, Ponzer S, Söderqvist A, Tidermark J. Internal fixation versus hemiarthroplasty for displaced fractures of the femoral neck in elderly patients with severe cognitive impairment. J Bone Joint Surg Br. 2005;87:523–9.

32. El-Abed K, McGuinness A, Brunner J, Dallovedova P, O'Connor P, Kennedy JG. Comparison of outcomes following uncemented hemiarthroplasty and dynamic hip screw in the treatment of displaced subcapital hip fractures in patients aged greater than 70 years. Acta Orthop Belg. 2005;71:48–54.

33. Hedbeck CJ, Inngul C, Blomfeldt R, Ponzer S, Törnkvist H, Enocson A. Internal fixation versus cemented hemiarthroplasty for displaced femoral neck fractures in patients with severe cognitive dysfunction: a randomized controlled trial. J Orthop Trauma. 2013;27:690–5.

34. Heetveld MJ, Raaymakers EL, Luitse JS, Nijhof M, Gouma DJ. Femoral neck fractures: can physiologic status determine treatment choice? Clin Orthop Relat Res. 2007;461:203–12.

35. Puolakka TJ, Laine HJ, Tarvainen T, Aho H. Thompson hemiarthroplasty is superior to Ullevaal screws in treating displaced femoral neck fractures in patients over 75 years. A prospective randomized study with two-year follow-up. Ann Chir Gynaecol. 2001;90:225–8.

36. Rödén M, Schön M, Fredin H. Treatment of displaced femoral neck fractures: a randomized minimum 5-year follow-up study of screws and bipolar hemiprostheses in 100 patients. Acta Orthop Scand. 2003;74:42–4.

37. Sikorski JM, Barrington R. Internal fixation versus hemiarthroplasty for the displaced subcapital fracture of the femur. A prospective randomised study. J Bone Joint Surg Br. 1981;63-B:357–61.

38. van Dortmont LM, Douw CM, van Breukelen AM, Laurens DR, Mulder PG, Wereldsma JC, van Vugt AB. Cannulated screws versus hemiarthroplasty for displaced intracapsular femoral neck fractures in demented patients. Ann Chir Gynaecol. 2000;89:132–7.

39. van Vugt AB, Oosterwijk WM, Goris RJ. Osteosynthesis versus endoprosthesis in the treatment of unstable intracapsular hip fractures in the elderly. A randomized clinical trial. Arch Orthop Trauma Surg. 1993;113:39–45.

40. Waaler Bjørnelv GM, Frihagen F, Madsen JE, Nordsletten L, Aas E. Hemiarthroplasty compared to internal fixation with percutaneous cannulated screws as treatment of displaced femoral neck fractures in the elderly: cost-utility analysis performed alongside a randomized, controlled trial. Osteoporos Int. 2012;23:1711–9.

41. Frihagen F, Nordsletten L, Madsen JE. Hemiarthroplasty or internal fixation for intracapsular displaced femoral neck fractures: randomised controlled trial. BMJ. 2007;335:1251–4.

42. Støen RØ, Lofthus CM, Nordsletten L, Madsen JE, Frihagen F. Randomized trial of hemiarthroplasty versus internal fixation for femoral neck fractures: no differences at 6 years. Clin Orthop Relat Res. 2014;472:360–7.

43. Parker MJ, Pryor G, Gurusamy K. Hemiarthroplasty versus internal fixation for displaced intracapsular hip fractures: a long-term follow-up of a randomised trial. Injury. 2010;41:370–3.

44. Parker MJ, Khan RJ, Crawford J, Pryor GA. Hemiarthroplasty versus internal fixation for displaced intracapsular hip fractures in the elderly. A randomised trial of 455 patients. J Bone Joint Surg Br. 2002;84:1150–5.

45. Avery PP, Baker RP, Walton MJ, Rooker JC, Squires B, Gargan MF, et al. Total hip replacement and hemiarthroplasty in mobile, independent patients with a displaced intracapsular fracture of the femoral neck: a seven- to ten-year follow-up report of a prospective randomised controlled trial. J Bone Joint Surg Br. 2011;93:1045–8.

46. Baker RP, Squires B, Gargan MF, Bannister GC. Total hip arthroplasty and hemiarthroplasty in mobile, independent patients with a displaced intracapsular fracture of the femoral neck. A randomized, controlled trial. J Bone Joint Surg Am. 2006;88:2583–9.

47. Blomfeldt R, Törnkvist H, Eriksson K, Söderqvist A, Ponzer S, Tidermark J. A randomised controlled trial comparing bipolar hemiarthroplasty with total hip replacement for displaced intracapsular fractures of the femoral neck in elderly patients. J Bone Joint Surg Br. 2007;89:160–5.

48. Hedbeck CJ, Enocson A, Lapidus G, Blomfeldt R, Törnkvist H, Ponzer S, et al. Comparison of bipolar hemiarthroplasty with total hip arthroplasty for displaced femoral neck fractures: a concise four-year follow-up of a randomized trial. J Bone Joint Surg Am. 2011;93:445–50.

49. Cadossi M, Chiarello E, Savarino L, Tedesco G, Baldini N, Faldini C, et al. A comparison of hemiarthroplasty with a novel polycarbonate-urethane acetabular component for displaced intracapsular fractures of the femoral neck: a randomised controlled trial in elderly patients. Bone Joint J. 2013;95-B:609–15.

50. Keating JF, Grant A, Masson M, Scott NW, Forbes JF. Displaced intracapsular hip fractures in fit, older people: a randomised comparison of reduction and fixation, bipolar hemiarthroplasty and total hip arthroplasty. Health Technol Assess. 2005;9(41):iii-iv, ix-x, 1-65.

51. Keating JF, Grant A, Masson M, Scott NW, Forbes JF. Randomized comparison of reduction and fixation, bipolar hemiarthroplasty, and total hip arthroplasty. Treatment of displaced intracapsular hip fractures in healthy older patients. J Bone Joint Surg Am. 2006;88:249–60.

52. Macaulay W, Nellans KW, Garvin KL, Iorio R, Healy WL, Rosenwasser MP, other members of the DFACTO Consortium. Prospective randomized clinical trial comparing hemiarthroplasty to total hip arthroplasty in the treatment of displaced femoral neck fractures: winner of the Dorr Award. J Arthroplasty. 2008;23:2–8.

53. Ravikumar KJ, Marsh G. Internal fixation versus hemiarthroplasty versus total hip arthroplasty for displaced subcapital fractures of femur—13 year results of a prospective randomised study. Injury. 2000;31:793–7.

54. Skinner P, Riley D, Ellery J, Beaumont A, Coumine R, Shafighian B. Displaced subcapital fractures of the femur: a prospective randomized comparison of internal fixation, hemiarthroplasty and total hip replacement. Injury. 1989;20:291–3.

55. van den Bekerom MP, Hilverdink EF, Sierevelt IN, Reuling EM, Schnater JM, Bonke H, et al. A comparison of hemiarthroplasty with total hip replacement for displaced intracapsular fracture of the femoral neck: a randomised controlled multicentre trial in patients aged 70 years and over. J Bone Joint Surg Br. 2010;92:1422–8.

56. Fisher MA, Matthei JD, Obirieze A, Ortega G, Tran DD, Carnegie DA, et al. Open reduction internal fixation versus hemiarthroplasty versus total hip arthroplasty in the elderly: a review of the National Surgical Quality Improvement Program database. J Surg Res. 2013;181:193–8.

57. Burgers PT, Van Geene AR, Van den Bekerom MP, Van Lieshout EM, Blom B, Aleem IS, et al. Total hip arthroplasty versus hemiarthroplasty for displaced femoral neck fractures in the healthy elderly: a meta-analysis and systematic review of randomized trials. Int Orthop. 2012;36:1549–60.

58. Cummings SR, Nevitt MC, Browner WS, Stone K, Fox KM, Ensrud KE, et al. Risk factors for hip fracture in white women. Study of Osteoporotic Fractures Research Group. N Engl J Med. 1995;332:767–73.

59. Hernandez-Avila M, Colditz GA, Stampfer MJ, Rosner B, Speizer FE, Willett WC. Caffeine, moderate alcohol intake, and risk of fractures of the hip and forearm in middle-aged women. Am J Clin Nutr. 1991;54:157–63.

60. Paganini-Hill A, Chao A, Ross RK, Henderson BE. Exercise and other factors in the prevention of hip fracture: the Leisure World study. Epidemiology. 1991;2:16–25.

15

Comparison of the efficacy of static versus articular spacers in two-stage revision surgery for the treatment of infection following total knee arthroplasty

Hai Ding[*], Jian Yao, Wenju Chang and Fendou Liu

Abstract

Background: The aim of this study was to compare the outcomes of static versus articular spacers in two-stage reimplantation for the treatment of infected total knee arthroplasty (TKA).

Methods: The literature regarding the articulating and static spacers for treating infected TKA were searched in PubMed, Embase, Cochrane Library, Chinese Periodical Full-Text Database of CNKI, and Wanfang database. Data were extracted according to the inclusion and exclusion criteria and analyzed by Review Manager 5.3.

Results: Ten studies were included to this meta-analysis (nine retrospective studies, one prospective study) according to the principle of PICOS. There was no significant difference regarding the eradication rate ($P = 0.28$) and the American Knee Society knee score (KSS) pain score ($P = 0.11$) between the articulating and static spacers in the two-stage revision surgery. There was no significant difference regarding quadriceps femoroplasty and tibial tubercle osteotomy between the two groups ($P = 0.50$). The knee range of motion (ROM), Hospital for Special Surgery (HSS) score, and KSS function score in the articulating group were significantly higher than those in the static group ($P < 0.00001$).

Conclusion: Articulating spacers can provide better ROM and knee function scores after revision surgery when compared to static spacer while not compromising the infection eradication rate, soft tissue contracture during exclusion period, and knee pain scores.

Keywords: Total knee arthroplasty, Periprosthetic infection, Two-stage revision arthroplasty, Antibiotic bone cement spacer, Meta-analysis

Background

The prosthetic joint infection (PJI) is a devastating and complex complication after total knee arthroplasty (TKA). Although the incidence was only 1 to 2% [1–3], the number of the joint arthroplasties being performed is increasing. It can lead to serious consequences such as bone defect and necrosis; thus, the diagnosis and effective treatment of postoperative infection are very important. The two-stage revision surgery is the "gold standard" for patients with infection following TKA, especially for patients with chronic infection. The implantation of antibiotic-containing bone cement spacers can be used to eradicate infected microbes before prosthesis implantation [4, 5]. In addition, spacers maintain length of involved limbs and prevent muscle and soft tissue contracture via simple bone cement blocks inserting into the joint space [6–8]. Two types of antibiotic bone cement spacer are available, including articulating spacers and statics spacers. The articulating antibiotic-loaded cement spacer can be used to make femoral and tibial prosthesis via the artificial plastic method. This type of spacer is similar to the anatomical structure of the normal knee joint, and thus has a good match with the residual bone surface. Meanwhile, it can

---

* Correspondence: dinghai_66@163.com
Department of Orthopedics, The First Affiliated Hospital of Bengbu Medical College, No. 287 Changhuai Road, Bengbu, Anhui 233004, People's Republic of China

maintain joint space and joint activity, reduce soft tissue adhesion, atrophy and scar formation, and reduce the recurrence rate of infection [6, 9–11]. The static spacers can not only effectively deliver high concentration of antibiotic to control infection, but also maintain the joint space and limb length. However, the flexion and extension of the knee joint can result in soft tissue contracture around the joint and difficulty with reimplantation [1, 12]. The use of articular bone cement spacer is becoming increasingly widespread. However, some researchers reported higher risks of complications and the infection rate for the articular bone cement spacers compared to static spacers [13, 14]. Currently, there exists controversy regarding which antibiotic spacers are superior in the treatment of infection following total knee arthroplasty. The aim of the present meta-analysis was to compare the clinical outcomes of static spacers with mobile spacers for the treatment of infection following TKA. This paper was conducted in strict accordance with the PICOS principle of formulating the inclusion criteria, and the related literatures were collected and retrieved at home and abroad.

Methods

Search strategy

We searched the ("Total knee arthroplasty" OR "TKA" OR "joint replacement") AND ("periprosthetic joint infection" OR "infection") AND ("two-stage revision" OR "revision") AND ("antibiotic bone cement spacer" OR "Spacers" OR "articulating Spacer" OR "static Spacer") in PubMed, EMBASE and the Cochrane Library during January 1960 and October 2016. No regional and ethnic restriction was employed. All the subjects were humans. The detailed search process is shown in Fig. 1.

Inclusion and exclusion criteria

Studies were considered to be eligible if they met the following criteria: (1) randomized controlled study, retrospective case-control study, or prospective cohort study of the two-stage revision of the first complete knee arthroplasty (which may include a small number of patients after knee revision surgery); (2) the study contains articulating group and static group; (3) the studies contains at least one of the following measured indicators: number of infection eradication, soft tissue contracture after the two-stage of surgery, recurrence of infection during the period of postoperative follow-up, range of motion after operation, postoperative follow-up joint function scores, and the complications (bone loss, mechanical complications, etc.).

Studies were excluded if they met the following criteria: (1) the total number of samples less than 20 cases of the study; (2) review literature, no control group literature, medical records reported literature; (3) the mean follow-up time less than 12 months; (4) studies

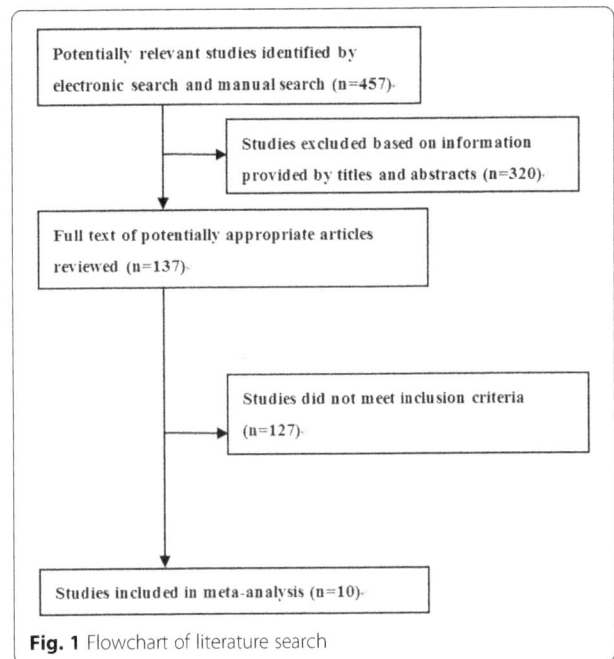

Fig. 1 Flowchart of literature search

from the same authors or repetitive reports; (5) poor quality observational studies; (6) non-English literature.

Data extraction

Literature data were extracted by Professor Ding Hai independently, and another two assistants validated these literatures. Any disagreement between reviewers was resolved by Professor Ding Hai. The data extracted included the first author, publication time, the type of study, the sample size, the patient's age, the average follow-up time, the type of antibiotic, the type of arthroplasty, the degree of preoperative joint activity, the degree of joint activity after revision at the final follow-up, number of recurrent infection at the final follow-up, knee score at the final follow-up, number of soft tissue angioplasty in the two stages of surgery, and postoperative complications (e.g., loss of bone loss and mechanical complications) at the final follow-up.

Quality evaluation

Among the ten included studies, nine were retrospective case-control and one was a prospective cohort study. Newcastle-Ottawa Scale (NOS) scale was used to evaluate the literature quality [15]. NOS adopt the semi-quantitative principle of the star system. Nine stars represented the highest quality followed by high quality (5 to 9 stars), and low quality between zero and four stars.

Statistical analysis

Review Manager 5.3 software was used for data analysis. The count data was expressed as the rates or the composition ratio. The odds ratio (OR) and 95% confidence interval (CI) were used to calculate the effect size. The measurement data were recorded by the mean and standard deviation (SD). The difference of the postoperative curative effect was based on the mean difference (MD) and the 95% CI. Then, we drew the forest map. $P < 0.05$ was considered to be statistically significant. Heterogeneity was assessed with the chi-square test value and I^2 value. Chi-square value of less than 0.1 and $I^2 > 50\%$ denoted a large heterogeneity among the included literatures, and the random effects model (RE) can be used to calculate the effect indicators. Conversely, the fixed effect model (FE) will apply. It should be noted that the heterogeneity of the source should be assessed if there is significant heterogeneity among the subjects.

Results
Study selection
Four hundred fifty-seven potentially eligible literatures were identified based on electronic databases search. After reviewing the titles and abstracts, 320 literatures did not meet the inclusion criteria. Subsequently, the full texts of the remaining 137 literatures were examined carefully. After excluding literatures with incomplete data, non-controls and those which are duplicated, a

total of ten studies were finally included in this study [6–8, 16–22]. All the included literatures were deemed suitable for our inclusion criteria in this meta-analysis. The search process is shown in Fig. 1.

Literature characteristics
The characteristics of the included studies were summarized in Table 1. There were 236 spacers in the articulating group and 256 in the static group. The number of samples ranged from 29 to 115, the mean postoperative follow-up period was more than 12 months. The antibiotic type of bone cement is mainly vancomycin or tobramycin, and then gentamicin or erythromycin. Articulating spacers can be divided into three types according to the production process: bone cement-bone cement type, metal-polyethylene type, and original pseudo-body type. Among the ten literatures, there was cement-bone cement type in six literatures, metal-polyethylene type in one literature, original pseudo-type in two literatures, and three coexisting type 1 literature. The NOS scores for these documents showed greater than 5 points, belonging to higher quality literature. The baseline information of the specific documents is shown in Table 1.

Table 1 Study characteristics

| Study | Type of study | Number of knees | | Age (A/S years) | M/F | Follow-up (months) | Type of antibiotic | Type of articulating positioner | Literature quality (NOS) |
		Articulating spacer group(A)	Static spacer group(S)						
Brunnekreef J 2013	Retrospective	26	9	61/58	15/20	12	Gentamycin/erythromycin	Metal-polyethylene	8
Johnson AJ 2012	Retrospective	34	81	62/61	NA	27/66	Vancomycin/tobramycin	Three different types	7
Choi HR 2012	Retrospective	14 (10)	33 (31)	64	23/24	58	Vancomycin/tobramycin	Original implant-bone cement	7
Chiang ER 2011	Prospective	23 (22)	22 (21)	71/72	22/23	41/40	Vancomycin	Bone cement-bone cement	7
Park SJ 2010	Retrospective	16	20	66.5/60.2	4/32	36/29	Vancomycin/erythromycin	Bone cement-bone cement	8
Freeman MG 2007	Retrospective	48	28	64.9/71.2	NA	Total 71.2 62.2/86.6	Vancomycin/tobramycin	Bone cement-bone cement	6
Hsu YC 2007	Retrospective	21	7	–	NA	58/101	Vancomycin/tobramycin or gentamicin	Bone cement-bone cement	8
Jämsen E 2006	Retrospective	24 (22)	10 (8)	68/70	11/23	32	NA	Original implant-bone cement	8
Emerson RH 2002	Retrospective	22	26	65.1/65.7	17/31	45.6/90	Vancomycin/tobramycin	Bone cement-bone cement	8
Fehring TK 2000	Retrospective	30 (15)[a]	25	NA	NA	27/36	Tobramycin	Bone cement-bone cement	7

Note: (1) The number in brackets in the sample size is the actual number of patients who completed the second revision and implantation of the new prosthesis (excluding the last document); (2) "NA" indicates that no information is available in the literature
[a]Fifteen is the number of patients who have actually completed follow-up

Clinical outcomes

Infection eradication

Among ten articles were evaluated by the infection eradication [6–8, 16–22]. There was no significant heterogeneity among these included subjects (χ^2 = 3.68, i^2 = 0, P = 0.88). The fixed effect model was used for data analysis, and the results showed that there was no significant difference regarding the eradication rate between the articulating and statics spacers in the two-stage revision surgery of postoperative infection after TKA (OR = 1.18, 95% CI: 0.66~2.11, P = 0.59) Fig. 2).

The release rate of soft tissue in two-stage revision (lengthening of the femoral quadriceps)

Among five literatures [7, 8, 18, 19, 21] were reported the release rate of soft tissue in two-stage revision (lengthening of the femoral quadriceps). There was moderate heterogeneity among the objects of study (χ^2 = 7.95, I^2 = 50%, P = 0.09) and using a random effects model. The results showed no significant difference regarding the release rate of soft tissue between articulating and static spacers in the two-stage revision of infection after TKA (OR = 0.65, 95% CI: 0.19~2.29, P = 0.50) (Fig. 3).

The release rate of soft tissue in two-stage revision (tibial tubercle osteotomy)

Among three literatures were evaluated the release rate of soft tissue (tibial tubercle osteotomy) in two-stage revision of infection after TKA [8, 16, 18]. There was a big heterogeneity between the object of these studies (χ^2 = 6.44, I^2 = 69%, P = 0.04). Random effects model was used for analysis. The results showed no significant difference between articulating and static spacers in the two-stage revision of infection after TKA regarding soft tissue release rate (tibial tubercle osteotomy) (OR = 0.55, 95% CI 0.10 to 3.13, P = 0.50) (Fig. 4).

Range of motion

Eight studies [6–8, 16–18, 21, 22] assessed the range of motion in this meta-analysis. There was a moderate heterogeneity among the subject in these studies (χ^2 = 16.73, I^2 = 52%, P = 0.03). Random effects model was used for analysis. The articulating group had greater postoperative ROM than the static group (MD = 12.19°, 95% CI 6.80~17.58, P < 0.00001) (Fig. 5).

KSS (function) score

Four studies assessed KSS (function) score [8, 20–22]. There was no significant heterogeneity between the object of these studies (χ^2 = 3.61, I^2 = 17%, P = 0.31). The fixed effect model was used for data analysis. There was a statistically significant difference between the articulating and static groups regarding KSS (function) score, and the articulating group had higher postoperative KSS (function) score than the static group (MD = 9.17, 95% CI 2.29~16.04, P = 0.009) (Fig. 6).

KSS (pain) score

Only three studies reported KSS (pain) score [8, 20, 22]. There was no significant heterogeneity between the object of these studies (χ^2 = 1.51, I^2 = 0%, P = 0.47). The fixed effect model was used for data analysis. There was no statistically significant difference between the articulating and static groups regarding KSS (pain) score (MD = 2.90, 95% CI: – 6.48~0.67, P = 0.11) (Fig. 7).

Hospital for Special Surgery (HSS) score

Three studies assessed HHS score [7, 8, 19] in the two-stage revision of infection after TKA. There was no significant heterogeneity between the object of these studies (χ^2 = 1.84, I^2 = 0%, P = 0.40). The fixed effect model was used for data analysis. There was a statistically significant difference between the articulating and static groups regarding HSS score, and the articulating group

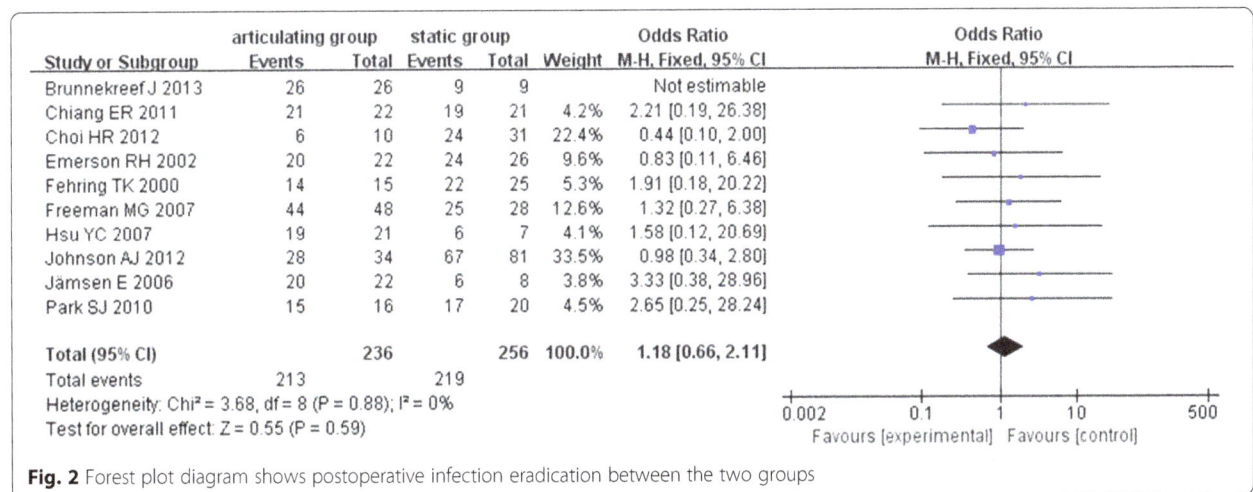

Fig. 2 Forest plot diagram shows postoperative infection eradication between the two groups

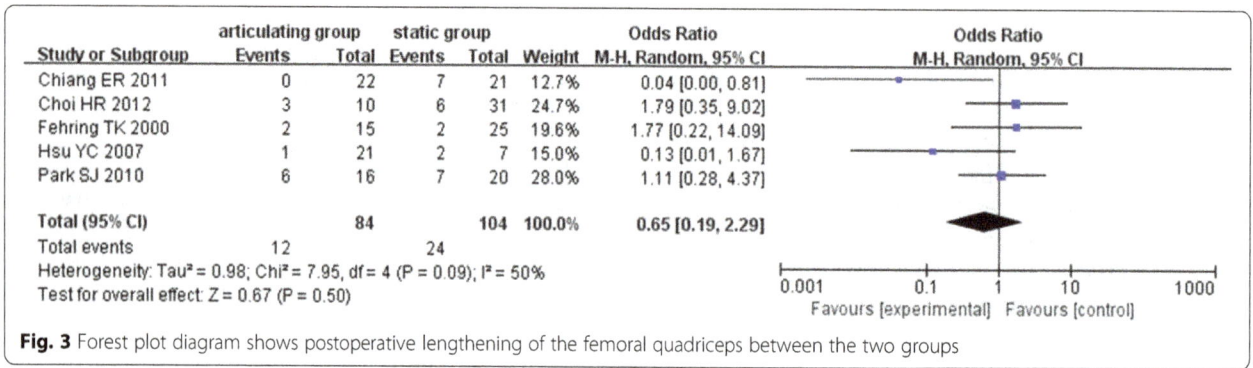

Fig. 3 Forest plot diagram shows postoperative lengthening of the femoral quadriceps between the two groups

had higher postoperative HSS score than the static group (MD = 7.00, 95% CI: 3.91~10.10, P < 0.00001) (Fig. 8).

Bone loss

There was less bone loss in the articulating group than in the static group [7, 8, 17, 21]. Fehring and Park reported that there was no bone loss in the articulating group [7, 8]. And Johnson and his colleague [17] demonstrated that more patients had severe bone loss in the static group (80%) than in the articulating group (53%). Femoral and tibial bone loss was 100% of the knees in the static group, while in the articulating group, only 28.6% of the knees with femoral bone loss, 47.6% of the knees with tibial bone loss [21].

Publication bias

The graphical funnel plot may of included studies for outcome measurements appeared to be symmetrical (Fig. 9). The spots are evenly distributed on both sides of the inverted funnel, suggesting that there was no significant publication bias in the retrieved documents.

Discussion

TKA has been regarded as an effective way to treat knee joint osteoarthritis, rheumatoid arthritis, and other advanced knee disorders since 1968. With the continuous improvement of surgical techniques and prosthetic design, TKA has become one of the most successful techniques in orthopedics. With the aging of the

population, the demand for total knee replacement is still increasing. The increase in the amount of surgery is associated with increasing postoperative complications, of which PJI is one of the greatest complications. The current "gold standard" for the treatment of periprosthetic infection is still the two-stage revision surgery, which can fundamentally eliminate the infection and create healthy and vigorous tissue for the preparation of new prosthesis implantation [23]. During the two-stage revision, the doctor's main goal is to prevent soft tissue contracture around the joint, which may lead to second operation exposure and refurbished prosthetic implant difficulties, and thus increased the surgical difficulties [24]. Therefore, it is crucial to maintain the stability of the knee joint and the balance of the soft tissue around the joint during the exclusion period of antibiotic bone cement. Moreover, there was a certain concentration of antibiotics in the knee joint to eradicate the infection [25, 26]. Currently, the antibiotic bone cement spacer can be divided into two categories, articulating type (hinge type) and static type (fixed type), and there was a significant controversy about whether articulating or static spacers can provide better outcomes. In this meta-analysis, we analyzed the difference of the two spacers regarding postoperative effects, including the infection eradication rate, the soft tissue release rate during the two-stage revision surgery, the ROM after the revision surgery, and function scores.

There was no significant difference between the two spacers regarding eradicate rate of infection in this

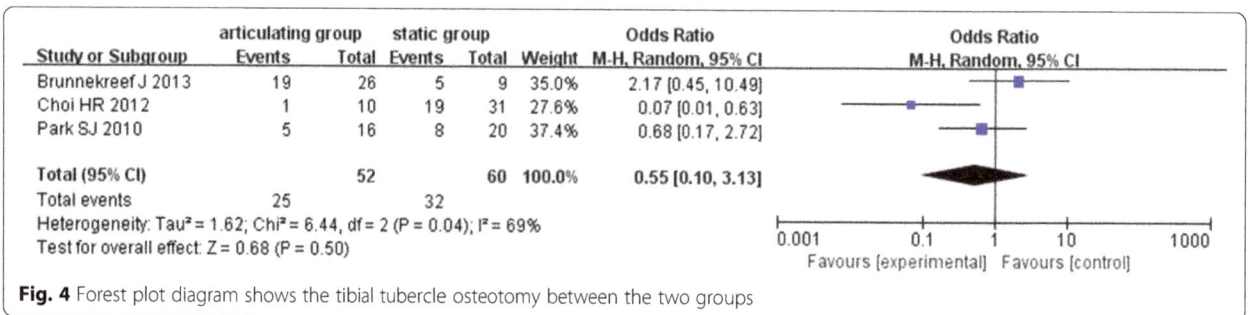

Fig. 4 Forest plot diagram shows the tibial tubercle osteotomy between the two groups

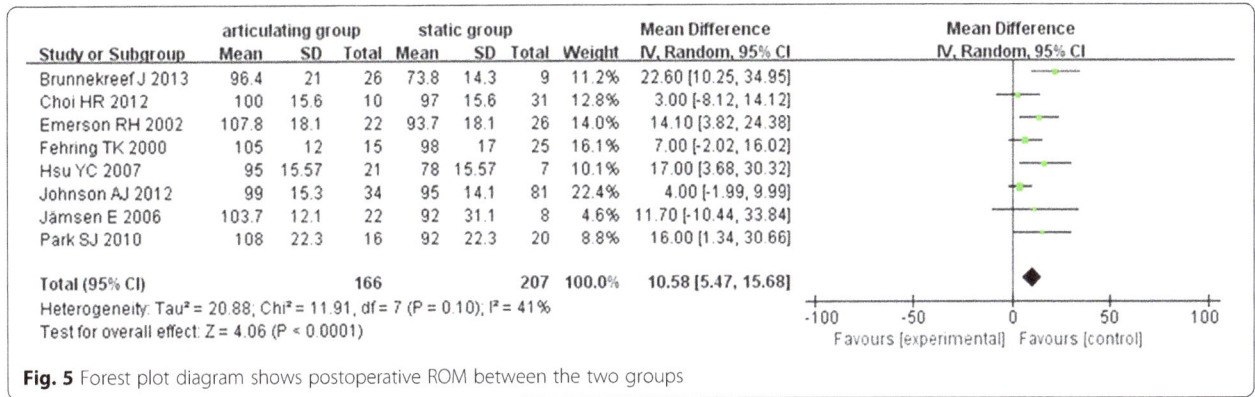

Fig. 5 Forest plot diagram shows postoperative ROM between the two groups

study. The majority of the included articles reported the similar antibiotic use time, antibiotics for at least 6 weeks in vivo during the period of spacers [6–8, 16–18, 20–22]. There is no consistent standard for the best mix of methods for preparing high-dose antibiotic bone cement spacers. Most of the antibiotics associated with spacers mainly vancomycin (1~4 g of added 40 g bone cement) or gentamicin, tobramycin (2.4~4.8 g of added 40 g bone cement) [25]. Bone cement spacers should have a sufficiently high level of antibiotic to provide a relatively high concentration of local tissue release levels, while the dose of antibiotics should be low enough to prevent the mechanical properties of bone cement spacers weakened [27]. John F. Nettrour et al. [28] reported that there was no dose-dependent of antibiotic bone cement. Voleti et al. [29] compared the clinical effects between the articulating and static groups, 1526 patients were included in their systematic review (872 cases of articulating spacers and 654 cases of statics spacers). Their findings indicated no statistical significance difference regarding the infection eradication. The results of Voleti et al. study are consistent with Piver et al. [30] study. In contrast, Romano et al. [31] showed that the articulating spacers can achieve higher infection eradication than the static spacers (91.2 versus 87%). However, some authors suggested that the static spacer can provide greater release and space for the soft tissue around the joint infection or blood transfusion and can better eliminate the infection [32].

ROM and functional recovery are indicators of postoperative efficacy. In this meta-analysis, the results of ROM and KSS (function) score in articulating group significance were higher than in the static group. However, there was no significant difference regarding HSS and KSS (pain) score between the two groups. Dr. Javad Parvizi and Thorsten Gehrke concluded that there was an encouraging postoperative function in patients which were treated with articulating spacers in the two-stage revision of the knee surgery. In contrast, the increasing trend of ROM in statics spacers was higher than those patients with articulating spacers after follow-up for 2 years. Their results were consistent with some larger scale systematical reviews [29, 30, 33].

In this study, the soft tissue release rate during the two-stage revision surgery was used to assess whether there were differences regarding soft tissue contracture between the two different spacers. The results showed that there was no significant difference between either quadriceps or tibial tubercle osteotomy in two different spacers. However, Guild et al. [33] found that the patients with articulating spacers were less associated with the assistive technology than those with static spacers. The reason may be that knee activities during the exclusion period helps to maintain the length and flexibility of the extensor device and prevent the formation of scar tissue around the knee, quadriceps shortening, and joint capsule thickening and contracture [34]. The results of our study suggest no significant difference regarding the

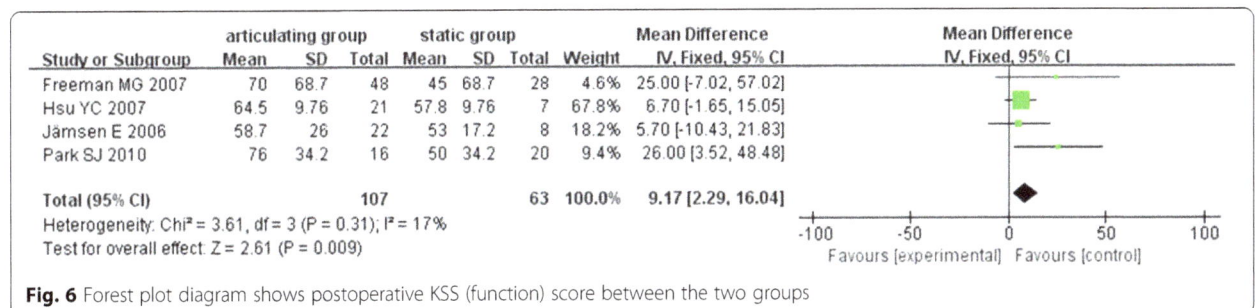

Fig. 6 Forest plot diagram shows postoperative KSS (function) score between the two groups

| Study or Subgroup | articulating group | | | static group | | | | Mean Difference | Mean Difference |
	Mean	SD	Total	Mean	SD	Total	Weight	IV, Fixed, 95% CI	IV, Fixed, 95% CI
Freeman MG 2007	45	18.9	48	50	18.9	28	16.5%	-5.00 [-13.81, 3.81]	
Jämsen E 2006	46.8	7.8	22	46	8.9	8	26.3%	0.80 [-6.18, 7.78]	
Park SJ 2010	42	8.14	16	46	5.79	20	57.2%	-4.00 [-8.73, 0.73]	
Total (95% CI)			**86**			**56**	**100.0%**	**-2.90 [-6.48, 0.67]**	
Heterogeneity: Chi² = 1.51, df = 2 (P = 0.47); I² = 0%									
Test for overall effect: Z = 1.59 (P = 0.11)									

Favours [experimental] Favours [control]

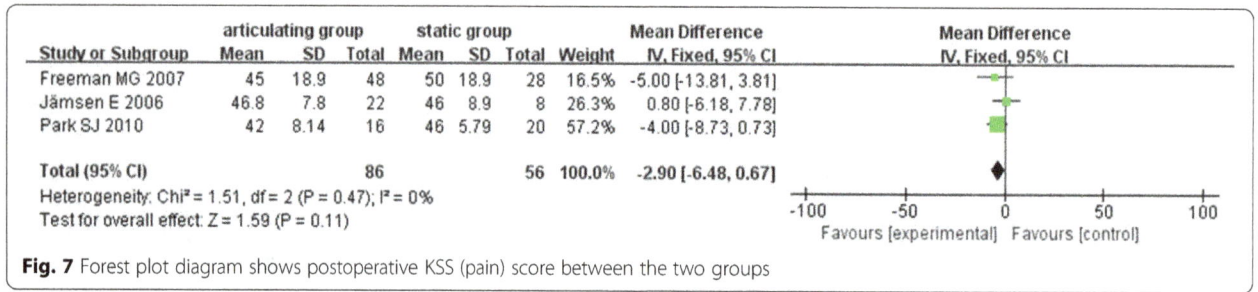

Fig. 7 Forest plot diagram shows postoperative KSS (pain) score between the two groups

soft tissue release rate, which may be due to the relatively small number of participants and sample size. Randomized controlled studies with larger number of samples are still required.

Bone loss is also a common complication during the exclusion period. Guild et al. [33] reported that there was less bone loss in articulating group than the static group. A retrospective case-control study [8] reported that 15 (75%) patients had pre-existing tibial or femoral bone loss in the static group, 10 cases (65%) had pre-existing tibial bone loss, 13 (65%) patients had femoral bone loss, and 8 patients had tibial bone loss. However, there was no bone loss in the articulating group. Some researchers demonstrated that the static spacers did not restore the normal knee anatomical profile [35]. In the traditional "block" static spacers, the bone cement surface and the bone surface are in point-like contact; the uneven pressure distribution and the local high point pressure lead to a large amount of bone loss during the exclusion period. However, with the continuous updating of the static type of the design of the spacers, there has been "internal skeleton" type static spacer, and the stability of the knee joint will be further strengthened. Yoo et al. [36] reported that the four patients using an internal skeleton-type static spacer showed excellent clinical outcomes and no bone loss, and noted that this technique may be more suitable for patients with suspected bone loss after removal of the prosthesis. For these patients, the articulating spacers cannot provide sufficient stability. Most of the included literatures did not provide sufficient data for the bone loss in our research.

There are several limitations in this meta-analysis. (1) There were no RCTs in this article, and retrospective case-control studies inevitably lead to the recall bias and the confounding bias between subjects and will lead to objectivity influences. (2) The length of follow-up period in patients with static and articulating groups was different in some literatures. Each article had different follow-up time. Although the duration of follow-up was greater than 12 months, the deviation caused by different follow-up time may also affect the objectivity of the results. (3) All included studies did not specify any inclusion or exclusion criteria to determine which patients would receive the articulating spacers or the static spacers, resulting in considerable selection bias. (4) All the included patients in this study had larger age span. The differences in medical and health levels will lead to greater differences in postoperative efficacy. (5) During the data extraction of some continuous variable data, only the mean values were available in the literature; therefore, the standard deviation was obtained by averaging and the P value or 95% CI [37], which may lead to bias in the outcome and affect the objectivity. (6) Due to the limited number of literature, it was not possible to provide sufficient data for subgroup analysis, which may be one of the sources of heterogeneity.

Conclusion

In this meta-analysis, we found no significant difference between articulating and static spacers in terms of infection eradication, the soft tissue contracture, and the knee pain scores. The patients with articulating spacers were able to achieve better ROM and limb function, but there

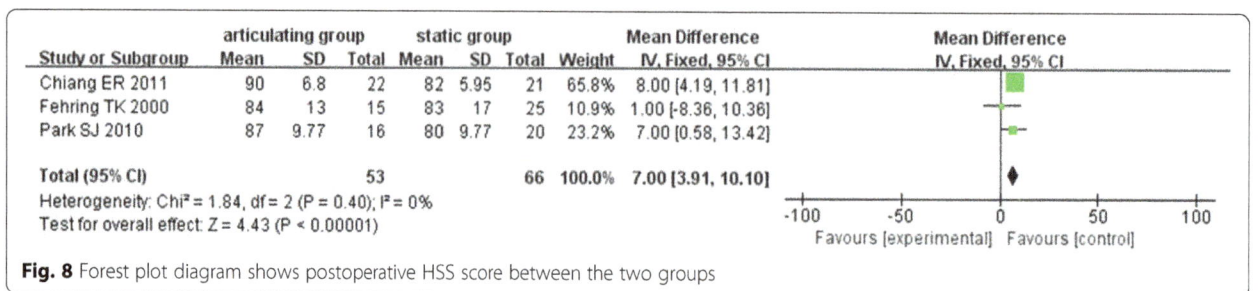

| Study or Subgroup | articulating group | | | static group | | | | Mean Difference | Mean Difference |
	Mean	SD	Total	Mean	SD	Total	Weight	IV, Fixed, 95% CI	IV, Fixed, 95% CI
Chiang ER 2011	90	6.8	22	82	5.95	21	65.8%	8.00 [4.19, 11.81]	
Fehring TK 2000	84	13	15	83	17	25	10.9%	1.00 [-8.36, 10.36]	
Park SJ 2010	87	9.77	16	80	9.77	20	23.2%	7.00 [0.58, 13.42]	
Total (95% CI)			**53**			**66**	**100.0%**	**7.00 [3.91, 10.10]**	
Heterogeneity: Chi² = 1.84, df = 2 (P = 0.40); I² = 0%									
Test for overall effect: Z = 4.43 (P < 0.00001)									

Favours [experimental] Favours [control]

Fig. 8 Forest plot diagram shows postoperative HSS score between the two groups

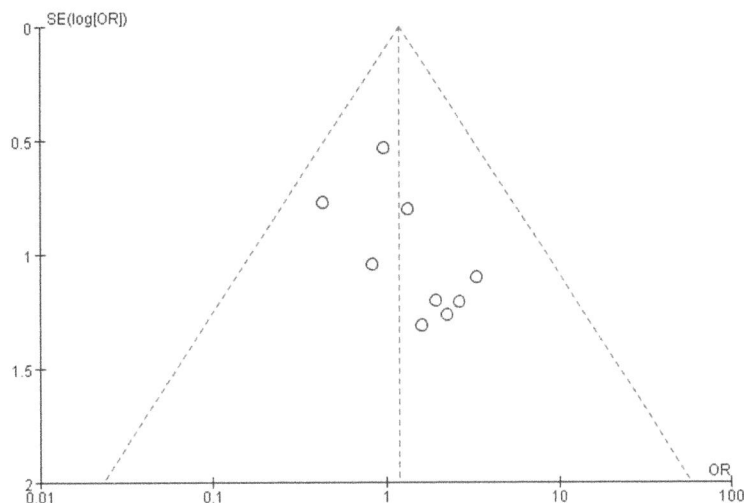

Fig. 9 The graphical funnel plot

was no significant difference in postoperative pain between the static and articulating spacers. Further randomized controlled studies on these two different spacers are still required to be carried out to provide more accurate and objective data for a comprehensive and accurate analysis.

Abbreviations
CI: Confidence interval; FE: Fixed effect model; HSS: Hospital for special surgery knee score; KSS: American Knee Society knee score; MD: Mean difference; NOS: Newcastle-Ottawa Scale; OR: Odds ratio; PJI: Prosthetic joint infection; RE: Random effects; SD: Standard deviation; TKA: Total knee arthroplasty

Acknowledgements
None

Funding
None.

Authors' contributions
HD conceived the manuscript and wrote the manuscript. JY interpreted the patient data. WC collected and analyzed the patient data. FL searched literatures. All authors read and approved the final manuscript.

Competing interests
The authors declare that they have no competing interests.

References
1. Kurtz SM, Lau E, Schmier J, Ong KL, Zhao K, Parvizi J. Infection burden for hip and knee arthroplasty in the United States. J Arthroplast. 2008;23(7):984–91. https://doi.org/10.1016/j.arth.2007.10.017.
2. Kurtz SM, Ong KL, Lau E, Bozic KJ, Berry D, Parvizi J. Prosthetic joint infection risk after TKA in the Medicare population. Clin Orthop Relat Res. 2010;468(1):52–6. https://doi.org/10.1007/s11999-009-1013-5.
3. Sherrell JC, Fehring TK, Odum S, Hansen E, Zmistowski B, Dennos A, et al. The Chitranjan Ranawat Award: fate of two-stage reimplantation after failed irrigation and debridement for periprosthetic knee infection. Clin Orthop Relat Res. 2011;469(1):18–25. https://doi.org/10.1007/s11999-010-1434-1.
4. Parvizi J, Della Valle CJ. AAOS Clinical Practice Guideline: diagnosis and treatment of periprosthetic joint infections of the hip and knee. J Am Acad Orthop Surg. 2010;18(12):771–2.
5. Lonner JH, Barrack R, Fitzgerald RH Jr, Hanssen AD, Windsor ER. Infection in total knee arthroplasty: part I. Classification, prophylaxis, and diagnosis. American journal of orthopedics (Belle Mead, NJ) 1999;28(9):530-535.
6. Jr ER, Muncie M, Tarbox TR, Higgins LL. Comparison of a static with a mobile spacer in total knee infection. Clin Orthop Relat Res. 2002;404(404): 132.
7. Fehring TK, Odum S, Calton TF, Mason JB. Articulating versus static spacers in revision total knee arthroplasty for sepsis. The Ranawat Award. Clin Orthop Relat Res. 2000;380(380):9–16.
8. Park SJ, Song EK, Seon JK, Yoon TR, Park GH. Comparison of static and mobile antibiotic-impregnated cement spacers for the treatment of infected total knee arthroplasty. Int Orthop. 2010;34(8):1181–6.
9. Toms AD, Davidson D, Masri BA, Duncan CP. The management of periprosthetic infection in total joint arthroplasty. J Bone Joint Surg. 2006;88(88): 149–55.
10. Pitto RP, Castelli CC, Ferrari R, Munro J. Pre-formed articulating knee spacer in two-stage revision for the infected total knee arthroplasty. Int Orthop. 2005;29(5):305–8.
11. Kraay MJ, Goldberg VM, Fitzgerald SJ, Salata MJ. Cementless two-staged total hip arthroplasty for deep periprosthetic infection. Clin Orthop Relat Res. 2006;441(441):243–9.
12. Calton TF, Fehring TK, Griffin WL. Bone loss associated with the use of spacer blocks in infected total knee arthroplasty. Clin Orthop Relat Res. 1997;345(345):148–54.
13. Klekamp J, Dawson JM, Haas DW, Deboer D, Christie M. The use of vancomycin and tobramycin in acrylic bone cement: biomechanical effects and elution kinetics for use in joint arthroplasty. J Arthroplast. 1999;14(3): 339–46.
14. Pietsch M, Hofmann S, Wenisch C. Zweizeitiger Prothesenwechsel bei infizierter Knieendoprothese. Oper Orthop Traumatol. 2006;18(1):66–87.
15. Asadollahi S, Sorial R, Coffey S, Gupta M, Eslick GD. Total knee arthroplasty after patellectomy: a meta-analysis of case-control studies. Knee. 2017;24(2): 191–6. https://doi.org/10.1016/j.knee.2017.01.004.
16. Brunnekreef J, Hannink G, Malefijt MW. Recovery of knee mobility after a static or mobile spacer in total knee infection. Acta Orthop Belg. 2013;79(1):83–9.
17. Johnson AJ, Sayeed SA, Naziri Q, Khanuja HS, Mont MA. Minimizing dynamic knee spacer complications in infected revision arthroplasty. Clin Orthop Relat Res. 2012;470(1):220–7.
18. Choi HR, Malchau H, Bedair H. Are prosthetic spacers safe to use in 2-stage treatment for infected total knee arthroplasty? J Arthroplast. 2012;27(8):1474–9.e1.
19. Chiang ER, Su YP, Chen TH, Chiu FY, Chen WM. Comparison of articulating and static spacers regarding infection with resistant organisms in total knee arthroplasty. Acta Orthop. 2011;82(4):460.

20. Freeman MG, Fehring TK, Odum SM, Fehring K, Griffin WL, Mason JB. Functional advantage of articulating versus static spacers in 2-stage revision for total knee arthroplasty infection. J Arthroplast. 2007;22(8):1116.
21. Hsu YC, Cheng HC, Ng TP, Chiu KY. Antibiotic-loaded cement articulating spacer for 2-stage reimplantation in infected total knee arthroplasty : a simple and economic method. J Arthroplast. 2007;22(7):1060–6.
22. Jämsen PS E, Halonen P, Lehto MUK, Moilanen T, Pajamäki J, Puolakka T, Konttinen YT. Spacer prostheses in two-stage revision of infected knee arthroplasty. Int Orthop. 2006;30(4):257–61.
23. Iarikov D, Demian H, Rubin D, Alexander J, Nambiar S. Choice and doses of antibacterial agents for cement spacers in treatment of prosthetic joint infections: review of published studies. Clin Infect Dis. 2012;55(11):1474.
24. Antoci V, Phillips MJ, Krackow KA. The treatment of recurrent chronic infected knee arthroplasty with a 2-stage procedure. J Arthroplast. 2009; 24(1):13–7.
25. Jacobs C, Christensen CP, Berend ME. Static and mobile antibiotic-impregnated cement spacers for the management of prosthetic joint infection. J Am Acad Orthop Surg. 2009;17(6):356–68.
26. Incavo SJ, Russell RD, Mathis KB, Adams H. Initial results of managing severe bone loss in infected total joint arthroplasty using customized articulating spacers. J Arthroplast. 2009;24(4):607–13.
27. Paz E, Sanzruiz P, Abenojar J, Vaqueromartín J, Forriol F, Del Real JC. Evaluation of elution and mechanical properties of high-dose antibiotic-loaded bone cement: comparative "in vitro" study of the influence of vancomycin and cefazolin. J Arthroplast. 2015;30(8):1423–9.
28. Nettrour JF, Polikandriotis JA, Bernasek TL, Gustke KA, Lyons ST. Articulating spacers for the treatment of infected total knee arthroplasty: effect of antibiotic combinations and concentrations. Orthopedics. 2013;36(1):19–24.
29. Voleti PB, Baldwin KD, Lee GC. Use of static or articulating spacers for infection following total knee arthroplasty: a systematic literature review. J Bone Joint Surg (Am Vol). 2013;95(17):1594–9.
30. Pivec R, Naziri Q, Issa K, Banerjee S, Mont MA. Systematic review comparing static and articulating spacers used for revision of infected total knee arthroplasty. J Arthroplast. 2014;29(3):553–7.
31. Romanò CL, Gala L, Logoluso N, Romanò D, Drago L. Two-stage revision of septic knee prosthesis with articulating knee spacers yields better infection eradication rate than one-stage or two-stage revision with static spacers. Knee Surgery Sports Traumatology Arthroscopy Official Journal of the Esska. 2012;20(12):2445–53.
32. Faschingbauer M, Bieger R, Reichel H, Weiner C, Kappe T. Complications associated with 133 static, antibiotic-laden spacers after TKA. Knee Surg Sports Traumatol Arthrosc. 2015;24(10):1–4.
33. Rd GG, Wu B, Scuderi GR. Articulating vs. static antibiotic impregnated spacers in revision total knee arthroplasty for sepsis. A systematic review. J Arthroplast. 2014;29(3):558–63.
34. Thabe H, Schill S. Two-stage reimplantation with an application spacer and combined with delivery of antibiotics in the management of prosthetic joint infection. Oper Orthop Traumatol. 2007;19(1):78–100.
35. Shen H, Zhang X, Jiang Y, Wang Q, Chen Y, Wang Q et al. Intraoperatively-made cement-on-cement antibiotic-loaded articulating spacer for infected total knee arthroplasty 2010;17(6):407–11.
36. Yoo J, Lee S, Han C, Chang J. The modified static spacers using antibiotic-impregnated cement rod in two-stage revision for infected total knee arthroplasty. Clinics in Orthopedic Surgery. 2011;3(3):245–8.
37. Higgins JP, Green S. Cochrane handbook of systematic reviews of interventions. Wiley-Blackwell. 2008;5(14):102–8.

16

Comparison of the clinical effectiveness of US grading scoring system vs MRI in the diagnosis of early rheumatoid arthritis (RA)

Huajun Xu[1,2], Yingchun Zhang[1*], Huimei Zhang[3], Caishan Wang[1] and Pan Mao[1]

Abstract

Background: As an irreversible disease, a treatment delay can negatively affect treatment response in rheumatoid arthritis (RA). Ultrasound and MRI have played an important role in assessing disease progression and response to treatment in RA for many years. The present study was designed to compare the diagnostic efficacy of ultrasound grading and MRI in early RA.

Methods: In this retrospective study, 62 early RA patients within 12 months of symptom onset were included. DAS28, rheumatoid factor (RF), CRP, ESR, and anti-cyclic citrullinated peptide antibody (CCP) of the patients were measured. Bilateral hand joints and wrists were examined by ultrasonography (US) and MRI; diagnosis outcome was compared. Relationship between DAS28 scores, laboratory parameters, and ultrasound findings were analyzed.

Results: Ultrasound and MRI had an equivalent diagnosis value in synovitis, joint effusion, and tenosynovitis. The detection rate of synovitis, arthroedema, and tenosynovitis on ultrasound and MRI was very close ($P > 0.05$). The detection rate of bone erosion was lower in ultrasonography than that in MRI ($P < 0.05$). There were significant differences between power Doppler ultrasonography (PDUS) and gray-scale ultrasonography (GSUS) in the diagnosis of synovitis ($x^2 = 3.92$, $P < 0.05$); the sensitivity of GSUS was better than that of PDUS ($P < 0.05$). PDUS was positively correlated with DAS28, ESR, CRP, and CCP ($P < 0.01$), but not correlated with RF and disease duration ($P > 0.05$). GSUS was positively correlated with RF and CRP ($P < 0.01$), but not correlated with DAS28, CCP, ESR, and disease duration ($P > 0.05$). Bone erosion was positively correlated with disease duration, CCP, and RF ($P < 0.01$) and was not correlated with DAS28, ESR, and CRP ($P > 0.05$).

Conclusion: Ultrasonography has a high reliability in the diagnosis of early RA in synovitis, joint effusion, tenosynovitis, and bone erosion. Ultrasonography and clinical and laboratory parameters had a great correlativity. Both ultrasound and MRI are effective techniques. In view of the advantages of low cost and convenience, ultrasound may be a better choice during early RA diagnosis.

Keywords: Ultrasound, Early rheumatoid arthritis, MRI, DAS28 score

Background

Rheumatoid arthritis (RA) is a chronic, systemic inflammatory disorder that can inflict joint destruction and malformation resulting in functional disability [1, 2]. A delay in initiating therapy could adversely affect treatment outcomes such as disease activity, remission, functional capacity, and radiographic progression [3–5]. The pathophysiology of RA is not completely understood, and no single test or gold standard exists to confirm the diagnosis. Hence, the diagnosis is made based on a set of findings and symptoms typical for the RA phenotype rather than measurement of the specific pathogenic processes that lead to this phenotype [3]. Early RA is most likely to erode wrist, metacarpophalangeal, and interphalangeal joints [6, 7]; synovial pannus may cause gradual erosion of the articular cartilage and bone cortex after its formation, so early diagnosis and effective treatment is very important [8, 9].

* Correspondence: zhangyingchun_88@126.com
[1]Department of Ultrasound, The Second Affiliated Hospital of Soochow University, San Xiang Road 1055, Suzhou 215004, China
Full list of author information is available at the end of the article

Conventional radiography remains the mainstay for evaluation of RA patients in daily practice [10, 11]. However, as the X-ray shows late signs of disease activity and destruction of cartilage or bone, other medical imaging techniques such as ultrasonography (US) and MRI are used in RA in order to assess the earlier signs [12]. Musculoskeletal ultrasound is a readily available, useful, and versatile imaging modality with high patient acceptability [13]. In patients with arthritis, gray-scale ultrasonography (GSUS) is more sensitive than clinical examination for detecting synovitis [14, 15] and more sensitive than conventional radiography for detecting bone erosions [15, 16]. Power Doppler (PD) has been introduced for the assessment of synovitis and may provide additional information [17, 18]. Musculoskeletal ultrasound has been confirmed to be more accurate than clinical inspection in detecting synovitis and tenosynovitis [19]. The initiation of synovial inflammation is characterized by periarticular vasodilatation followed by synovial proliferation, which is accompanied by angiogenesis resulting in intra-articular new blood vessel formation. Power Doppler US (PDUS) makes it possible to discriminate between peri- and intra-articular blood flow in microvessels and to demonstrate synovial proliferation [20], while GSUS mainly assess the abnormalities of synovial morphology caused by synovitis [21].

Previously, some simplified ultrasound scoring methods have been reported and analyzed correlatively with clinical manifestations [22]. But there is a lack of contrast between clinical, laboratory, and radiologic imaging. The sensitivity and specificity of ultrasound inflammatory parameters (GSUS and PDUS) for the diagnosis of synovitis are not yet clear [23]. Magnetic resonance imaging (MRI) can directly visualize the bone and soft tissues in three dimensions and has the potential to measure inflammatory activity and joint destruction [24]. The sensitivity of ultrasound for detecting joint inflammation relative to MRI is yet to be determined.

The primary objective of this study was to investigate the sensitivity and specificity of ultrasonography (GSUS and PDUS) compared to MRI in early RA diagnosis and to compare the detection rate between ultrasound and MRI in terms of synovitis, joint effusion, tenosynovitis, and bone erosion. The secondary objective was to analyze the correlation between laboratory parameters and ultrasound findings and to analyze the reliability of each parameter of ultrasound in early RA diagnosis.

The present study was designed to compare the diagnostic efficacy of ultrasound grading and MRI in early RA. In this study, the wrist, metacarpophalangeal, and proximal interphalangeal joints were examined by ultrasound grading; the ultrasonographic features of the lesions were observed and compared with MRI and clinical and laboratory parameters; relationship between DAS28 scores, laboratory parameters, and ultrasound findings were analyzed.

Methods
Patients

From January 2012 to June 2016, 62 early RA patients in the outpatient department and inpatient department of Rheumatology in our hospital were enrolled in our study. This study was approved by the ethics committee of the local hospital, and informed consent was obtained from all patients. All patients underwent routine medical history inquiry, physical examination, and laboratory examination such as ESR, CRP rheumatoid factor (RF), and anti-cyclic citrullinated peptide antibody (CCP). In these 62 patients, 1364 joints of the wrist, metacarpophalangeal, and proximal interphalangeal were both examined by color Doppler ultrasonography and MRI.

Inclusion criteria include the following: within 12 months of RA symptom onset and diagnosis of RA was based on 2010 ACR/EULAR Early RA Classification and Scoring Criteria [25]. The selection of the early RA patients was supervised by two experienced rheumatologists.

The exclusion criteria were as follows: age < 18; history of rheumatoid arthritis > 2 years; been treated with anti-rheumatic drugs (methotrexate, chloroquine, leflunomide, NSAIDs, and salazosulfadimidine) previously; history of glucocorticoid usage in the past 3 months; and history of joint trauma, bacterial infection (such as purulent arthritis), or surgery.

Clinical data collection

General clinical data including gender, age, course of disease, and laboratory parameters such as ESR, CRP, RF, and CCP were collected. Clinical physical examination was conducted by the same doctor attending the Department of Rheumatism, to simplify the examination of 28 joints. TJC28 and SJC28 were recorded and DAS28 was calculated.

DAS28 was calculated as follows. (1) TJC28 (tender joint count): a total of 28 cases of bilateral metacarpophalangeal joint, proximal interphalangeal joint, wrist joint, elbow joint, shoulder joint, and knee joint were examined and TJC28 was calculated; (2) SJC28 (swollen joint count): check the swelling situation of the above 28 joints and calculate the SJC28. DAS28 = [0.56 × SQRT (TJC28) + 0.28 × SQRT (SJC28) + 0.70 × Ln (ESR)] × 1.08 + 0.16. DAS value > 5.1 indicates high disease activity; DAS < 3.2 indicates low disease activity; and DAS < 2.6 indicates disease remission [26].

Ultrasonography

MyLab70 (Biosound Easote), PHILIPS iU 22 high-grade color ultrasonic diagnostic apparatus, and a 10~18-MHz linear array probe were used for ultrasonic inspection. Low-pass filter, pulse repetition frequency (1000~1800 Hz), and no Doppler signal which appear behind the bone cortex are regarded as the advisable maximum gain. The inspection was performed by two ultrasound doctors who had more than 5 years of experience with musculoskeletal ultrasonography, and the two doctors had similar musculoskeletal experience. The transducer was placed in the wrist region, metacarpophalangeal (MCP), and proximal interphalangeal (PIP) joints on the dorsal and palmar view, bilaterally. All the joints were assessed in transversal and longitudinal scans. A total of 1364 joints of the wrist, metacarpophalangeal, and proximal interphalangeal joints of the 62 patients were examined. Inflammatory changes and joint structural damage of ultrasound were recorded; GSUS synovial hyperplasia, PDUS color signal, and bone erosion were graded with a semi-quantitative method. A higher score between the scores of metacarpophalangeal and proximal interphalangeal joints was taken as a representative. The ultrasound images were assessed by the above ultrasound doctors. The interrater reliability of the two ultrasonographers during the obtainment of the GSUS and PDUS was evaluated by κ statistics ($\kappa = 0.75$–0.85). Once divergence occurred during the ultrasound grading evaluation, the two parties shall solve the difference through consultation.

The following are the US classification standards [22]:

1) Synovial thickening (GSUS)

Synovial thickening was analyzed as follows: grade 0 (absence), grade 1 (small hypoechoic/anechoic line beneath joint capsule), grade 2 (joint capsule elevated parallel to joint area), and grade 3 (strong distension of joint capsule) [27, 28].

2) PDUS

PDUS was performed for synovitis and tenosynovitis in each scanning plane described above. The semi-quantitative findings of PDUS activity for synovitis were scored as follows: grade 0 = no intra-articular color signal; grade 1 = up to three single color signals or two single color signals and one confluent color signal representing only low flow; grade 2 = < 50% of the intra-articular area filled with color signals representing clear flow; and grade 3 = 50% of the intra-articular area filled with color signals.

3) Bone erosion score

The following are the bone erosion scores: grade 0 = continuous cortical bone; grade 1 = the surface of the bone cortex was not smooth, but there was no obvious bone defect in two perpendicular sections; grade 2 = cortical bone defects can be seen in two perpendicular sections; and grade 3 = extensive bone defects on the surface of the cortical bone.

4) Tenosynovitis

The sonogram showed a thickening of the tendon, reduced and uneven echo, unclear normal fibrous structure, irregular margin, and edema in the surrounding tissues. Blood flow signal in the tendon sheath can be detected by power Doppler US (PDUS) [29]. Ultrasound showed normal tendon sheaths were recorded as negative (0 points) and the abnormality was recorded as positive (1 point).

5) Joint effusion

The ultrasound of the joint effusion showed no echo or hypoechoic area in the articular cavity, to be compressible, and no color Doppler flow signal. The thickness of articular cavity effusion < 2 mm was recorded as negative (0 points) and > 2 mm was recorded as positive (1 point).

MRI examination

GE Signa HDX 3.0 T MRI scanner (GE, USA) was used for MRI examination. All 62 patients were placed in a prone position with hands flat over the head and placed in the wrist joint coil; the hand back was fixed with a tape, so that the metacarpal and phalanx were placed in a same plane. MRI scanning sequences included SE T1WI coronal plane (TR 300 ms, TE 14 ms, matrix 512 × 256, layer thickness 3 mm, interval 0.5 mm), FastSE (FSE) T2WI coronal plane (TR 2000 ms, TE 42 ms, matrix 384 × 224, layer thickness 4 mm, interval 0.5 mm), and axial plane. Sixty-two patients underwent bilateral wrist MRI, and the MRI tablets were diagnosed by two Deputy Chief MRI diagnostic physicians. Once divergence occurred during MRI examination, the two parties shall solve the difference through consultation.

Statistical analysis

Quantitative data for normal distribution were expressed as means ± standard (SD); the skew distribution data were expressed as median (M) and quartile spacing (Q); qualitative data was expressed as rate. SPSS 22.0 (SPSS Inc., USA) was used for statistical analysis. The detection rates of synovitis, tenosynovitis, joint effusion, and bone erosion were compared by paired chi-square test. The differences in the assessment of synovial fluid between GSUS and

Table 1 General clinical data of all patients

Item	
Gender (male/female)	13/49
Mean age (years)	42.5 ± 12.1
Mean duration of disease (months)	7.6 ± 3.5
DAS28 score	4.14 ± 1.24
CRP (mg/L)	31.12 ± 11.25
ESR (mm/h)	42 ± 12.05
RF (n/%)	38/61.29%
CCP (+) (n/%)	33/53.23%
Tenosynovitis (n/%)	19/31.23%
Joint effusion (n/%)	18/29.55%
GSUS score (M/Q)	2.0/1.75
PDUS score (M/Q)	1.0/0.75
Bone erosion score (M/Q)	1.0/1

Data presented as means ± SD, or n patients
ESR erythrocyte sedimentation rate, *CRP* C-reactive protein, *CPP* anti-cyclic citrullinated peptide antibody, *GSUS* gray-scale ultrasonography, *PDUS* power Doppler ultrasonography

Table 2 Ultrasonic classification index (joint number: $n = 1364$)

Ultrasonic indicators	Points	Constituent ratio
GSUS score	0	290 (21.26%)
	1	285 (20.89%)
	2	708 (51.91%)
	3	81 (5.94%)
PDUS score	0	352 (25.81%)
	1	652 (47.80%)
	2	283 (20.75%)
	3	77 (5.65%)
Bone erosion score	0	792 (58.06%)
	1	306 (22.43%)
	2	218 (15.98%)
	3	48 (3.52%)
Tenosynovitis	0	938 (68.77%)
	1	426 (31.23%)
Joint effusion	0	961 (70.45%)
	1	403 (29.55%)

GSUS gray-scale ultrasonography, *PDUS* power Doppler ultrasonography

PDUS were compared using the paired chi-square test. Spearman rank correlation analysis was used to evaluate the correlation between the indexes of ultrasonic grading and clinical and laboratory parameters. $P < 0.05$ indicated that the difference was statistically significant.

Results

General clinical data of all patients

Sixty-two early RA patients (13 males/49 females) were included in our experiment. The general clinical data of all patients and the ultrasonic classification index are listed in Tables 1 and 2, respectively.

Comparison of ultrasonography and MRI examination in the diagnosis of RA

When the PDUS or GSUS score is ≥ 1, the diagnostic result is considered positive for early RA.

The detection rates of synovitis, tenosynovitis, arthroedema, and bone erosion were compared. The detection rates of synovitis, arthroedema, and tenosynovitis on ultrasound and MRI were very close ($P > 0.05$). The

Table 3 Comparison of ultrasonography and MRI examination in the diagnosis of RA (joint number: $n = 1364$)

Method	Synovitis	Joint effusion	Tenosynovitis	Bone erosion
US	1074 (78.74%)	403 (29.55%)	426 (31.23%)	572 (41.94%)
MRI	1053 (77.20%)	420 (30.79%)	446 (32.70%)	886 (64.96%)
χ^2	0.94	0.50	0.67	145.26
P	0.33	0.48	0.41	0.0001

When the PDUS or GSUS score is ≥ 1, the diagnostic result is considered positive for early RA

Table 4 Comparison of GSUS and PDUS in the evaluation of synovitis

Ultrasonic indicators	Positive/negative	Positive rate	χ^2	P
GSUS	1074/290	78.74%	7.83	< 0.05
PDUS	1012/352	74.20%		

detection rate of bone erosion was lower in ultrasonography than in MRI ($P < 0.05$) (Table 3).

Analysis of the evaluation of synovitis by ultrasonography

As is shown in Table 4 and Fig. 1, there were 1074 GSUS-positive and 1012 PDUS-positive joints among all 1364 joints, with a positive rate of 78.74 and 74.20%, respectively. There were significant differences between PDUS and GSUS in the diagnosis of synovitis ($\chi^2 = 3.92$, $P < 0.05$); the sensitivity of GSUS was better than PDUS ($P < 0.05$).

Correlation between ultrasonography and clinical and laboratory parameters

According to the results of Spearman rank correlation analysis, PDUS was significantly positively correlated with DAS28, ESR, CRP, and CCP ($P < 0.01$), while no significant correlation was found between PDUS, RF, and course of disease. GSUS was positively correlated with RF and CRP ($P < 0.01$), and there was no significant correlation with DAS28, CCP, ESR, and course of disease. Significant positive correlation was found between bone erosion and duration of disease, CCP, and RF ($P < 0.01$), and there was no significant correlation with DAS28, ESR, and CRP ($P > 0.05$) (Table 5).

Discussion

With the development of high-frequency ultrasound technology, ultrasound plays an increasingly important role in the early radiographic imaging of RA. The thickened

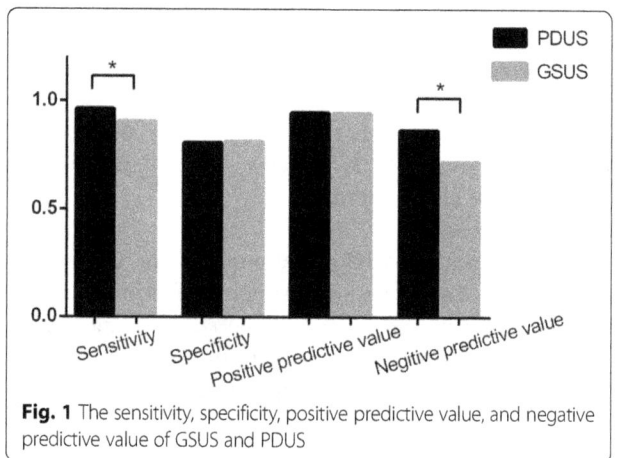

Fig. 1 The sensitivity, specificity, positive predictive value, and negative predictive value of GSUS and PDUS

Table 5 Correlation between the indexes of ultrasonic grading and clinical and laboratory parameters

Clinical and laboratory parameters	r (GSUS)	r (PDUS)	r (bone erosion)
Duration of disease	0.09	0.16	0.40*
DAS28	0.13	0.39*	− 0.15
CRP	0.31*	0.39*	0.16
ESR	0.13	0.41*	− 0.05
RF	0.30*	0.12	0.35*
CCP	0.18	0.29*	0.37*

*$P < 0.05$, statistically significant

synovial tissue can be observed by GSUS, and the low velocity blood flow signal in synovial tissue can be displayed by PDUS, which is of great significance for clinical diagnosis and treatment of RA [30]. Previously, some simplified ultrasound scoring methods have been reported and analyzed correlatively with clinical manifestations. Luz et al. proposed a novel ultrasound scoring system for hand and wrist joints (US10) and for evaluation of patients with early RA and correlated the US10 with clinical, laboratory, and functional variables. The proposed US10 scoring system proved to be a useful tool for monitoring inflammation and joint damage in early RA [31].

As the joint capsule, synovial membrane, tendons, ligaments, and other soft tissue attached to the bone surface, in the relatively simple anatomy of the limb joints, these soft tissues are easy to be scanned by ultrasound. At present, ultrasound has a high reliability in the diagnosis of inflammatory lesions of RA. The application value of ultrasound diagnosis has been widely recognized by rheumatologists [32–34]. In the evaluation of joint structure, our study showed that 572 cases of bone destruction were detected by ultrasound, while 886 cases were detected by MRI (Figs. 2 and 3). The comparison of GSUS and PDUS in synovitis evaluation showed that GSUS was superior to PDUS in diagnostic sensitivity and negative predictive values; the diagnostic specificity and positive predictive value were not significantly different between GSUS and PDUS. The results of GSUS and PDUS confirmed the synovial tissue congestion and inflammatory thickening changes of early RA. Studies have shown that this subclinical synovitis is closely related to the structural damage of RA patients [35, 36]. Effective treatment can eliminate the blood flow signal in PDUS, which has a positive effect on prolonging the remission of disease in RA patients.

The presentation of ultrasound on synovial inflammation was related to RA disease activity; PDUS can better reflect the disease activity [37]. No significant correlation was found between GSUS and DAS28, CCP, ESR, and course of disease ($P > 0.05$); this may be related to the slow thickening of synovial membrane and regression of inflammation during early RA. Significant positive correlation was found between bone erosion and duration of disease, CCP, and RF; this suggested that bone erosion is a progressive destructive process in rheumatoid arthritis and it is irreversible once it appears. Traditional X-ray lacks sensitivity to early bone erosion [38, 39].

Although it has been proven that MRI has a strong correlation with histological data and provides a predictive value in structural joint damage, MRI is rather expensive, time-consuming, not always available

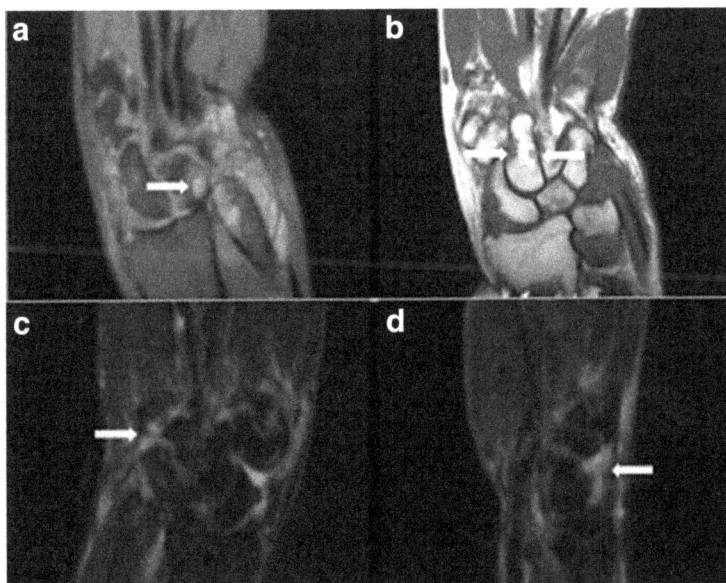

Fig. 2 Typical case: 52-year-old female diagnosed with RA for 1 year. MRI: carpal synovitis with bone destruction. **a** T2WI: oval high signal within the lunare bone—pannus formation. **b** T1WI: carpal bones showed low signal loss—bone destruction. **c, d** T2WI: carpal synovitis

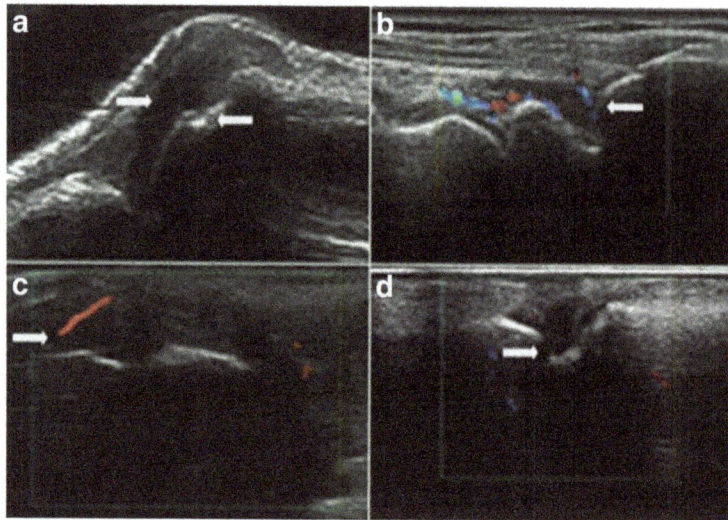

Fig. 3 Typical case: 52-year-old female diagnosed with RA for 1 year. US: synovial hyperplasia, synovitis with bone destruction. **a** Synovial hyperplasia (2 points) and bone erosion (1 point) of the radiocarpal joint. **b** Synovitis of the scapholunate joint (PDUS: 1 point). **c, d** Synovial hyperplasia (GSUS: 2 points), synovitis (PDUS: 1 point), and bone erosion (2 points) of the scapholunate joint

for routine examinations, and difficult to reproduce [40, 41]. US, by its increased degree of resolution due to high-frequency transducers, constitutes a reliable and compulsory method to diagnose and monitor RA patients. Unlike MRI, US is relatively cheap, is available, and can be used as many times as necessary during patient examination, improving the exactitude of clinical examination [42–44]. Ultrasound and MRI have similar effects on the diagnosis of characteristic RA lesions [45]. Because of the advantages of economy, convenience, no radiation, good repeatability, and so on, ultrasound has been widely used in the limb joints. The value of ultrasound in early RA diagnosis and disease surveillance was highly emphasized in the guidelines for the early diagnosis of RA in 2013 [46, 47].

There are some limitations in this study: (1) the group was limited in the number of patients; a larger group of patients would probably have strengthened the results. (2) Due to its physical properties, acoustic waves cannot effectively penetrate the cortex, so ultrasound cannot assess the true situation of bone marrow edema. (3) Unlike X-ray, CT, and MRI, ultrasound cannot provide complete information about the structure of the joint due to its spatial resolution; thus, the reliability of ultrasonic diagnostic information is subject to the doctor's operating experience to a certain extent. (4) The assessment of a single selected US image instead of a real-time examination of the joints performed by the second rheumatologist obviously introduces bias into the study. However, this is the standard way to record US examination in daily practice, and the images for a second reading were chosen by an experienced sonographer.

Conclusion

Ultrasonography has a high reliability in the diagnosis of early RA in synovitis, joint effusion, tenosynovitis, and bone erosion. There was a good correlation between ultrasonography and clinical and laboratory parameters. Both ultrasound and MRI are effective techniques. In view of the advantages of low cost and convenience, ultrasound may be a better choice during early RA diagnosis.

Abbreviations
CCP: Anti-cyclic citrullinated peptide antibody; GSUS: Gray-scale ultrasonography; PD: Power Doppler; RA: Rheumatoid arthritis; RF: Rheumatoid factor

Acknowledgements
Not applicable.

Funding
None.

Authors' contributions
YZ designed the study. HZ, CW, and PM performed the experimental work. HX and HZ evaluated the data. HX wrote the manuscript. All authors read and approved the final manuscript.

Competing interests
The authors declare that they have no competing interests.

Author details
[1]Department of Ultrasound, The Second Affiliated Hospital of Soochow University, San Xiang Road 1055, Suzhou 215004, China. [2]Department of Ultrasound, Huzhou Central Hospital, Hong Qi Road 198, Huzhou 313000, China. [3]Department of Radiology, Huzhou Central Hospital, Hong Qi Road 198, Huzhou 313000, China.

References

1. Fuchs HA, Kaye JJ, Callahan LF, Nance EP, Pincus T. Evidence of significant radiographic damage in rheumatoid arthritis within the first 2 years of disease. J Rheumatol. 1989;16:585–91.
2. van der Heijde DM. Joint erosions and patients with early rheumatoid arthritis. Br J Rheumatol. 1995;34(Suppl 2):74–8.
3. Finckh A, Liang MH, van Herckenrode CM, de Pablo P. Long-term impact of early treatment on radiographic progression in rheumatoid arthritis: a meta-analysis. Arthritis Rheum. 2006;55:864–72.
4. Kyburz D, Gabay C, Michel BA, Finckh A. Physicians of S-R. The long-term impact of early treatment of rheumatoid arthritis on radiographic progression: a population-based cohort study. Rheumatology (Oxford). 2011; 50:1106–10.
5. Nell VP, Machold KP, Eberl G, Stamm TA, Uffmann M, Smolen JS. Benefit of very early referral and very early therapy with disease-modifying anti-rheumatic drugs in patients with early rheumatoid arthritis. Rheumatology (Oxford). 2004;43:906–14.
6. Bi YN, Xiao CH, Pan C, Zhao XF, Cao YY, Yuan Y, Zuo FF. The correlation study on syndrome differentiation of rheumatoid arthritis and joint high frequency ultrasound performance. Zhongguo Zhong Xi Yi Jie He Za Zhi. 2015;35:19–24.
7. Zhang H, Jin D, Sun E. The early and late stages of crowned dens syndrome: two case reports. Spine J. 2015;15:e65–8.
8. Bruyn GA, Hanova P, Iagnocco A, d'Agostino MA, Moller I, Terslev L, Backhaus M, Balint PV, Filippucci E, Baudoin P, van Vugt R, Pineda C, Wakefield R, Garrido J, Pecha O, Naredo E, Force OUT. Ultrasound definition of tendon damage in patients with rheumatoid arthritis. Results of a OMERACT consensus-based ultrasound score focussing on the diagnostic reliability. Ann Rheum Dis. 2014;73:1929–34.
9. Fiehn C, Kruger K. Management of rheumatoid arthritis. Internist (Berl). 2016; 57:1042–51.
10. Sommer OJ, Kladosek A, Weiler V, Czembirek H, Boeck M, Stiskal M. Rheumatoid arthritis: a practical guide to state-of-the-art imaging, image interpretation, and clinical implications. Radiographics. 2005;25:381–98.
11. Wakefield RJ, Gibbon WW, Conaghan PG, O'Connor P, McGonagle D, Pease C, Green MJ, Veale DJ, Isaacs JD, Emery P. The value of sonography in the detection of bone erosions in patients with rheumatoid arthritis: a comparison with conventional radiography. Arthritis Rheum. 2000;43:2762–70.
12. Botar-Jid C, Bolboaca S, Fodor D, Bocsa C, Tamas MM, Micu M, Dudea SM, Vasilescu D, Badea R. Gray scale and power Doppler ultrasonography in evaluation of early rheumatoid arthritis. Med Ultrason. 2010;12:300–5.
13. Smolen JS, Robert L, Breedveld FC, Maya B, Gerd B, Maxime D, Paul E, Cécile GV, Laure G, Jackie N. EULAR recommendations for the management of rheumatoid arthritis with synthetic and biological disease-modifying antirheumatic drugs: 2013 update. Ann Rheum Dis. 2010;69:964–75.
14. Wakefield RJ. Should oligoarthritis be reclassified? Ultrasound reveals a high prevalence of subclinical disease. Ann Rheum Dis. 2004;63:382–5.
15. Szkudlarek M, Klarlund M, Narvestad E, Court-Payen M, Strandberg C, Jensen KE, Thomsen HS, Østergaard M. Ultrasonography of the metacarpophalangeal and proximal interphalangeal joints in rheumatoid arthritis: a comparison with magnetic resonance imaging, conventional radiography and clinical examination. Arthritis Research & Therapy. 2006;50: 2103–12.
16. Baillet A, Gaujoux-Viala C, Mouterde G, Pham T, Tebib J, Saraux A, Fautrel B, Cantagrel A, Le Loet X, Gaudin P. Comparison of the efficacy of sonography, magnetic resonance imaging and conventional radiography for the detection of bone erosions in rheumatoid arthritis patients: a systematic review and meta-analysis. Rheumatology (Oxford). 2011;50:1137–47.
17. Szkudlarek M, Court-Payen M, Strandberg C, Klarlund M, Klausen T, Ostergaard M. Power Doppler ultrasonography for assessment of synovitis in the metacarpophalangeal joints of patients with rheumatoid arthritis: a comparison with dynamic magnetic resonance imaging. Arthritis & Rheumatism. 2001;44:2018.
18. Terslev L, Torp-Pedersen S, Savnik A, Von der Recke P, Qvistgaard E, Bliddal H. Doppler ultrasound and magnetic resonance imaging of synovial inflammation of the hand in rheumatoid arthritis: a comparative study. Arthritis & Rheumatism. 2003;48:2434–41.
19. Naredo E. Assessment of inflammatory activity in rheumatoid arthritis: a comparative study of clinical evaluation with grey scale and power Doppler ultrasonography. Ann Rheum Dis. 2005;64:375–81.
20. Martinoli C, Pretolesi F, Crespi G, Bianchi S, Gandolfo N, Valle M, Derchi LE. Power Doppler sonography: clinical applications. Eur J Radiol. 1998; 27(Suppl 2):S133–40.
21. Tian J, Chen J, Li F, Xie X, Du J, Mao N, Gao J. Grey scale and power Doppler ultrasonographic assessment of bone erosion and disease activity in early rheumatoid arthritis. Zhong Nan Da Xue Xue Bao Yi Xue Ban. 2013;38:1270–4.
22. Luz KR, Pinheiro MM, Petterle GS, Dos Santos MF, Fernandes AR, Natour J, Furtado RN. A new musculoskeletal ultrasound scoring system (US10) of the hands and wrist joints for evaluation of early rheumatoid arthritis patients. Rev Bras Reumatol Engl Ed. 2016;56:421–31.
23. Scheel AK, Hermann KG, Kahler E, Pasewaldt D, Fritz J, Hamm B, Brunner E, Muller GA, Burmester GR, Backhaus MA. Novel ultrasonographic synovitis scoring system suitable for analyzing finger joint inflammation in rheumatoid arthritis. Arthritis Rheum. 2005;52:733–43.
24. Backhaus M, Burmester GR, Sandrock D, Loreck D, Hess D, Scholz A, Blind S, Hamm B, Bollow M. Prospective two year follow up study comparing novel and conventional imaging procedures in patients with arthritic finger joints. Ann Rheum Dis. 2002;61:895–904.
25. Aletaha D, Neogi T, Silman AJ, Funovits J, Felson DT, Bingham CO, 3rd, Birnbaum NS, Burmester GR, Bykerk VP, Cohen MD, Combe B, Costenbader KH, Dougados M, Emery P, Ferraccioli G, Hazes JM, Hobbs K, Huizinga TW, Kavanaugh A, Kay J, Kvien TK, Laing T, Mease P, Menard HA, Moreland LW, Naden RL, Pincus T, Smolen JS, Stanislawska-Biernat E, Symmons D, Tak PP, Upchurch KS, Vencovsky J, Wolfe F, Hawker G. 2010 rheumatoid arthritis classification criteria: an American College of Rheumatology/European League Against Rheumatism collaborative initiative. Arthritis Rheum 2010; 62: 2569-2581.
26. van Riel PL, Renskers L. The disease activity score (DAS) and the disease activity score using 28 joint counts (DAS28) in the management of rheumatoid arthritis. Clin Exp Rheumatol. 2016;34(Suppl 101):40–4.
27. Luz KR, Furtado R, Mitraud SV, Porglhof J, Nunes C, Fernandes AR, Natour J. Interobserver reliability in ultrasound assessment of rheumatoid wrist joints. Acta Reumatol Port. 2011;36:245–50.
28. Szkudlarek M, Court-Payen M, Jacobsen S, Klarlund M, Thomsen HS, Ostergaard M. Interobserver agreement in ultrasonography of the finger and toe joints in rheumatoid arthritis. Arthritis Rheum. 2003;48:955–62.
29. Saran S, Bagarhatta M, Saigal R. Diagnostic accuracy of ultrasonography in detection of destructive changes in small joints of hands in patients of rheumatoid arthritis: a comparison with magnetic resonance imaging. J Assoc Physicians India. 2016;64:26–30.
30. Tamas MM, Bondor CI, Rednic N, Ghib LJ, Rednic S. The evolution of time-intensity curves of contrast enhanced ultrasonography in early arthritis patients with wrist involvement. Med Ultrason. 2015;17:345–51.
31. Luz KR, Pinheiro MM, Petterle GS, Santos MFD, Fernandes ARC, Natour J, Furtado RNVA. New musculoskeletal ultrasound scoring system (US10) of the hands and wrist joints for evaluation of early rheumatoid arthritis patients. Rev Bras Reumatol. 2016;56:421–31.
32. Dasgupta B, Cimmino MA, Kremers HM, Schmidt WA, Schirmer M, Salvarani C, Bachta A, Dejaco C, Duftner C, Jensen HS, Duhaut P, Poor G, Kaposi NP, Mandl P, Balint PV, Schmidt Z, Iagnocco A, Nannini C, Cantini F, Macchioni P, Pipitone N, Del Amo M, Espigol-Frigole G, Cid MC, Martinez-Taboada VM, Nordborg E, Direskeneli H, Aydin SZ, Ahmed K, Hazleman B, Silverman B, Pease C, Wakefield RJ, Luqmani R, Abril A, Michet CJ, Marcus R, Gonter NJ, Maz M, Carter RE, Crowson CS, Matteson EL. 2012 provisional classification criteria for polymyalgia rheumatica: a European League Against Rheumatism/American College of Rheumatology collaborative initiative. Arthritis Rheum. 2012;64:943–54.
33. Micu MC, Berghea F, Fodor D. Concepts in diagnosing, scoring, and monitoring tenosynovitis and other tendon abnormalities in patients with rheumatoid arthritis—the role of musculoskeletal ultrasound. Med Ultrason. 2016;18:370–7.
34. Lage-Hansen PR, Lindegaard H, Chrysidis S, Terslev L. The role of ultrasound in diagnosing rheumatoid arthritis, what do we know? An updated review. Rheumatol Int. 2017;37:179–87.
35. Lai KL, Chen DY, Chen YH, Huang WN, Hsieh TY, Hsieh CW, Chen YM, Hung WT, Chen HH. Assessment of wrist joint inflammation in patients with rheumatoid arthritis by quantitative two- and three-dimensional power Doppler ultrasonography. Clin Exp Rheumatol. 2014;32:674–9.
36. Cheung PP, Kong KO, Chew LC, Chia FL, Law WG, Lian TY, Tan YK, Cheng YK. Achieving consensus in ultrasonography synovitis scoring in rheumatoid arthritis. Int J Rheum Dis. 2014;17:776–81.
37. Dejaco C, Duftner C, Wipfler-Freissmuth E, Weiss H, Graninger WB, Schirmer M. Ultrasound-defined remission and active disease in rheumatoid arthritis:

association with clinical and serologic parameters. Semin Arthritis Rheum. 2012;41:761–7.

38. Ikeda K, Sanayama Y, Nakagomi D, Nakajima H. Evaluation of joint damage with conventional radiograph and synovitis with musculoskeletal ultrasonography in rheumatoid arthritis. Nihon Rinsho. 2013;71:1185–92.

39. Wang Y, Geng Y, Deng XR, Zhang ZL. Relationship between wrist bone mineral density and synovitis, erosion by ultrasonography in female rheumatoid arthritis patients. Beijing Da Xue Xue Bao. 2015;47:774–80.

40. Mcgonagle D, Conaghan PG, O'Connor P, Gibbon W, Green M, Wakefield R, Ridgway J, Emery P. The relationship between synovitis and bone changes in early untreated rheumatoid arthritis: a controlled magnetic resonance imaging study. Arthritis & Rheumatology. 1999;42:1706.

41. Ostendorf B, Peters R, Dann P, Becker A, Scherer A, Wedekind F, Friemann J, Schulitz KP, Modder U, Schneider M. Magnetic resonance imaging and miniarthroscopy of metacarpophalangeal joints: sensitive detection of morphologic changes in rheumatoid arthritis. Arthritis Rheum. 2001;44:2492–502.

42. Chakr RM, Mendonca JA, Brenol CV, Xavier RM, Brenol JC. Assessing rheumatoid arthritis disease activity with ultrasound. Clin Rheumatol. 2013; 32:1249–54.

43. Damjanov N, Radunovic G, Prodanovic S, Vukovic V, Milic V, Simic Pasalic K, Jablanovic D, Seric S, Milutinovic S, Gavrilov N. Construct validity and reliability of ultrasound disease activity score in assessing joint inflammation in RA: comparison with DAS-28. Rheumatology (Oxford). 2012;51:120–8.

44. Mitran C, Barbulescu A, Vreju FA, Criveanu C, Rosu A, Ciurea P. Musculoskeletal Ultrasound in Early Rheumatoid Arthritis - Correlations with Disease Activity Score. Current Health Sciences Journal. 2015;41:213-8.

45. Krohn M, Ohrndorf S, Werner SG, Schicke B, Burmester GR, Hamm B, Backhaus M, Hermann KG. Near-infrared fluorescence optical imaging in early rheumatoid arthritis: a comparison to magnetic resonance imaging and ultrasonography. J Rheumatol. 2015;42:1112–8.

46. Plaza M, Nowakowska-Plaza A, Pracon G, Sudol-Szopinska I. Role of ultrasonography in the diagnosis of rheumatic diseases in light of ACR/EULAR guidelines. J Ultrason. 2016;16:55–64.

47. Kelly S, Bombardieri M, Humby F, Ng N, Marrelli A, Riahi S, DiCicco M, Mahto A, Zou L, Pyne D, Hands RE, Pitzalis C. Angiogenic gene expression and vascular density are reflected in ultrasonographic features of synovitis in early rheumatoid arthritis: an observational study. Arthritis Res Ther. 2015;17:58.

17

Circuit training enhances function in patients undergoing total knee arthroplasty: a retrospective cohort study

Wei-Hsiu Hsu[1,2†], Wei-Bin Hsu[1†], Wun-Jer Shen[3], Zin-Rong Lin[4], Shr-Hsin Chang[1] and Robert Wen-Wei Hsu[1,2*]

Abstract

Background: The number of patients receiving total knee arthroplasty (TKA) has been rising every year due to the aging population and the obesity epidemic. Post-operative rehabilitation is important for the outcome of TKA.

Methods: A series of 34 patients who underwent primary unilateral TKA was retrospectively collected and divided into either exercise group (n = 16) and control group (n = 18). The exercise group underwent a 24-week course of circuit training beginning 3 months after total knee arthroplasty (TKA). The effect of circuit training on TKA patients in terms of motion analysis, muscle strength testing, Knee injury and Osteoarthritis Outcomes Score (KOOS) questionnaire and patient-reported outcome measurement Short-Form Health Survey (SF-36) at the pre-operation, pre-exercise, mid-exercise, and post-exercise.

Results: Motion analysis revealed the stride length, step velocity, and excursion of active knee range of motion significantly improved in the exercise group when compared to those in the control group. KOOS questionnaire showed a greater improvement in pain, ADL, and total scores in the exercise group. The SF-36 questionnaire revealed a significant improvement in general health, bodily pain, social function, and physical components score in the exercise group.

Conclusions: The post-operative circuit training intervention can facilitate recovery of knee function and decrease the degree of pain in the TKA and might be considered a useful adjunct rehabilitative modality. The ultimate influence of circuit training on TKA needs further a prospective randomized clinical trial study and long-term investigation.

Trial registration: NCT02928562

Keywords: Circuit training, Total knee arthroplasty, Motion analysis, KOOS, SF-36

Background

Total knee arthroplasty (TKA) is a well-accepted procedure for the treatment of advanced osteoarthritis of the knee joint [1], with good long-term survivorship of the implants and satisfactory surgical outcome [2]. The number of patients receiving TKA has been rising every year due to the aging population and the obesity

epidemic [3–5]. Enhancing the recovery process after TKAs is an important issue. Physical exercise was suggested to enhance muscular strength, muscular endurance, cardiovascular fitness, flexibility, agility, balance, and coordination in the healthy aged population [6]. Physical exercise could further increase the range of motion and quadriceps strength in TKA patients [7]. However, these effects of post-operative exercise were usually limited by a short hospital stay, impaired exercise adherence, and in compliance to exercise regimens [8–10].

A more balanced exercise approach is therefore recommended for TKA patients [11]. Circuit training comprised of different exercise principles, including stretching exercise, aerobic training, and resistant

* Correspondence: wwh@cgmh.org.tw
†Equal contributors
[1]Sports Medicine Center, Chang Gung Memorial Hospital, No. 6, West Section, Chia-Pu Road, Putz City 61363, Chiayi Country, Taiwan, Republic of China
[2]Department of Orthopaedic Surgery, Chang Gung Memorial Hospital, No. 6, West Section, Chia-Pu Road, Putz City 61363, Chiayi Country, Taiwan, Republic of China
Full list of author information is available at the end of the article

training. Multiple stations for training different muscle groups, stretching exercise, and aerobic exercise was employed to progress towards cardiovascular fitness and muscle strength [12]. We had previously reported its positive effect on body composition improvement in overweight women [9]. Meanwhile, good exercise adherences were also observed with concomitant increases in the mental domain of functional score, since the incidence of female osteoarthritis (OA) is twice that of men [13] and the number undergoing TKA in the female is about twice in men between 2001 and 2010 [14]. The retrospective study focused on the female and assessed the feasibility and effect of post-operative circuit training intervention on TKA. The circuit training intervention would carry out at 3 months after the operation for 6 months. The assessments of this intervention were measured using motion analysis and muscle strength testing, KOOS questionnaire, and patient-reported outcome measurement Short-Form Health Survey (SF-36). The goal was to demonstrate the effect, if any, that circuit training intervention might have on post-operative knee functional recovery and daily activities.

Methods
Participants
The aim was to demonstrate the effect, if any, that circuit training intervention might have on post-operative knee functional recovery and daily activities in female TKA.

The inclusion criteria of the study included end-stage OA and female. Patients with diabetes, neuromusculoskeletal disorders, severe chronic medical disease, history of fracture of a lower limb, artificial limb, and being otherwise unsuitable for exercise training were excluded.

From October 2013 to August 2015, a consecutive cohort of 34 patients underwent TKA (16 in the exercise group and 18 in the control group) at Chang Gung Memorial Hospital Chiayi branch was included in the current study.

The participants in the exercise group practiced a 24-week circuit training intervention while the control group followed the routine post-operative rehabilitation protocol, including quadriceps training and range of motion exercise during the same time period.

Intervention
The circuit training program included stretching, aerobic training, and resistance training. The order of practice was performed in the following pattern: stretching/aerobic training/resistance training/aerobic training/resistance training/stretching. Each exercise was performed for 10 min, with a 30 s rest period between each exercise, and the program was carried out three times a week for 24 weeks. Aerobic training consisted of riding

an exercise bike with the intensity of 60–80% target heart rate, and the resistance training was performed on hydraulic resistance equipment (AGOSS, Taipei, Taiwan) set at an intensity of 60–80% one repetition maximum. Six exercise machines were randomly chosen from ten exercise machines which included six types of equipment for the upper limbs and four for the lower limbs. The program was hospital-based and supervised by one exercise therapist at the Sports Medicine Center of Chang Gung Memorial Hospital Chiayi branch.

Objectives
The aim of the study was to assess the feasibility and effect of post-operative circuit training intervention on TKA women. The effect of this intervention was measured using motion analysis, muscle strength testing, Knee injury and Osteoarthritis Outcome Score (KOOS) questionnaire and Short-Form Health Survey (SF-36) measurement patient-reported outcome. The goal was to demonstrate the effect, if any, that circuit training intervention might have on post-operative knee functional recovery and daily activities.

Outcomes
All measurements in both the exercise group and control group were performed at the following time points, i.e., before TKA operation (pre-operation), before exercise (pre-exercise), at 12 weeks after the beginning of the circuit training program (mid-exercise), and after completion of the circuit training (post-exercise).

Gait analysis
Gait analysis was performed by a three-dimensional, eight-camera motion capture system (VICON, Oxford Metrics, London, England) synchronized with two force platforms (OR6, AMTI, Watertown, Massachusetts) to record ground reaction force. Marker data were sampled at 100 Hz. Force platform data were sampled at 1000 Hz. Data collection starts with standing calibration to identify joint centers and create a segment impeded coordinate system. After calibration, subjects practiced walking until reaching a constant self-selected speed. The collected trials fell within 5% of the practiced speed with clear contact of only one foot on each force plate. Five walking trials were collected for each subject. While kinematics and kinetics of the segments are calculated, the whole body is modeled as a segment-linkage system consisting of the head, trunk, pelvis, bilateral upper arms, forearms, hands, thighs, shanks, and feet. Reflective markers attached on the segments were used to establish coordinate systems representing each segment. Data were processed utilizing the Nexus motion analysis system (VICON; Oxford Metrics Ltd. Ver.1.6.5), which was integrated with data recording software.

Muscle strength

Lower extremity muscle strength (including extension and flexion of the hip and knee, dorsi, and plantar flexion of the ankle) was measured using the HUMAC NORM system (CSMi, Stoughton, MA) with the concentric/eccentric contraction mode at an angular velocity of 60° per second. All measurements were evaluated with the participant in a sitting position. Isokinetic tests were performed five times for each participant, and each test was separated by a rest period of 3 min. The participants received verbal encouragement during the exertion of peak torque. The muscle strength was presented as a peak torque which was normalized to body weight [15].

KOOS assessment

Clinical knee scoring using the Chinese version KOOS scale was performed in the outpatient self-explanatory assessment [16]. The KOOS is a 42-item self-administered knee-specific questionnaire assessing pain (9 items), symptoms (7 items), activities of daily living (ADL, 17 items), function, sports and recreational activities (sports/rec, 5 items), and knee-related quality of life (QOL, 4 items) in five separate subscales. All items are scored 0 to 4; for each subscale, the scores are transformed to a 0 to 100 scales (0 representing extreme knee problems and 100 representing no knee problems) [17].

Quality of life

Quality of life was assessed using the Short-Form Health Survey (SF-36, Taiwan version [18]). The SF-36 questionnaire is a multi-purpose and short-form health survey, which is commonly used to evaluate patients' quality of life in clinical practice. A total of eight domains were evaluated in this questionnaire including physical functioning (PF), role limitation due to physical problems (RP), bodily pain (BP), general health (GH), vitality (VT), social functioning (SF), role limitation due to emotional problem (RE), and mental health (MH). Additionally, the eight health domains can be used to provide physical component summary (PCS) and mental component summary (MCS) scores.

Statistical analysis

All data analysis was done using the Statistical Package for the Social Sciences, Windows version 17.0 (SPSS, Chicago, IL, USA). All continuous data are presented as the mean ± standard deviation. Generalized estimating equations (GEEs) [19] were used for determining the differences between the exercise and control groups across the time period. A p value of < 0.05 was considered statistically significant.

Results

The demographic data, including age, height, and weight was similar in the exercise and control groups (Table 1). The mean age was 72 and 70 years old for the exercise and control groups, respectively.

In gait analysis, it was noted both exercise and control group were shown similar in gait parameters at pre-operation and pre-exercise evaluation. Three months after beginning exercise interventions, the stride length for exercise and control group were 101.6 ± 3.4 and 85.0 ± 5.5 cm, respectively (p = 0.01). Similarly, step length and step velocity were greater in the exercise group than those in control group. ($p < 0.05$) (Table 2). Meanwhile, the excursion of knee range of motion was 48.6 ± 1.2 and 44.5 ± 1.6 degree for exercise and control group, respectively ($p < 0.05$). The differences in stride length and excursion of knee range of motion (ROM) lasted till the post-exercise evaluation (Table 2). When comparison was performed within the individual group in temporal fashion, it was shown that stride length, stride velocity, step length, and step velocity increased in mid-excise assessment in the exercise group, while no such difference was noted in control group. The control group demonstrated increases in these parameters at post-exercise assessment ($p < 0.05$). Circuit training improved gait pattern at an earlier time point compared with the control group.

In isokinetic muscle strength assessment, it was shown that the maximal knee extensor torque for the exercise group was 24.4 ± 5.2, 31.4 ± 3.3, 44.0 ± 4.8, and 51.0 ± 5.9 N-m/Kg for pre-operation, pre-exercise, mid-exercise, and post-exercise, respectively ($p < 0.05$). Similar increases were demonstrated in the control group for knee extensor (Table 3). Indeed, it was shown that maximal muscle strength in hip extensor, hip flexor, knee extensor and knee flexor, ankle plantar flexor, and dorsiflexor all increased after TKA surgery in a temporal fashion for both exercise and control group ($p < 0.05$). Meanwhile, it was shown that there were no differences between the exercise and control group at all time point (Table 3). Meanwhile, we measured the muscular strength of lower extremity since previous studies have shown that knee extensor strength is closely correlated to functional performance, especially after TKA [20, 21].

Table 1 Demography of participants

	Exercise group (n = 16)	Control group (n = 18)
Age (years)	72.1 ± 6.7	69.6 ± 8.2
Height (cm)	152.6 ± 5.6	154.3 ± 6.4
Weight (kg)	63.7 ± 6.0	63.2 ± 11.9
BMI (kg/m^2)	27.5 ± 3.3	26.5 ± 4.0

Data presented as mean ± SD

Table 2 Comparison of gait kinematics between two groups of the TKA patients

	Pre-operation			Pre-exercise			Mid-exercise			Post-exercise		
	Exercise	Control	p	Exercise	Control	p	Exercise	Control	p	Exercise	Control	p
Stride time (sec)	1.2 ± 0.1	1.2 ± 0.1	.709	1.2 ± 0.1	1.2 ± 0.1	.716	1.1 ± 0.1	1.1 ± 0.1	.988	1.1 ± 0.1*****,***	1.1 ± 0.1**	.270
Stride length (cm)	85.6 ± 5.7	82.0 ± 5.8	.663	92.0 ± 5.0	81.5 ± 4.9	.136	101.6 ± 3.4**,*****,***	85.0 ± 5.5	.010*	100.0 ± 4.3**,*****,***	85.1 ± 5.2	.027*
Stride velocity (cm/s)	72.6 ± 6.0	70.4 ± 6.7	.808	78.2 ± 5.9	69.8 ± 5.5	.295	90.4 ± 4.8**,*****,***	76.1 ± 5.8	.060	91.0 ± 5.8**,*****,***b	80.5 ± 5.7**,*****	.198
Step time (sec)	0.6 ± 0.1	0.6 ± 0.1	.633	0.6 ± 0.1	0.6 ± 0.1	.938	0.6 ± 0.1**,*****	0.6 ± 0.1	.959	0.6 ± 0.1**,*****	0.5 ± 0.1**,*****	.383
Step length (cm)	42.6 ± 2.9	39.3 ± 3.0	.436	45.7 ± 2.6	40.5 ± 2.7	.158	50.9 ± 1.9**,*****,***	42.6 ± 2.8	.013*	50.8 ± 2.3**,*****	44.8 ± 2.9**,*****,***	.102
Step velocity (cm/s)	69.6 ± 5.8	68.9 ± 7.0	.937	78.0 ± 5.4	71.1 ± 6.1	.400	92.2 ± 5.1**,*****,***	77.0 ± 5.7	.046*	93.5 ± 5.8**,*****	80.5 ± 6.6**,*****	.136
Excursion of active knee ROM (°)	34.9 ± 2.8	35.7 ± 2.7	.836	44.0 ± 1.9**,*****	40.2 ± 1.5	.112	48.6 ± 1.2**,*****	44.5 ± 1.6**,*****	.045*	51.0 ± 1.4**,*****	44.8 ± 2.6**,*****,***	.037*

Data presented as mean ± SD

A significant difference (p < 0.05) between two groups is calculated by GEEs

*p < .05, difference between groups; **p < .05, difference with pre-operation; ***p < .05, difference with pre-exercise

Table 3 Comparison of muscle strength between the two groups of the TKA patient

(Nm/kg)	Pre-operation			Pre-exercise			Mid-exercise			Post-exercise		
	Exercise	Control	p	Exercise	Control	p	Exercise	Control	p	Exercise	Control	p
HE	40.9 ± 5.5	44.2 ± 10.3	.733	56.0 ± 5.2**	58.1 ± 5.0	.774	66.9 ± 7.2**	74.1 ± 9.4**	.543	80.4 ± 10.4*******	84.0 ± 7.0******	.773
HF	14.6 ± 2.5	16.7 ± 3.5	.615	17.8 ± 2.4	23.1 ± 2.2**	.109	26.0 ± 3.0******	27.2 ± 3.6**	.807	26.2 ± 3.6******	33.3 ± 2.6******	.114
KE	24.4 ± 5.2	32.5 ± 7.2	.363	31.4 ± 3.3	38.2 ± 6.4	.345	44.0 ± 4.8*******	56.2 ± 8.4*******	.207	51.0 ± 5.9******	61.5 ± 6.6******	.236
KF	26.1 ± 3.5	23.2 ± 4.3	.608	34.2 ± 2.4**	39.1 ± 5.9**	.444	48.6 ± 4.0******	52.0 ± 8.3*******	.705	49.8 ± 3.7******	55.3 ± 5.6*******	.413
PF	20.0 ± 2.6	20.8 ± 4.7	.888	24.6 ± 3.0	23.6 ± 3.1	.805	34.6 ± 4.0*******	34.0 ± 6.6	.939	32.7 ± 2.9******	41.7 ± 5.4******	.145
DF	2.5 ± 0.6	3.3 ± 1.1	.568	3.7 ± 0.7*****b	4.3 ± 1.5	.718	5.3 ± 0.8*******	7.8 ± 1.8******	.204	6.6 ± 1.2**	7.6 ± 1.8******	.309

Data presented as mean ± SD

A significant difference (p < 0.05) between two groups is calculated by GEEs

HE hip extension, HF hip flexion, KE knee extension, KF knee flexion, PF plantarflexion, DF dorsiflexion

*p < .05, difference between groups; **p < .05, difference with pre-operation; ***p < .05, difference with pre-exercise

In post-exercise KOOS assessment, KOOS total score was 78.7 ± 3.2 and 66.4 ± 4.1 for exercise and control group, respectively ($p = 0.018$). In the subcategorical assessment, these differences were observed in pain and ADL ($p < 0.05$) (Table 4). When comparison of KOOS was performed within the individual group, the temporal improvement was observed in symptoms, pain, ADL, QOL, and total score for both exercise and control group ($p < 0.05$) (Table 4). Interestingly, the sports subcategory was shown significantly improved from 17.1 ± 5.4 at pre-operative assessment to 48.3 ± 7.8 at post-exercise assessment in the exercise group ($p < 0.05$), while no such difference was shown in the control group.

In the SF-36 questionnaire which included physical and mental domains, it was shown a significant increase in the domains of GH, SF, and PCS at the mid-exercise point in the exercise group compared to the control group ($p < 0.05$) (Table 5). The circuit training efficiently improved the GH, SF, and PCS at the earlier time point. At the post-exercise assessment, only SF and BP were shown a significant increase in the exercise group compared with the control group (Table 5). When comparison was performed within the individual group in temporal fashion, it was shown that exercise improved all mental domains in mid-exercise assessment, and these improvements lasted to the post-exercise assessment, while no such improvement was observed in the control group. In the physical domain, it seemed both groups were shown improvement.

Discussion

The most significant findings in the present study were that 24-week circuit training resulted in a decrease of pain and an increase of ADL and SF, along with an increase in stride length and excursion of knee ROM in gait analysis [8, 22, 23]. Second, the increases in all muscle strength were demonstrated in a temporal fashion in both exercise and control group [24]. Circuit training seemed not further increase the maximal muscle strength. Third, earlier recoveries in gait parameters, KOOS, and SF-36 at mid-exercise assessment for exercise group were well demonstrated. Although circuit training did not result in a further increase in maximal isokinetic muscle strength, it was postulated to enhance the muscle coordination which facilitated the performance of walking and daily function [25]. The improvement in pain after circuit training both in the KOOS and SF-36 further provided an important basis that knee can undergo unlimited swing and hence to increase the stride length [23].

In gait analysis, stride length and excursion of knee ROM in the exercise group were shown significant increases as compared to control group at the mid-

exercise assessment, and these differences lasted to the post-exercise assessment (Table 2). It is well demonstrated that faster restoration of gait patterns in exercise group as compared to the control group. None of the subjects enrolled in the exercise group reported discomfort or injury, and none needed further management. This indicates that our circuit training intervention is safe for TKA patients and feasible to perform following the TKA surgery.

The function of quadriceps strength relied on maximal muscular strength and muscular coordination in TKA patients, which could be improved by post-operative progressive strengthening protocol [24, 26–29]. Quadriceps weakness is a hallmark characteristic of knee osteoarthritis [24, 27, 30, 31]. Post-operatively, quadriceps strength was not comparable to their age-matched counterparts in the mid- or long-term follow-up [29]. Muscle strength recovery in those aging patients underwent TKA followed a temporary pattern [24]. The current study displayed a simultaneous trend in pain and muscle function recovery. Actually, as the pain improved 3 months after TKA, the patient was able to load their knees and hence improve the lower extremity muscle force. As the pain improved more, it was shown that lower leg muscle strength has a corresponding further increase. We have previously demonstrated the progress of both cardiovascular fitness and muscle strength by circuit training and 12-week circuit training in healthy middle-aged women (aged 45–75) [12]. However, the circuit training in the current study did not result in a further increase in the maximal isokinetic muscle strength. Two possibilities existed. First, the intensity of resistant training in the current study could be inadequate and would not result in a further increase as compared to the daily activities [23]. Second, the maximal strength has plateaued. Further study was warranted to delineate the mechanism underlying the findings in the current study. On the other hand, the muscle coordination and performance were improved by circuit training as shown in gait parameters. This finding paralleled literature that modified gait efficacy scale was improved by exercise [23]. In this laboratory study, it was further shown a 15% increase in stride length, accompanied by 10% increase in excursion of knee ROM during walking. These results provided a solid basis to explain the positive effect of exercise on gait function. It was possible that the decrease in pain and a more coordinated muscle function improved the gait function.

Decreased exercise adherence usually endangered the effect of exercise intervention [10, 32]. The motives for exercise participation among patients with knee OA was suggested mainly as positive outcome expectation [10]. Other factors such as social interaction and enjoyment of exercise have been described as important facilitators

Table 4 Comparison of KOOS subscales between two groups of the TKA patients

	Pre-operation			Pre-exercise			Mid-exercise			Post-exercise		
	Exercise	Control	p	Exercise	Control	p	Exercise	Control	p	Exercise	Control	p
Symptom	45.9 ± 5.3	49.4 ± 4.8	.628	61.6 ± 3.1**	67.4 ± 3.8**	.240	72.9 ± 3.2**,***	71.0 ± 3.6**	.700	82.7 ± 3.2**,***	72.4 ± 4.5**	.059
Pain	46.8 ± 9.1	47.3 ± 6.4	.964	71.6 ± 4.5**	70.5 ± 4.8**	.866	76.3 ± 4.2**	77.8 ± 5.0**	.813	84.0 ± 2.5**,***	73.8 ± 4.5**	.048*
ADL	48.8 ± 7.5	48.5 ± 5.7	.980	72.6 ± 5.1**	70.8 ± 4.8**	.792	77.1 ± 4.2**	73.5 ± 5.0**	.570	84.5 ± 2.7**,***	71.2 ± 5.1**	.020*
Sport	17.1 ± 5.4	28.6 ± 6.7	.182	51.3 ± 8.6**	38.8 ± 6.1	.240	38.7 ± 4.9**	34.8 ± 5.9	.607	48.3 ± 7.8**	33.7 ± 5.4	.123
QOL	38.1 ± 6.0	40.2 ± 4.0	.775	53.9 ± 5.1**	48.3 ± 3.6	.367	63.5 ± 4.6**	61.7 ± 4.2**,***	.778	67.6 ± 4.3**,***	60.7 ± 4.7**,****	.277
Total score	43.3 ± 6.3	44.7 ± 4.9	.856	66.2 ± 4.1**	64.2 ± 3.9**	.715	70.4 ± 3.0**	68.3 ± 4.4**	.698	78.7 ± 3.2**,***	66.4 ± 4.1**	.018*

Data presented as mean ± SD

A significant difference ($p < 0.05$) between two groups is calculated by GEEs

*$p < .05$, difference between groups; **$p < .05$, difference with pre-operation; ***$p < .05$, difference with pre-exercise

Table 5 Comparison of perceived health (SF-36) between two groups of the TKA patients

	Pre-operation			Pre-exercise			Mid-exercise			Post-exercise		
	Exercise	Control	p	Exercise	Control	p	Exercise	Control	p	Exercise	Control	p
PF	40.0 ± 4.8	35.2 ± 4.9	.487	49.1 ± 6.7	42.1 ± 6.3	.444	58.9 ± 4.5**	45.8 ± 5.5	.065	54.4 ± 6.5**	45.4 ± 6.6	.330
RP	31.7 ± 10.4	19.0 ± 9.2	.362	31.4 ± 10.4	50.2 ± 10.5**	.203	76.3 ± 9.***·***	48.0 ± 11.5**	.058	58.4 ± 12.9	51.4 ± 12.9**	.702
BP	36.0 ± 4.5	34.0 ± 4.6	.761	52.1 ± 5.0**	54.2 ± 5.0**	.763	64.1 ± 3.2**·***	57.7 ± 4.5**	.244	76.8 ± 3.7**·***	65.4 ± 4.1**	.038*
GH	49.9 ± 6.8	44.3 ± 5.3	.519	53.0 ± 5.3	50.5 ± 4.3	.715	62.5 ± 4.9***	46.1 ± 5.3	.022*	56.8 ± 5.8	49.3 ± 5.4	.340
VT	60.2 ± 4.5	55.5 ± 4.9	.477	65.5 ± 3.6	58.8 ± 4.4	.237	63.9 ± 3.9	63.9 ± 4.0	.986	71.2 ± 4.5**	64.1 ± 3.7	.220
SF	65.1 ± 7.4	61.4 ± 7.1	.715	66.5 ± 5.3	63.9 ± 4.6	.709	80.6 ± 3.6**·***	65.3 ± 4.7	.010*	82.8 ± 3.7**·***	68.6 ± 3.8	.008*
RE	43.8 ± 10.9	43.1 ± 10.7	.964	46.6 ± 11.2	65.5 ± 9.6	.138	75.5 ± 9.2**·***	62.7 ± 10.3	.352	76.1 ± 10.9**·***	64.3 ± 11.9	.465
MH	57.5 ± 4.3	56.2 ± 3.9	.823	64.9 ± 2.7	62.1 ± 2.9	.489	65.4 ± 3.6	65.5 ± 3.6	.995	68.5 ± 3.9**	63.0 ± 4.3	.343
PCS	35.5 ± 1.7	32.6 ± 1.7	.230	38.6 ± 2.1**	38.2 ± 1.4**	.874	45.6 ± 1.5**·***	38.5 ± 2.2**	.008*	43.9 ± 2.5**	40.4 ± 2.3**	.309
MCS	45.3 ± 2.4	44.8 ± 2.7	.900	46.9 ± 2.0	48.0 ± 1.8	.675	49.3 ± 2.1	48.4 ± 2.3	.766	51.8 ± 2.2**	48.6 ± 2.3	.318

Data presented as mean ± SD
A significant difference ($p < 0.05$) between two groups is calculated by GEEs
*$p < .05$, difference between groups; **$p < .05$, difference with pre-operation; ***$p < .05$, difference with pre-exercise

of exercise behavior [22, 32]. The present study demonstrated the improvement in social function which could result in exercise adherence to 80%, which was comparable in OA patient without TKA [10, 22]. Our results supported that a more balanced exercise program in patients with TKA to achieve a better exercise adherence and consequent improvement in gait and function [11]. Furthermore, the present study provided a quantitative data regarding the exercise prescription with efficacy and efficiency, which could be practiced for months. These results could be the basis for developing home exercise regimens.

Several limitations in this study must be acknowledged. First, the small sample size (34 patients) in this study resulted in under power to show a statistical difference between two groups in head-to-head comparisons. However, comparisons in repeated measure provided a better statistical power. Comparisons of repeated measurements in the same patient demonstrated the effect of exercise in a time sequence. Second, the study is limited to the Asian experience of knee arthroplasty. Third, this was a short-term study; thus, we were unable to assess the effect post-operative circuit training in long-term functional outcomes. The resistance training, though might be submaximal, in combination with aerobic exercise and stretching exercise help faster recovery in gait, functional score, and social function. Fourth, this study is a retrospective study. The results of circuit training on TKAs should be further proved by a prospective randomized clinical trial design. Fifth, there was a heterogeneous effect among the patients in the exercise. The previous investigation has shown that the carrier with polymorphism of monocarboxylate transporter 1 gene (A1470T) exhibits a worse lactate transport and influences the performance with high-intensity circuit training [33]. The genetic variance may be responsible

for the heterogeneity of circuit training effect on the individual patients. The further study focused on the genetic test before training intervention was suggested.

Conclusions

Our post-operative circuit training intervention is safe and effective in improving and hastening the functional recovery after TKA surgery, even without enhancement of lower limb muscle strength. This circuit training intervention might be incorporated into the standard post-operative rehabilitation protocol for TKA patients. The ultimate influence of circuit training on TKA needs further long-term investigation.

Abbreviations
ADL: Activities of daily living; BP: Bodily pain; GEE: Generalized estimating equations; GH: General health; KOOS: Knee injury and Osteoarthritis Outcome Score; MCS: Mental component summary; MH: Mental health; OA: Osteoarthritis; PCS: Physical component summary; PF: Physical functioning; RE: Role Limitation due to emotional problem; ROM: Range of motion; RP: Role Limitation due to physical problems; SF: Social functioning; SF-36: Short-Form Health Survey; VT: Vitality

Acknowledgements
The authors thank Chao-Ling Lai and Chia-Fang Chang for collecting the participants' data.

Funding
Financial support from Chang Gung Memorial Hospital Grant CORPG6C0021-23 is appreciated. There was no external funding.

Authors' contributions
WHH and WBH drafted the manuscript and revised it critically for important intellectual content. WHH and WBH contributed equally to the work. SHC performed statistical analysis. WJS, ZRL, and RWWH contributed substantially to the conception and design of the study. All authors read and approved the final manuscript.

Competing interests
The authors declare that they have no competing interests.

Author details
[1]Sports Medicine Center, Chang Gung Memorial Hospital, No. 6, West Section, Chia-Pu Road, Putz City 61363, Chiayi Country, Taiwan, Republic of China. [2]Department of Orthopaedic Surgery, Chang Gung Memorial Hospital, No. 6, West Section, Chia-Pu Road, Putz City 61363, Chiayi Country, Taiwan, Republic of China. [3]PO CHENG Orthopedic Institute, No. 100, Bo-ai 2nd Road, Kaohsiung 81357, Zuoying District, Taiwan, Republic of China. [4]Department of Athletic Sports, National Chung Cheng University, No.168, University Road, Minhsiung Township 62102, Chiayi Country, Taiwan, Republic of China.

References
1. Daigle ME, Weinstein AM, Katz JN, Losina E. The cost-effectiveness of total joint arthroplasty: a systematic review of published literature. Best Pract Res Clin Rheumatol. 2012;26(5):649–58.
2. Ranawat CS, Flynn WF Jr, Saddler S, Hansraj KK, Maynard MJ. Long-term results of the total condylar knee arthroplasty. A 15-year survivorship study. Clin Orthop Relat Res. 1993;286:94–102.
3. Crowninshield RD, Rosenberg AG, Sporer SM. Changing demographics of patients with total joint replacement. Clin Orthop Relat Res. 2006;443:266–72.
4. Gillespie GN, Porteous AJ. Obesity and knee arthroplasty. Knee. 2007;14(2):81–6.
5. Kurtz S, Ong K, Lau E, Mowat F, Halpern M. Projections of primary and revision hip and knee arthroplasty in the United States from 2005 to 2030. J Bone Joint Surg Am. 2007;89(4):780–5.
6. Physical Activity Guidelines Advisory Committee Report. 2008.https://health.gov/paguidelines/pdf/paguide.pdf.
7. Pozzi F, Snyder-Mackler L, Zeni J. Physical exercise after knee arthroplasty: a systematic review of controlled trials. Eur J Phys Rehabil Med. 2013;49(6):877–92.
8. Hiyama Y, Kamitani T, Wada O, Mizuno K, Yamada M. Effects of group-based exercise on range of motion, muscle strength, functional ability, and pain during the acute phase after total knee arthroplasty: a controlled clinical trial. J Orthop Sports Phys Ther. 2016;46(9):742–8.
9. Han AS, Nairn L, Harmer AR, Crosbie J, March L, Parker D, Crawford R, Fransen M. Early rehabilitation after total knee replacement surgery: a multicenter, noninferiority, randomized clinical trial comparing a home exercise program with usual outpatient care. Arthritis Care Res (Hoboken). 2015;67(2):196–202.
10. Chen M, Li P, Lin F. Influence of structured telephone follow-up on patient compliance with rehabilitation after total knee arthroplasty. Patient Prefer Adherence. 2016;10:257–64.
11. Piva SR, Gil AB, Almeida GJ, DiGioia AM 3rd, Levison TJ, Fitzgerald GK. A balance exercise program appears to improve function for patients with total knee arthroplasty: a randomized clinical trial. Phys Ther. 2010;90(6):880–94.
12. Hsu WH, Hsu RW, Lin ZR, Fan CH. Effects of circuit exercise and tai chi on body composition in middle-aged and older women. Geriatr Gerontol Int. 2015;15(3):282–8.
13. Hame SL, Alexander RA. Knee osteoarthritis in women. Curr Rev Musculoskelet Med. 2013;6(2):182–7.
14. Whitlock KG, Piponov HI, Shah SH, Wang OJ, Gonzalez MH. Gender role in total knee arthroplasty: a retrospective analysis of perioperative outcomes in US patients. J Arthroplast. 2016;31(12):2736–40.
15. Song R, Roberts BL, Lee EO, Lam P, Bae SC. A randomized study of the effects of t'ai chi on muscle strength, bone mineral density, and fear of falling in women with osteoarthritis. J Altern Complement Med. 2010;16(3):227–33.
16. Xie F, Li SC, Roos EM, Fong KY, Lo NN, Yeo SJ, Yang KY, Yeo W, Chong HC, Thumboo J. Cross-cultural adaptation and validation of Singapore English and Chinese versions of the Knee injury and Osteoarthritis Outcome Score (KOOS) in Asians with knee osteoarthritis in Singapore. Osteoarthr Cartil. 2006;14(11):1098–103.
17. Roos EM, Roos HP, Lohmander LS, Ekdahl C, Beynnon BD. Knee injury and Osteoarthritis Outcome Score (KOOS)—development of a self-administered outcome measure. J Orthop Sports Phys Ther. 1998;28(2):88–96.
18. Tsai SY, Chi LY, Lee LS, Chou P. Health-related quality of life among urban, rural, and island community elderly in Taiwan. J Formos Med Assoc. 2004; 103(3):196–204.
19. K-Y LIANG, ZEGER SL. Longitudinal data analysis using generalized linear models. Biometrika. 1986;73(1):13–22.
20. Maly MR, Costigan PA, Olney SJ. Determinants of self-report outcome measures in people with knee osteoarthritis. Arch Phys Med Rehabil. 2006;87(1):96–104.
21. Yoshida Y, Mizner RL, Ramsey DK, Snyder-Mackler L. Examining outcomes from total knee arthroplasty and the relationship between quadriceps strength and knee function over time. Clin Biomech (Bristol, Avon). 2008;23(3):320–8.
22. Fransen M, McConnell S, Harmer AR, Van der Esch M, Simic M, Bennell KL. Exercise for osteoarthritis of the knee. Cochrane Database Syst Rev. 2015;1:CD004376.
23. Taniguchi M, Sawano S, Kugo M, Maegawa S, Kawasaki T, Ichihashi N. Physical activity promotes gait improvement in patients with total knee arthroplasty. J Arthroplast. 2016;31(5):984–8.
24. Mizner RL, Petterson SC, Snyder-Mackler L. Quadriceps strength and the time course of functional recovery after total knee arthroplasty. J Orthop Sports Phys Ther. 2005;35(7):424–36.
25. Kuntze G, von Tscharner V, Hutchison C, Ronsky JL. Alterations in lower limb multimuscle activation patterns during stair climbing in female total knee arthroplasty patients. J Neurophysiol. 2015;114(5):2718–25.
26. Mizner RL, Petterson SC, Stevens JE, Axe MJ, Snyder-Mackler L. Preoperative quadriceps strength predicts functional ability one year after total knee arthroplasty. J Rheumatol. 2005;32(8):1533–9.
27. Mizner RL, Petterson SC, Stevens JE, Vandenborne K, Snyder-Mackler L. Early quadriceps strength loss after total knee arthroplasty. The contributions of muscle atrophy and failure of voluntary muscle activation. J Bone Joint Surg Am. 2005;87(5):1047–53.
28. Mizner RL, Snyder-Mackler L. Altered loading during walking and sit-to-stand is affected by quadriceps weakness after total knee arthroplasty. J Orthop Res. 2005;23(5):1083–90.
29. Ishii Y, Noguchi H, Sato J, Sakurai T. Toyabe SI. Knee Surg Sports Traumatol Arthrosc: Quadriceps strength impairment in the mid- to long-term follow-up period after total knee arthroplasty; 2016.
30. Stevens JE, Mizner RL, Snyder-Mackler L. Quadriceps strength and volitional activation before and after total knee arthroplasty for osteoarthritis. J Orthop Res. 2003;21(5):775–9.
31. Meier W, Mizner RL, Marcus RL, Dibble LE, Peters C, Lastayo PC. Total knee arthroplasty: muscle impairments, functional limitations, and recommended rehabilitation approaches. J Orthop Sports Phys Ther. 2008;38(5):246–56.
32. Bennell K, Dobson F. Review: exercise interventions improve pain and function in people with knee osteoarthritis compared with no exercise. Evid Based Nurs. 2014;17(4):109.
33. Cupeiro R, Benito PJ, Maffulli N, Calderon FJ, Gonzalez-Lamuno D. MCT1 genetic polymorphism influence in high intensity circuit training: a pilot study. J Sci Med Sport. 2010;13(5):526–30.

18

The efficacy of tranexamic acid using oral administration in total knee arthroplasty

Lu-kai Zhang[1,2†], Jian-xiong Ma[1†], Ming-jie Kuang[1], Jie Zhao[1], Bin Lu[1], Ying Wang[1], Xin-long Ma[1,3*] and Zheng-rui Fan[1]

Abstract

Background: Total knee arthroplasty (TKA) is gradually regarded as an effective choice for end-stage osteoarthritis or rheumatic arthritis. In the past, the management of tranexamic acid (TXA) using intravenous injection or topical application has been extensively researched. However, several studies have reported that oral TXA has an effect on blood loss. Therefore, a meta-analysis should be performed to determine whether oral TXA helps to prevent blood loss.

Methods: Randomized controlled trials or retrospective cohort studies about relevant studies were searched in PubMed (1996–April 2017), Embase (1980–April 2017), and the Cochrane Library (CENTRAL, April 2017). Six studies that compared oral TXA to non-TXA were included in our meta-analysis. Meta-analyses (PRISMA) guidelines, the Cochrane Handbook, and the Jadad scale were used to evaluate the included studies and the results to ensure that the meta-analysis was viable.

Results: In accordance with inclusion and exclusion, six studies with 2553 patients (oral TXA = 1386, without TXA = 1167) were eligible and accepted into this meta-analysis. Pooled data indicated that the oral TXA group was effective compared to the without TXA group in terms of hemoglobin (Hb) drop ($P < 0.05$), blood loss at 24 h ($P < 0.05$), total blood loss ($P < 0.05$), and the transfusion rate ($P < 0.05$). No significant differences were found in the length of hospital stay ($P = 0.96$) and complications ($P = 0.39$).

Conclusion: Compared to the non-TXA group, the oral TXA group showed effects of blood sparing. Considering the cost and effectiveness, oral TXA is useful for TKA.

Keywords: Tranexamic acid, Oral, Total knee arthroplasty, Blood loss, Meta-analysis

Background

Total knee arthroplasty (TKA) is recommended as an effective method for end-stage knee osteoarthritis or rheumatoid arthritis [1]. However, it may cause severe blood loss during the perioperative period. Tranexamic acid (TXA) is one of most important antifibrinolytic agents and is known to reduce blood loss, hemoglobin (Hb) drop, and blood transfusion [2–4]. While many meta-analyses and randomized controlled trials (RCTs) have focused on the efficacy of intravenous and topical TXA on TKA [5–7], few have demonstrated the safety and efficacy of oral administration [3, 8, 9]. While drug allergic reaction of anaphylactic shock have been reported in intravenous administration [10], topical administration has a risk of periprosthetic contamination due to infected needles that may cause septicopyemia [11]; in addition, the short duration of the topical form of the drug limits its application [11, 12]. Because oral TXA is administered gradually, a number of RCTs or retrospective controlled studies (RCSs) have been performed to investigate its efficacy and side effects [13–15]. Oral TXA application undergoes rapid and large absorption.

* Correspondence: ZLMM10@163.com

†Equal contributors

[1]Biomechanics Labs of Orthopaedics Institute, Tianjin Hospital, No. 155, Munan Road, Heping District, Tianjin 300050, People's Republic of China

[3]Department of Orthopedics, Tianjin Hospital, Tianjin 300211, People's Republic of China

Full list of author information is available at the end of the article

Furthermore, it is easy to use without special equipment compared to intravenous or topical injection, is less costly, and offers a less burdensome workload for medical personnel [16]. No conclusive evidence has been found regarding the efficacy of using oral TXA during the perioperative period in TKA. The purpose of this meta-analysis was to determine the blood-sparing efficacy of oral TXA administration in TKA.

Methods

Search strategy

We systemically searched randomized controlled trials or retrospective cohort studies, including PubMed (1996–April 2017), Embase (1980–April 2017), and the Cochrane Library (CENTRAL, April 2017). Trials were also found in related references of additional studies. Only English publications were included in our meta-analysis. The search terms "total knee arthroplasty," "total knee replacement," "oral tranexamic acid," and "oral TXA" were used as keywords with Boolean operators "AND" or "OR." The search results are presented in Fig. 1.

Inclusion criteria

Studies were eligible for the meta-analysis if they met the following PICOS (participants, intervention, comparison, outcomes, and study design) criteria: (1) participants: patients who received TKA for the first time; (2) intervention: oral administration of TXA; (3) comparison: non-TXA applied to TKA; (4) outcomes: hemoglobin drop, blood loss, transfusion rate, complications, and length of hospital stay; (5) study design: randomized controlled trials or retrospective cohort studies.

Data extraction and quality assessment

A standard data entry form was designed for the data extraction. Two reviewers independently extracted the available study data. The extracted data included author(s), patients (n), publication date, age, gender, study design, body mass index, and dose of TXA. The primary outcomes were Hb drop and blood loss. The secondary outcomes consisted of the transfusion rate, length of hospital stay, and complications. We emailed the corresponding authors of studies with incomplete or graphical data. Any disagreement between two reviewers was solved by a third reviewer. The Jadad scale was used to evaluate the risk of bias for RCTs, which consisted of random sequence generation, allocation concealment, the blinding of participants and personnel, incomplete outcome data, selective reporting, and other biases [17, 18]. The study was considered high quality if the Jadad score was more than 4 points. For non-RCTs, the risk of bias was evaluated using the Newcastle-Ottawa scale [19], and a score of more than 5 points was considered high quality.

Data synthesis

Outcomes were calculated using Windows Review Manager Software 5.3 (The Nordic Cochrane Center, The Collaboration, 2014, Copenhagen, Denmark). For continuous outcomes, we used mean difference (MD) with 95% confidence intervals (CIs) to weigh the effect interval. For noncontinuous outcomes, relative risk (RR), odds ratio (OR), or risk difference (RD) with 95% CIs were used to weigh the effect interval. The statistical heterogeneity was judged by the value of P and I^2 using the standard chi-squared test. $I^2 > 50\%$ and $P < 0.1$ were considered statistically significant in our results, and a random-effect model was applied for assessment; otherwise, a fixed-effect model was used for extracted data.

Subgroup analysis

When the data had high heterogeneity, we used the random-effect model to ensure the outcome was reliable and accurate, and we performed a subgroup analysis to investigate the causes of heterogeneity. Even when the random-effect model and subgroup analysis were used to decrease the heterogeneity, there was inevitable heterogeneity in the study design and the dose of oral administration, among other factors.

Results

Search results

A total of 224 studies were identified through the search strategy. Thirty-four studies were excluded by Endnote software. Overall, 178 studies were excluded due to the title and abstract. According to the inclusion criteria, 6 studies were included by reading the full text: 5 were RCTs [14, 15, 20–22] and 1 was an RCS [13]. The baseline characteristics of the included studies are summarized in Tables 1 and 2.

Study characteristics

Risk of bias in included studies

Publication bias was evaluated using a funnel plot diagram (Fig. 2). The funnel plot diagram of Hb drops, blood loss, transfusion rate, length of hospital stay, and complications was symmetrical, indicating a low risk of publication bias.

Meta-analysis results

Hemoglobin drop

Data from three studies including 2150 patients reported the Hb drops at the lowest postoperative Hb level during hospital stays. Compared to the control group, oral TXA significantly prevented Hb drop (MD = − 0.80; 95% CI, − 0.88, − 0.71; $P < 0.05$; Fig. 3). The fixed-effect model was used to find the statistical heterogeneity between the two groups ($x^2 = 0.17$; df = 2; $P = 0.92$; $I^2 = 0\%$; Fig. 3).

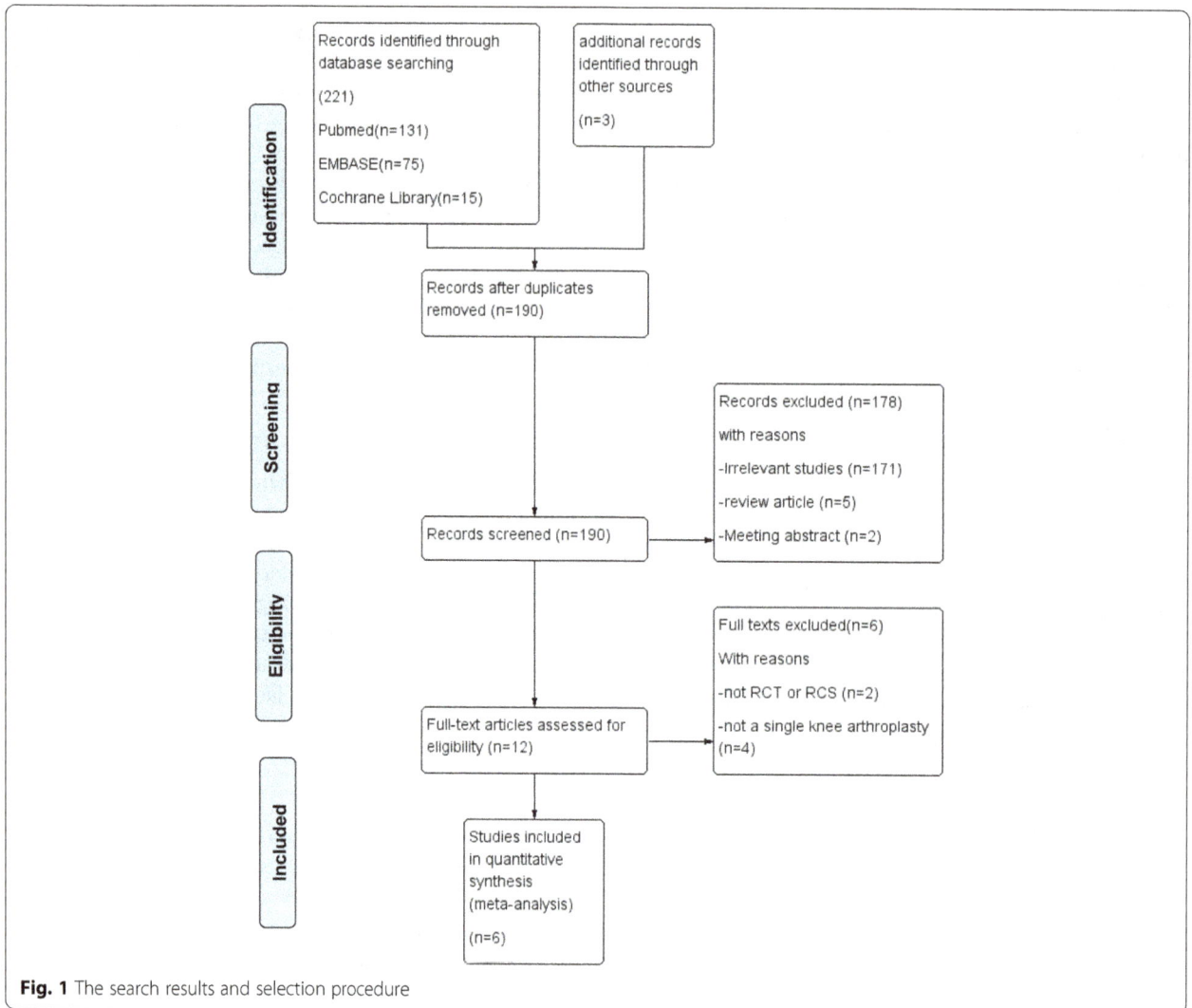

Fig. 1 The search results and selection procedure

Blood loss

The blood loss 12 h after surgery was reported in two studies totaling 93 patients. No significant difference was found between the oral TXA and the control groups (MD = − 36.15; 95% CI, − 141.99, 69.68; $P > 0.05$; Fig. 4). The blood loss 24 h after surgery was reported in two studies of 93 patients. Compared to the control groups, oral TXA significantly prevented blood loss 24 h after surgery (MD = − 144.66; 95% CI, − 201.56, − 87.76; $P < 0.05$; Fig. 4). Data from two studies including 235 patients recorded the total blood loss. The oral TXA groups had significantly less blood loss compared to the control groups (MD = − 231.55; 95% CI, − 290.70, − 172.39; $P < 0.05$; Fig. 4). Statistical heterogeneity was not found in blood loss 24 h after surgery ($x^2 = 0.25$; df = 1; $P = 0.62$; $I^2 = 0\%$) or total blood loss ($x^2 = 0.06$; df = 1; $P = 0.80$; $I^2 = 0\%$; Fig. 4). A random-effects model was applied in the study due to the statistical heterogeneity

found in blood loss 12 h after surgery ($x^2 = 3.28$; df = 1; $P = 0.07$; $I^2 = 69\%$; Fig. 4).

Transfusion rate

The transfusion rate was reported in three studies including 2384 patients. Compared to the control groups, the oral TXA groups had significantly reduced transfusion rates (OR = 0.40; 95% CI, 0.30, 0.52; $P < 0.05$; Fig. 5). A fixed-effect model was applied because no statistical heterogeneity was found in this meta-analysis ($x^2 = 0.25$; df = 2; $P = 0.88$; $I^2 = 0\%$; Fig. 5).

Complications

We extracted data on complications including deep vein thrombosis (DVT) and pulmonary embolism (PE) from five studies including 465 patients. There was no significant difference between the oral TXA and the control groups (RD = − 0.01; 95% CI, − 0.04, 0.02; $P > 0.05$; Fig.

Table 1 The characteristics of included studies

Studies (year)	Country	Cases	Ages (year)	Female gender (%)	Preoperative Hb (g/dL)	BMI (kg/m²)	Reference type	Preoperative diagnose	Preoperative thromboembolic events	Preoperative clotting disorder or anticoagulant therapy	QAS
						Oral TXA group/control group					
Lee et al. (2017) [15]	China	94/95	70/68	67/69.55	13.6 ± 1.3/13.8 ± 1.2	27.7/28.4	RCT	N/A	None	None	6
Yuan et al. (2017) [14]	China	140/40	63.2/64.6	51.4/53.5	13.2 ± 0.8/13.2 ± 0.8	22.69/22.68	RCT	OA or RA	N/A	None	6
Perreault et al. (2017) [13]	USA	1049/866	66.1/66.2	62.4/58.2	14 ± 1.4/14 ± 1.4	N/A	RCS	N/A	None	N/A	6
Zohar et al. (2004) [21]	Israel	20/20	69/73	60/65	N/A	N/A	RCT	N/A	N/A	None	5
Alipour et al. (2013) [22]	Iran	27/26	68.6/63.11	59.3/56.7	N/A	28.9/29.3	RCT	OA or RA	None	None	6
Bradshaw et al. (2012) [20]	Australia	26/20	67.1/68.2	46.2/35	13.4 ± 2.5/13.8 ± 3	32.4/32.5	RCT	OA	None	None	6

TXA tranexamic acid, Hb hemoglobin, BMI body mass index, QAS quality assessment score, RCT randomized controlled trial, RCS retrospective cohort study, N/A not applicable, USA the United States of America, OA osteoarthritis, RA rheumatoid arthritis

Table 2 Characteristics of included studies showing general intervention information

Studies (year)	Dosage of TXA (mg)	Surgical approach	Transfusion criteria	Postoperative anticoagulation	Surgery	Anesthesia	DVT screening method	Pneumatic tourniquet
Lee et al. (2017) [15]	3000	MP	Hb < 80 g/L	N/A	Primary TKA	General anesthesia	Doppler ultrasonography	Yes
Yuan et al. (2017) [14]	N/A	MP	Hb < 80 g/L or anemia symptoms	10 mg/day rivaroxaban	Primary TKA	General anesthesia	Doppler ultrasonography and chest computed tomography	Yes
Perreault et al. (2017) [13]	3900	N/A	Hb < 80 g/L or anemia symptoms	N/A	Primary TKA	N/A	N/A	N/A
Zohar et al. (2004) [21]	3000	N/A	Hematocrit < 28%	40 mg/day enoxaparin	Primary TKA	N/A	Doppler ultrasound imaging and signs of lower limb DVT(swelling or increase in calf diameter)	Yes
Alipour et al. (2013) [22]	3000	N/A	N/A	40 mg/day enoxaparin	Primary TKA	Standard general anesthesia	N/A	Yes
Bradshaw et al. (2012) [20]	6000	MP	Hb < 70 g/L or anemia symptoms	40 mg/day enoxaparin	Primary TKA	N/A	N/A	Yes

TXA tranexamic acid, *N/A* not applicable, *Hb* hemoglobin, *MP* medial parapatellar approach, *DVT* deep vein thrombosis, *TKA* total knee arthroplasty

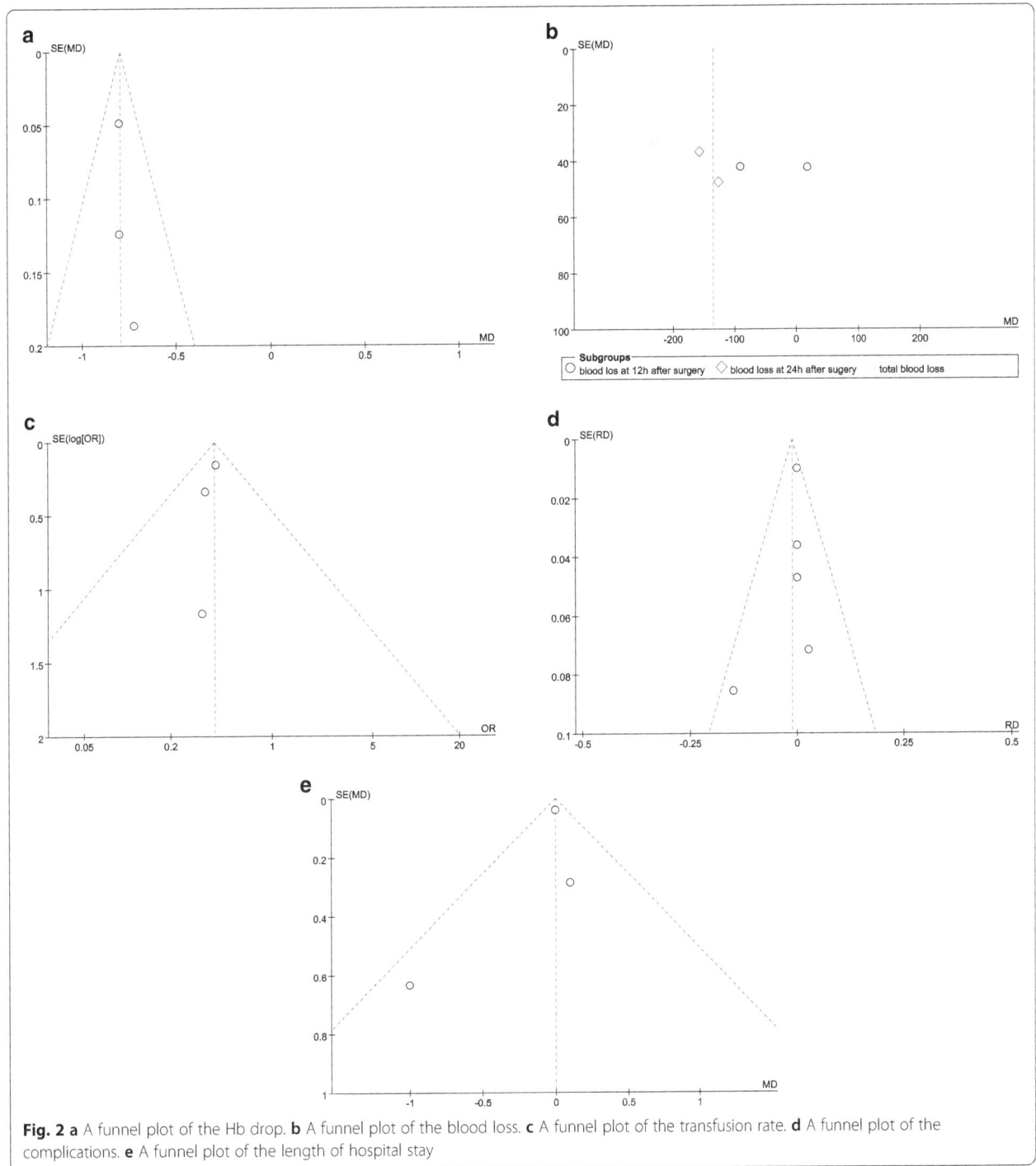

Fig. 2 a A funnel plot of the Hb drop. **b** A funnel plot of the blood loss. **c** A funnel plot of the transfusion rate. **d** A funnel plot of the complications. **e** A funnel plot of the length of hospital stay

6). Because of the low statistical heterogeneity, we used a fixed-effect model ($x^2 = 4.51$; df $=4$; $P = 0.34$; $I^2 = 11\%$; Fig. 6).

Length of hospital stay

Length of hospital stay was reported in three studies involving 2144 patients. No significant difference was found between the two groups (MD $= -0.00$; 95% CI, -0.08, 0.08; $P > 0.05$; Fig. 7). Because of the low statistical

heterogeneity, we used a fixed-effect model ($x^2 = 2.62$; df $= 2$; $P = 0.27$; $I^2 = 24\%$; Fig. 7).

Discussion

Recently, attention has been paid to oral TXA due to its rapid absorption, operability, and less cost [23, 24]. Applicable management during the perioperative period reduces both the recovery time and the transfusion rate. TXA as one of the most important antifibrinolytics has

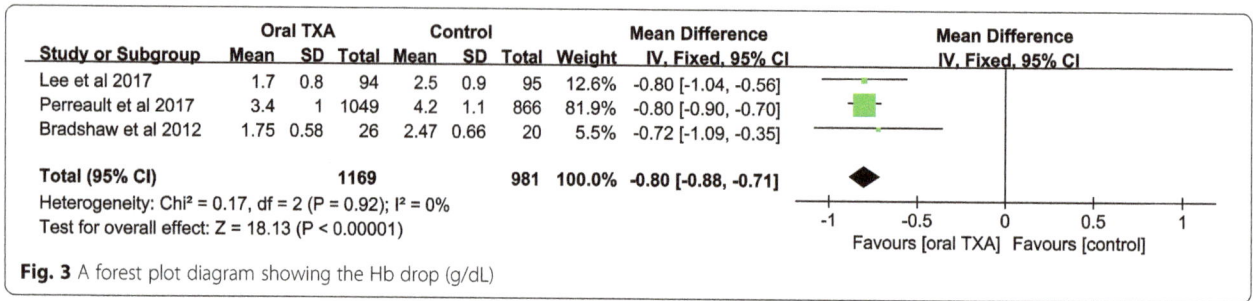

Fig. 3 A forest plot diagram showing the Hb drop (g/dL)

shown strong effects on reducing blood loss by blocking the lysine-binding sites of plasminogen. The two methods of topical application and intravenous injection administration prevented significant blood loss [25–27]. Anaphylactic shock was reported in patients using intravenous injection, and there was also a potential risk of periprosthetic infection once the needle was contaminated [11, 12]. It has recently been reported that oral TXA has the same effects in preventing blood loss, Hb drop, and the transfusion rate compared to intravenous or topical administration [28].

In our meta-analysis, all patients in the included studies had been diagnosed without preoperative coagulation disorders. Alipour et al. [22] excluded from the study patients with thromboembolic events and those who had recently taken anticoagulants or non-steroidal anti-inflammatory drugs. Bradshaw et al. [20] had exclusion criteria that included a history of thromboembolic events and/or anticoagulation that could not be ceased within the recommended time before surgery. Patients with thromboembolic

diseases, anticoagulation, or DVT prophylaxis were excluded by Lee et al [15]. Yuan et al. [14] excluded patients with coagulopathy or bleeding disorders. Zohar et al. [21] excluded patients with bleeding disorders or current anticoagulant therapy. Perreault et al. [13] excluded patients with a history of pulmonary embolus or DVT. Three of the included studies recorded preoperative hemoglobin levels. Lee et al. [15] reported preoperative Hb levels in the oral and control groups of 13.3 ± 1.3 g/dL and 13.8 ± 1.2 g/dL, respectively. Yuan et al. [14] reported preoperative Hb levels of 13.2 ± 0.8 g/dL and 13.2 ± 0.8 g/dL, respectively, in the oral and control groups. Bradshaw et al. [20] reported preoperative Hb levels of 13.4 ± 2.5 g/dL and 13.8 ± 3 g/dL in the oral and control groups, respectively. Perreault et al. [13] reported preoperative Hb levels of 14.1 ± 1.4 g/dL in the oral group and 14 ± 1.4 g/dL in the control group.

Concerning the surgical approach, the medial parapatellar method was performed by Lee et al. [15], Yuan et al. [14], and Bradshaw et al. [20]. Three of the included

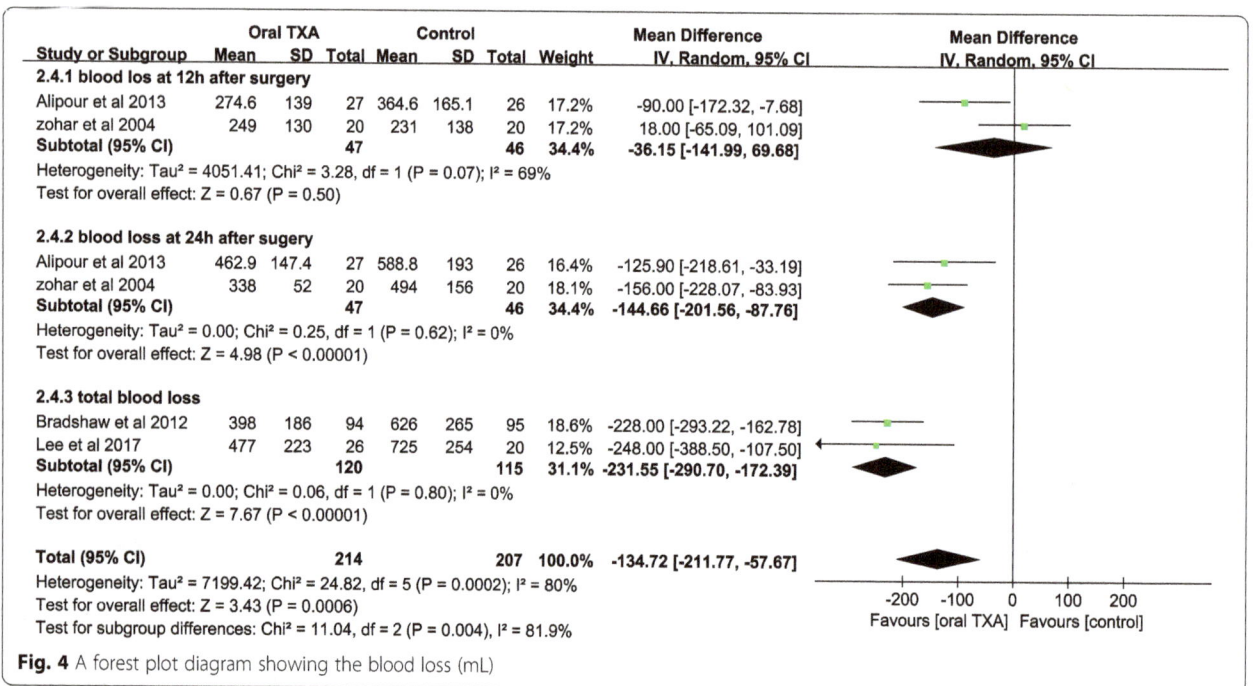

Fig. 4 A forest plot diagram showing the blood loss (mL)

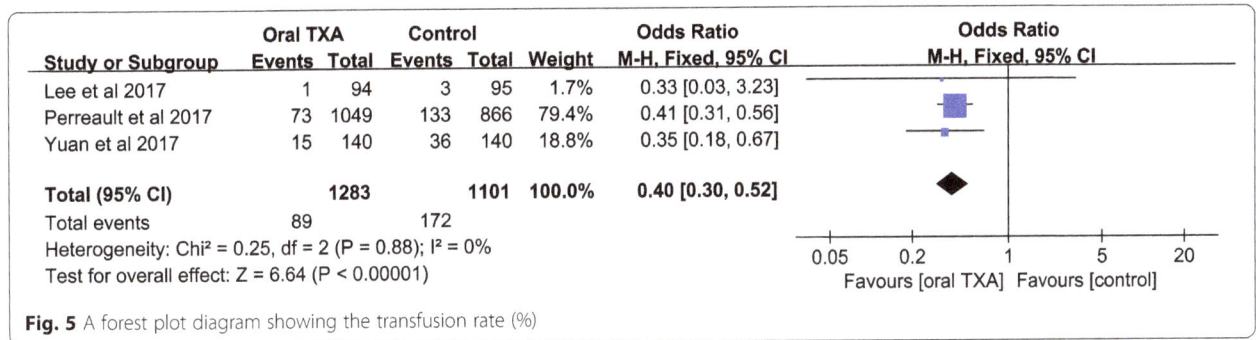

Study or Subgroup	Oral TXA Events	Total	Control Events	Total	Weight	Odds Ratio M-H, Fixed, 95% CI
Lee et al 2017	1	94	3	95	1.7%	0.33 [0.03, 3.23]
Perreault et al 2017	73	1049	133	866	79.4%	0.41 [0.31, 0.56]
Yuan et al 2017	15	140	36	140	18.8%	0.35 [0.18, 0.67]
Total (95% CI)		1283		1101	100.0%	0.40 [0.30, 0.52]
Total events	89		172			

Heterogeneity: Chi² = 0.25, df = 2 (P = 0.88); I² = 0%
Test for overall effect: Z = 6.64 (P < 0.00001)

Fig. 5 A forest plot diagram showing the transfusion rate (%)

studies did not record the surgical methods [13, 21, 22]. Bradshaw et al. [20] reported that the indications for blood transfusion were hemoglobin levels of less than 7 g/dL or clinical symptoms of anemia. Lee et al. [15] recorded that the serum Hb level for transfusion trigger was 8 g/dL. Yuan et al. [14] showed that blood transfusions were performed following a restrictive strategy (Hb < 8 g/dL) or symptoms of anemia. Zohar et al. [21] reported that hematocrit < 28% constituted the postoperative transfusion trigger. Perreault et al. [13] settled on a predefined protocol, with transfusion of Hb < 8 g/dL or Hb < 10 g/dL in patients with significant symptoms of anemia.

Concerning the anticoagulation method, rivaroxaban (10 mg/day) was taken orally until 21 days after hospital discharge in Yuan et al.'s research [14]. In Zohar et al.'s [21] study, subcutaneous enoxaparin (40 mg/day) was administered for DVT prophylaxis. Alipour et al. [22] reported that enoxaparin with a dose of 40 mg/day was prescribed from 1 day before surgery and maintained for 2 weeks. Bradshaw et al. [20] reported that anticoagulation consisted of 40 mg/day of enoxaparin was administered for 2 weeks starting at 12 h postoperatively. Lee et al. [15]reported all patients had Doppler ultrasonography on postoperative day 7 to detect any proximal DVT. In Zohar et al.'s [21] trial, all patients were examined daily for signs of lower limb DVT (swelling or an increase in the calf diameter) and underwent lower limb Doppler ultrasound imaging on the fifth postoperative day.

Hb drop was the primary outcome in our meta-analysis. Several high-quality RCTs and RCSs showed that oral TXA can prevent Hb drop postoperatively [13, 15]. Perreault et al. [13] found that there was less Hb drop in the oral TXA group compared to the untreated group. These results were consistent with our outcomes. Our pooled data demonstrated that oral TXA can prevent Hb drop postoperatively. Irwin et al. [29] demonstrated that oral TXA provided similar effects on lower Hb drop compared to intravenous TXA. In conclusion, oral TXA can effectively inhibit Hb drop.

Blood loss was also an important indicator for evaluating blood sparing. An RCT reported by Bradshaw et al. [20] showed that oral TXA prevented total blood loss significantly compared to the untreated group, and the same outcome was reported by Lee et al. [15]. Our meta-analysis was consistent with these results. In our meta-analysis, oral TXA significantly reduced total blood loss compared to the control group. Two high-quality RCTs showed that oral TXA could limit blood loss 24 h after surgery [21, 22]. This is consistent with our findings. As to blood loss at 12 h after surgery, Zohar et al. [21] reported that the amount of blood loss in the surgical drain was similar in the oral TXA group and the control group. This is also consistent with our findings. Our meta-analysis concluded that no significant differences were found between the oral TXA group and the control group. Meanwhile, risk of bias and high heterogeneity should be considered when interpreting the

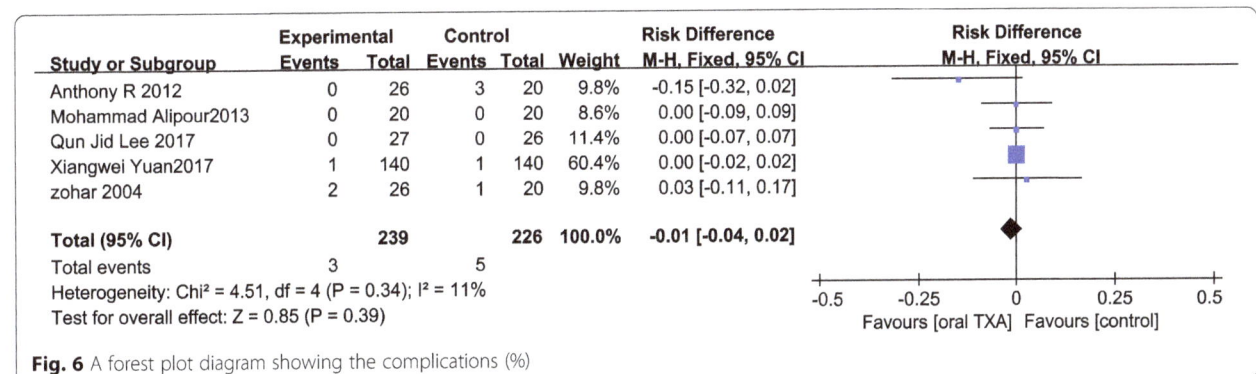

Study or Subgroup	Experimental Events	Total	Control Events	Total	Weight	Risk Difference M-H, Fixed, 95% CI
Anthony R 2012	0	26	3	20	9.8%	-0.15 [-0.32, 0.02]
Mohammad Alipour2013	0	20	0	20	8.6%	0.00 [-0.09, 0.09]
Qun Jid Lee 2017	0	27	0	26	11.4%	0.00 [-0.07, 0.07]
Xiangwei Yuan2017	1	140	1	140	60.4%	0.00 [-0.02, 0.02]
zohar 2004	2	26	1	20	9.8%	0.03 [-0.11, 0.17]
Total (95% CI)		239		226	100.0%	-0.01 [-0.04, 0.02]
Total events	3		5			

Heterogeneity: Chi² = 4.51, df = 4 (P = 0.34); I² = 11%
Test for overall effect: Z = 0.85 (P = 0.39)

Fig. 6 A forest plot diagram showing the complications (%)

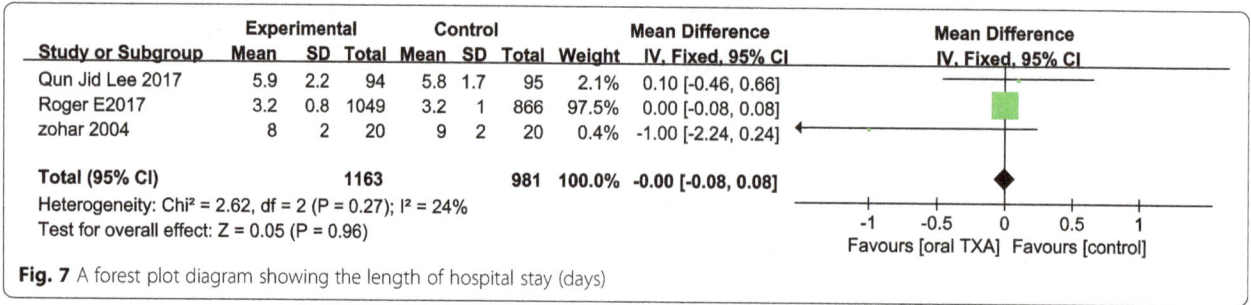

Study or Subgroup	Experimental			Control			Weight	Mean Difference IV, Fixed, 95% CI	Mean Difference IV, Fixed, 95% CI
	Mean	SD	Total	Mean	SD	Total			
Qun Jid Lee 2017	5.9	2.2	94	5.8	1.7	95	2.1%	0.10 [-0.46, 0.66]	
Roger E2017	3.2	0.8	1049	3.2	1	866	97.5%	0.00 [-0.08, 0.08]	
zohar 2004	8	2	20	9	2	20	0.4%	-1.00 [-2.24, 0.24]	
Total (95% CI)			**1163**			**981**	**100.0%**	**-0.00 [-0.08, 0.08]**	

Heterogeneity: Chi² = 2.62, df = 2 (P = 0.27); I² = 24%
Test for overall effect: Z = 0.05 (P = 0.96)

Favours [oral TXA]   Favours [control]

Fig. 7 A forest plot diagram showing the length of hospital stay (days)

findings. We considered that the imbalance between fibrinolysis and TXA-induced antifibrinolytics is due to the release of tourniquet. Tourniquet release can accelerate fibrinolysis, while the optimal effects of oral TXA appeared 2 h after ingestion [16, 30]. As a consequence, the oral TXA group did not have inhibited fibrinolysis caused by tourniquet release. Therefore, no significant differences in blood loss were found in the oral and control TXA groups 12 h after surgery. However, because of the small sample size (under 100 patients), the conclusion with respect to blood loss was limited compared to the findings on Hb drop and transfusion rate.

The blood-sparing efficacy was also reflected in the transfusion rate. Perreault et al. [13] used a large hospital database to assess the rate of transfusion among the oral TXA and control groups. The outcomes of this RCT demonstrated that the oral TXA group had a lower rate of transfusion compared to the control group. This is consistent with our findings. Lee et al. [15] reported that there were no significant differences in transfusion rates between the two groups. The possible reason for low transfusion rate in both groups was the high postoperative Hb level compared to the transfusion trigger [31]. Thus, we conclude that the oral TXA group has a lower transfusion rate compared to the control group. Postoperative DVT and PE were common complications in TKA patients who took TXA. Our meta-analysis failed to find any significant differences between the two groups. Similar findings were reported by Lee et al. [15]. The results of our pooled data indicated that there were no differences in length of hospital stay because of the low incidence in both groups. Taking these findings together, we considered that there were no obvious differences in complications and length of hospital stay in the oral TXA group and the control group. Moreover, it has been reported that the cost of oral TXA administration was much lower compared to intravenous or topical forms [14, 32, 33]. However, all patients of our included studies have been diagnosed without history of thromboembolic events or a higher thromboembolic risk, and there was less or even no data available dealing with the use of TXA with a higher thromboembolic risk. Taking

these into consideration, it may potentially limit the general use of TXA in elective surgeries.

Several reports have demonstrated that oral TXA helps reduce hematocrit drop [20, 22]. Our meta-analysis did not analyze hematocrit drop for two reasons: because of the small sample of included studies, and the ratio between Hb drop and hematocrit drop is always supposed to be 1/3. Patients with potential malfunctioning coagulation systems such as hemophilia, unknown bleeding disorders, active liver disease, and so on usually cannot be detected without preoperative diagnostics during preoperative blood management, while malfunctioning coagulation system can potentially cause postoperative DVT [34]. In our meta-analysis, Lee et al. [15] excluded 46 patients who had potentially malfunctioning coagulation systems and a history of thromboembolic disease and other disease. Yuan et al. [14] excluded three patients with clotting mechanism disorders throughout preoperative diagnostics. Remaining studies failed to carry out preoperative diagnostics on patients during preoperative blood management, which may increase the risk of thrombus.

Our meta-analysis and systematic review have several limitations: (1) Only five studies were included in our meta-analysis. The statistical results would be better if more RCTs had been included. (2) Outcomes such as hematocrit and cost were not analyzed due to the small sample size and/or insufficient data. (3) Only English publications were included in our meta-analysis, so there is publication bias. (4) Because of the significant heterogeneity of blood loss at 12 h ($I^2 = 69\%$), we attempted to investigate the source of heterogeneity. Throughout the full articles, the administrations time of TXA before surgery were different (1 and 2 h before surgery, respectively) and the length of enoxaparin use showed large differences (1 and 14 days, respectively) in two studies. Considering the short half-life of oral TXA and the anticoagulant effect of enoxaparin, we believe these differences were the major sources of the heterogeneity. Meta-analyses (PRISMA) guidelines and the Cochrane Handbook were used to assess the quality of the data published in the included studies to ensure that the results of our meta-analysis were reliable and receivable.

Conclusions

Compared to the control group, Hb drop, blood loss, and transfusion rates can be significantly reduced using oral TXA without increasing the risk of complications. Moreover, oral administration is cheaper and easier to use compared to IV and topical applications. Nevertheless, oral TXA should be restricted to selected patients after adequate preoperative blood management and surgeries with extensive blood loss, as there is no current clear recommendation for the general use of TXA in elective orthopedic surgeries such as TKA.

Abbreviations

CIs: Confidence intervals; DVT: Deep vein thrombosis; Ha: Hematocrit; Hb: Hemoglobin; LOS: Length of stay; MD: Mean difference; MP: Medial parapatellar approach; OA: Osteoarthritis; OR: Odds ratio; PE: Pulmonary embolism; PRISMA: Preferred Reporting Items for Systematic Review and Meta-Analyses; QAS: Quality assessment score; RA: Rheumatoid arthritis; RCSs: Retrospective cohort studies; RCTs: Randomized controlled trials; RD: Risk difference; RR: Relative risk; TKA: Total knee arthroplasty; TXA: Tranexamic acid

Acknowledgements

Not applicable.

Funding

No external funding was received for the study.

Authors' contributions

LKZ and JXM conceptualized the study. MJK and JZ contributed to the data curation. BL and YW carried out the formal analysis. LKZ and MJK provided the methodology. BL and ZRF finished the project administration. MJK was responsible for the software. LKZ supervised the study. XLM participated in the validation. LKZ wrote the original draft. XLM reviewed and edited the paper. All authors read and approved the final manuscript.

Competing interests

The authors declare that they have no competing interests.

Author details

[1]Biomechanics Labs of Orthopaedics Institute, Tianjin Hospital, No. 155, Munan Road, Heping District, Tianjin 300050, People's Republic of China. [2]Graduate School of Tianjin University of Traditional Chinese Medicine, Tianjin 300193, People's Republic of China. [3]Department of Orthopedics, Tianjin Hospital, Tianjin 300211, People's Republic of China.

References

1. Gidwani S, Fairbank A. The orthopaedic approach to managing osteoarthritis of the knee. BMJ. 2004;329(7476):1220–4.
2. Yang ZG, Chen WP, Wu LD. Effectiveness and safety of tranexamic acid in reducing blood loss in total knee arthroplasty: a meta-analysis. J Bone Joint Surg Am. 2012;94(13):1153–9.
3. Alshryda S, et al. A systematic review and meta-analysis of the topical administration of tranexamic acid in total hip and knee replacement. Bone Joint J. 2014;96-b(8):1005–15.
4. Poeran J, et al. Tranexamic acid use and postoperative outcomes in patients undergoing total hip or knee arthroplasty in the United States: retrospective analysis of effectiveness and safety. BMJ. 2014;349:g4829.
5. Chen TP, et al. Comparison of the effectiveness and safety of topical versus intravenous tranexamic acid in primary total knee arthroplasty: a meta-analysis of randomized controlled trials. J Orthop Surg Res. 2017;12(1):11.
6. Li JF, et al. Combined use of intravenous and topical versus intravenous tranexamic acid in primary total knee and hip arthroplasty: a meta-analysis of randomised controlled trials. J Orthop Surg Res. 2017;12(1):22.
7. Mi B, et al. Is combined use of intravenous and intraarticular tranexamic acid superior to intravenous or intraarticular tranexamic acid alone in total knee arthroplasty? A meta-analysis of randomized controlled trials. J Orthop Surg Res. 2017;12(1):61.
8. Alshryda S, et al. Tranexamic acid in total knee replacement: a systematic review and meta-analysis. J Bone Joint Surg Br. 2011;93(12):1577–85.
9. Panteli M, et al. Topical tranexamic acid in total knee replacement: a systematic review and meta-analysis. Knee. 2013;20(5):300–9.
10. Lucaspolomeni MM, et al. A case of anaphylactic shock with tranexamique acid (Exacyl). Ann Fr Anesth Reanim. 2004;23(6):607–9.
11. Klak M, et al. Tranexamic acid, an inhibitor of plasminogen activation, aggravates staphylococcal septic arthritis and sepsis. Scand J Infect Dis. 2010;42(5):351–8.
12. Zhang LK, et al. Comparison of oral versus intravenous application of tranexamic acid in total knee and hip arthroplasty: A systematic review and meta-analysis. Int J Surg. 2017;45:77–84.
13. Perreault RE, et al. Oral Tranexamic Acid Reduces Transfusions in Total Knee Arthroplasty. J Arthroplasty. 2017;32(10):2990–4.
14. Yuan X, et al. Comparison of 3 Routes of Administration of Tranexamic Acid on Primary Unilateral Total Knee Arthroplasty: A Prospective, Randomized, Controlled Study. J Arthroplasty. 2017;32(9):2738–43.
15. Lee QJ, Ching WY, Wong YC. Blood sparing efficacy of oral tranexamic acid in primary total knee arthroplasty: a randomized controlled trial. Knee Surg Relat Res. 2017;29(1):57–62.
16. Beckett AH, Taylor JF, Kourounakis P. The absorption, distribution and excretion of pentazocine in man after oral and intravenous administration. J Pharm Pharmacol. 1970;22(2):123–8.
17. Hartling L, et al. Risk of bias versus quality assessment of randomised controlled trials: cross sectional study. BMJ. 2009;339:b4012.
18. Jadad AR, et al. Assessing the quality of reports of randomized clinical trials: is blinding necessary? Control Clin Trials. 1996;17(1):1–12.
19. Wells GA, et al. The Newcastle–Ottawa scale (NOS) for assessing the quality of non-randomized studies in meta-analysis. Appl Eng Agric. 2000;18(6):727–34.
20. Bradshaw AR, et al. Oral tranexamic acid reduces blood loss in total knee replacement arthroplasty. Current Orthopaedic Practice. 2012;23(3):209–12.
21. Zohar E, et al. The postoperative blood-sparing efficacy of oral versus intravenous tranexamic acid after total knee replacement. Anesth Analg. 2004;99(6):1679–83. table of contents
22. Alipour M, et al. Effectiveness of oral Tranexamic acid administration on blood loss after knee artropslasty: a randomized clinical trial. Transfus Apher Sci. 2013;49(3):574–7.
23. Fillingham YA, et al. The James A. Rand Young Investigator's Award: a randomized controlled trial of oral and intravenous Tranexamic acid in total knee arthroplasty: the same efficacy at lower cost? J Arthroplast. 2016;31(9 Suppl):26–30.
24. Lee QJ, Chang WY, Wong YC. Blood-sparing efficacy of oral tranexamic acid in primary total hip arthroplasty. J Arthroplast. 2017;32(1):139–42.
25. Wang C, et al. Topical application of tranexamic acid in primary total hip arthroplasty: a systemic review and meta-analysis. Int J Surg. 2015;15:134–9.
26. Roy SP, et al. Efficacy of intra-articular tranexamic acid in blood loss reduction following primary unilateral total knee arthroplasty. Knee Surg Sports Traumatol Arthrosc. 2012;20(12):2494–501.
27. Konig G, Hamlin BR, Waters JH. Topical tranexamic acid reduces blood loss and transfusion rates in total hip and total knee arthroplasty. J Arthroplast. 2013;28(9):1473–6.
28. Mcgrath S, Yates P, Prosser G. Oral tranexamic acid in hip and knee arthroplasty: a prospective cohort study. Open J Orthopedics. 2014;04(8):215–20.
29. Irwin A, et al. Oral versus intravenous tranexamic acid in enhanced-recovery primary total hip and knee replacement: results of 3000 procedures. Bone Joint J. 2013;95-b(11):1556–61.
30. Tanaka N, et al. Timing of the administration of tranexamic acid for maximum reduction in blood loss in arthroplasty of the knee. J Bone Joint Surg Br. 2001;83(5):702–5.
31. Engel JM, et al. Regional hemostatic status and blood requirements after total knee arthroplasty with and without tranexamic acid or aprotinin. Anesth Analg. 2001;92(3):775–80.
32. Moskal JT, Harris RN, Capps SG. Transfusion cost savings with tranexamic acid in primary total knee arthroplasty from 2009 to 2012. J Arthroplast. 2015;30(3):365–8.

19

Selective medial soft tissue release combined with tibial reduction osteotomy in total knee arthroplasty

Qian Tang[1†], Hua-chen Yu[1†], Ping Shang[2], Shang-kun Tang[3], Hua-zi Xu[1], Hai-xiao Liu[1*] and Yu Zhang[1*]

Abstract

Background: To obtain the correct coronal alignment and balancing in flexion and extension, we established a selective medial release technique and investigated the effectiveness and safety of the technique during primary total knee arthroplasty (TKA).

Methods: Four hundred sixty-six primary TKAs with varus deformity were prospectively evaluated between June 2013 and June 2015. A knee joint position similar to Patrick's sign was used to release the medial structure. The medial release technique consisted of release of the capsule and the deep medial collateral ligament (dMCL) (step1), selective release of superficial medial collateral ligament (sMCL) or posterior oblique ligament (POL) (step 2), and selective tibial reduction osteotomy (step 3). Improvement of medial joint gap at each step and other clinical outcomes were evaluated.

Results: Among the 466 knees, symmetrical gaps could be achieved by the limited release of the capsule and the dMCcL in 276 (59%) knees. One hundred fifty-two (33%) required additional sMCL release with 2–5 cm from the joint line distally or POL release. Thirty-eight (8%) necessitated an additional tibial reduction osteotomy. Anterior-medial release and 4-mm medial osteotomy contributed to more improvement of medial gap in flexion than in extension (each $p < 0.01$). Posteromedial release and posteromedial osteotomy contributed to more improvement in extension than in flexion (each $p < 0.01$). No specific complication related to our technique was identified.

Conclusion: The technique of the tibial reduction osteotomy combined with medial soft structure release using Patrick's sign is effective, safe, and minimally invasive to obtain balanced mediolateral and extension-flexion gaps in primary TKA.

Keywords: Total knee arthroplasty, Medial collateral ligament, Tibial reduction osteotomy, Varus knee, Soft tissue release, Orthopedic surgery

Background

Varus deformity is a common problem in total knee arthroplasty (TKA), and an uncorrected deformity has a bad influence on the longevity of the implants [1–4]. To obtain the correct coronal alignment and balancing in flexion and extension, a soft tissue release of the medial structures is frequently needed in severe varus knee [5]. There is a consensus among authors that a medial release should be performed sequentially depending on the degree of varus deformity [6–9].

There exists a controversy in the methods and the order of soft tissue release to achieve balanced gap during TKA of varus deformed osteoarthritic knee [9, 10]. Most surgeons suggested deep layer of the medial collateral ligament (dMCL) release from the proximal tibial attachment as their first step of medial soft tissue release in varus knees. At the next step, various and complex protocols of medial release have been reported including release of superficial layer of the medial collateral ligament (sMCL), posterior oblique ligament (POL), posteromedial capsule, semimembranosus (SM), and pes anserinus, as well as tibial reduction osteotomy [11, 12].

* Correspondence: spineliu@163.com; drzhangyu@hotmail.com
†Equal contributors
[1]Department of Orthopaedic Surgery, The Second Affiliated Hospital and Yuying Children's Hospital of Wenzhou Medical University, 109, Xueyuanxi road, 325027 Wenzhou, China
Full list of author information is available at the end of the article

In knees with severe medial tightness, the possibility of complete detachment of the sMCL by an extensive subperiosteal release during primary TKA has been a concern [13]. Extensive release techniques can lead to instability and also seem to be less effective. The sMCL is the primary restraint to the valgus force of the medial side of the knee [11, 12, 14]. Conservation of the distal attachment of sMCL is considered to be critical to maintain the joint stability when possible. Reduction osteotomy is known as a soft tissue-sparing technique for achieving soft tissue balancing [15], and it is capable of reducing the amount of release required to balance the knee, minimizing the risk of medial over release.

As minimal and efficacious release is the prerequisite of the ideal soft tissue-balancing technique in TKA, we describe steps to release the medial elements mini-invasively by the method of the medial proximal tibial reduction osteotomy combined with soft tissue release during TKA in severely deformed knees. It consists of dMCL release, selective release of sMCL or POL, and selective tibial reduction osteotomy.

In addition, release of posteromedial corner structures, such as POL and SM tendon, are often cumbersome in severe varus knees [15]. In this study, we sought to (1) introduce a knee joint position similar to Patrick's sign in favor of sufficient exposure of the medial structure, (2) determine whether the technique of tibial reduction osteotomy combined with medial soft structure release is effective and minimally invasive, and (3) provide a fine control of mediolateral balance as well as extension-flexion balance by selective soft structure release and selective tibial reduction osteotomy.

Methods

Approval to conduct the study was gained from the local Human Research Ethics Committee. All patients involved in our study signed the informed consent.

The data of 504 consecutive varus knees of 436 patients who underwent primary TKAs was prospectively collected between June 2013 and June 2015. Knees of neutral alignment without any soft tissue release, valgus knees, extraarticular varus deformity, and primary TKAs with severe preoperative ligament instability that needed constrained TKAs were excluded. The cases with large defects after tibial resections were also excluded. The large defects, as defined by Dorr, may occupy 25% or more of the component undersurface and involve a deficit deeper than 5 mm [16].

Among them, 38 knees of 34 patients were lost to follow-up. Thus, 466 knees of 402 patients (92%) comprised the cohort of this study with a mean follow-up of 1.3 years (range, 1–2 years). The mean age of the patients was 63.7 years (range, 55–76 years). All patients diagnosed with knee osteoarthritis were included.

All the TKAs were performed by a senior author in our institute using a medial parapatellar approach. The bone resections were performed before any soft tissue release procedures. Both cruciate ligaments were removed for a posterior cruciate-substituting system (Smith & Nephew, Genesis II). Femoral distal resection was made at 5°–7° valgus by an intramedullary alignment guide with respect to the femoral anatomic axis. The femoral external rotation was decided using the transepicondylar axis and anteroposterior axis. A tibial cut was made perpendicularly to the mechanical axis of the tibia, approximately 9–11 mm in thickness from the lateral tibial cortex by extramedullary guided manner. If there were bone defects that require tibial resections of more than the planned, another 2-mm resection of the tibia was conducted with the joint line being slightly lower (1 mm).

A knee joint position similar to Patrick's sign was used to release the medial structure (Fig. 1), which is performed by having the knee flexed and the thigh abducted and externally rotated. In this position, the surgical procedures for releasing medial structure could be easily performed with pulling away the soft tissue by a retractor. The peripheral osteophytes of the distal femur

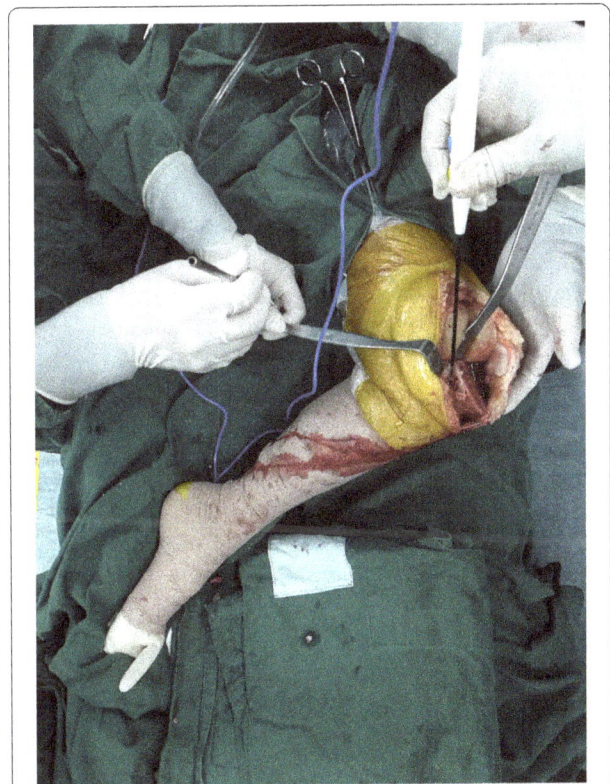

Fig. 1 A knee joint position similar to Patrick's sign was used by pushing the ankle joint to the medial side and the knee joint to the lateral side, which was in favor of exposing the medial structure of the knee

and proximal tibia were removed. The dMCL was released at the menisco-capsular junction, and the medial capsule was regionally released from the edge of the tibial joint surface, which was not beyond 2 cm from the joint line distally (step 1). If the medial gap is still tight, two different methods were further selected according to the medial tightness of flexion and extension gaps: release of anterior-medial or posteromedial structure. Accordingly, medial tightness in flexion only was addressed by releasing the anterior-medial portion of the capsule, anterior arm of SM tendon, and proximal division of the sMCL, while medial tightness in extension only was addressed by releasing the posteromedial structure including the posteromedial capsule, POL, anterior arm, and direct arm of SM tendon as well as proximal division of the sMCL [11, 12, 17, 18] (Fig. 2a, step 2). This release procedure was performed approximately 2–5 cm from the joint line distally.

If the medial gap was still tight, tibial reduction osteotomy was performed until balancing of the joint gap medially to laterally as well as in extension and flexion was achieved. The tibial component was placed along the line of the lateral margin of the tibial surface. After the size and the location of the tibial component were decided, 4-mm vertical osteotomy along the medial aspect of the uncapped tibial surface was performed. According to the medial tightness of flexion and extension gaps, two different regions of tibial reduction osteotomy were selected for medial release. Medial tightness in flexion was released by medial tibial reduction osteotomy, which was parallel to the anteroposterior axis. Medial tightness in extension was released by posteromedial tibial reduction osteotomy, which inclined to the anteroposterior axis at an angle of 30° (Fig. 2b, step 3).

Measurements of the medial and lateral femorotibial joint gap width were performed in full extension and 90° of flexion step-by-step during surgery by a spreader device with a torque meter (Fig. 3). The spreader device was inserted into the joint to adequately distract the joint with the same extrusion force by the thumb and forefinger. The amount of tightness in the joint gap was recorded twice at each step of medial release, and the average value was calculated. Clinical outcomes were also evaluated by the range of motion, knee alignment parameter, and Knee Society Scores (KSSs). The postoperative standing full-length lower limb radiographs were taken, and the knee alignment was recorded.

Statistical analysis was performed with SPSS 16 software (SPSS Inc., Chicago, IL, USA). For numeric data, mean ± SD was calculated. Chi-square test was used to compare the ratio of gender and outliers of alignment among different groups. Overall comparison of the age, range of motion, KSS, and knee alignment among three groups was conducted by the analysis of variance (ANOVA). Statistical heterogeneity was considered to be present at $p < 0.1$; data were analyzed using ANOVA as no heterogeneity existed. Differences were considered as statistically significant with a p value of less than 0.05.

Results

Patients' demographics, imaging parameters, and relevant clinical scores are presented in Table 1. According to the step-by-step release of the medial structure of the knee, the patients were divided into three groups. In 276 of the 466 (59%) primary TKAs, symmetrical gaps could be achieved by the limited release of the capsule and dMCL within 2 cm from the joint line distally (group 1). In 152 cases (33%), release of adhesive structure was performed approximately 2–5 cm from the joint line distally and the distal attachment of sMCL was not released (group 2). In 38 out of the 466 (8%), the medial tightness necessitated a reduction osteotomy after the above procedures (group 3). There was no significant difference in age and gender ratio among the three groups (each $p >$

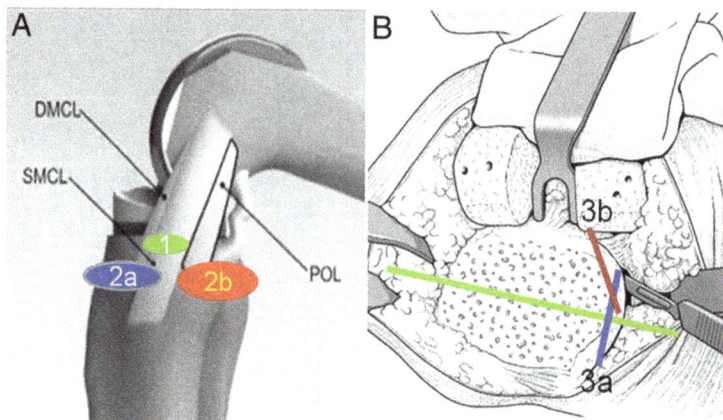

Fig. 2 A diagram illustrates the step by step procedures of medial structure release. **a** The release of medial soft tissue structures which are consisted of dMCL release (Step 1), selective release of anterior-medial (Step 2a) or posteromedial structure (Step 2b); **a** The selective reduction osteotomy which consisted of selective medial (Step 3a) or posteromedial tibia reduction osteotomy (Step 3b)

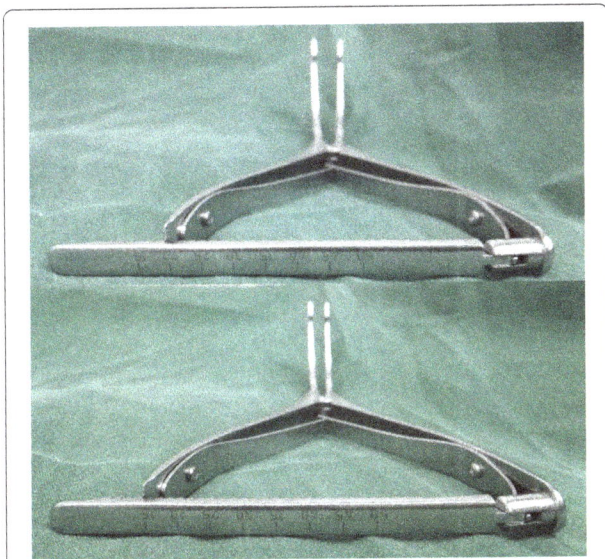

Fig. 3 The spreader device with a torque meter provides a stepwise spreading by detents, and the step size is 1 mm

0.05, Table 1). There were significant differences in the preoperative knee alignment, preoperative range of motion, and preoperative KSS among the three groups (each $p < 0.01$, Table 1).

The beneficial effects of medial soft tissue release and reduction osteotomy were evident on the analysis of joint gap kinematics. Medial gap width increased 1.6 ± 0.8 mm and 1.7 ± 0.6 mm at knee extension and flexion of 90°, respectively, following limited release of the capsula and dMCL (step 1). Medial gap width increased 1.0 ± 0.4 mm and 1.6 ± 0.5 mm at knee extension and flexion, respectively, following additional release of adhesive anterior-medial structure (step 2a). Likewise, the increase of the medial gap at knee extension and flexion was 1.7 ± 0.6 mm and 1.2 ± 0.5 mm, respectively, after release of adhesive posteromedial structure (step 2b). Regardless of the region of the reduction osteotomy

performed, the medial gap significantly increased in both extension and flexion. The increase of the medial gap at knee extension and flexion of 90° was 1.1 ± 0.5 mm and 2.0 ± 0.8 mm, respectively, following medial reduction osteotomy (step 3a). Likewise, following posteromedial reduction osteotomy, the increase of medial gap at knee extension and flexion of 90° was 1.5 ± 0.8 mm and 0.8 ± 0.4 mm, respectively (step 3b). The final amount of medial structure release is shown in Table 2.

The range of motion improved from $118.4 + 7.0°$, $112.1 + 10.6°$, and $109.4 + 8.9°$ preoperatively to $125.8 + 6.6°$, $124.3 + 5.9°$, and $123.5 + 6.4°$ postoperatively at the last follow-up for groups 1, 2, and 3, respectively. The mean preoperative knee mechanical alignment was varus of $5.2 + 2.1°$, $6.6 + 2.2°$, and $9.7 + 2.6°$ and was corrected to $0.6 + 1.6°$, $0.8 + 1.5°$, and $1.2 + 1.7°$ postoperatively for groups 1, 2, and 3, respectively. The KSS improved from $63.7 + 4.8$, $60.8 + 5.9$, and $56.8 + 6.4$ preoperatively to $89.7 + 3.4$, $88.4 + 4.1$, and $87.5 + 3.1$ postoperatively for groups 1, 2, and 3, respectively. There was significant difference in postoperative KSS at the last follow-up among the three groups ($p < 0.001$, Table 1). No difference was noted when comparing postoperative knee alignment and ratio of outliers in the three groups ($p = 0.222$, $p = 0.457$, respectively, Table 1). No specific complications related to the present technique, such as nerve injury, hematoma formation, subsidence of the tibial component, or conversion to a constrained prosthesis due to over release, were observed.

Discussion

We introduce a knee joint position similar to Patrick's sign in favor of exposing the medial structure and established a step-by-step selective release procedure, which consisted of dMCL release, selective release of medial soft structure, and selective tibial reduction osteotomy (Fig. 4). A refined technique of selective medial release was performed using anterior-medial soft tissue release and medial tibial reduction osteotomy for tightness in

Table 1 Comparisons of demographics of patients in each group

	Group 1 (n = 276) Mean ± SD	Group 2 (n = 152) Mean ± SD	Group 3 (n = 38) Mean ± SD	p value
Age (years)	63.8 ± 4.7	63.6 ± 5.7	63.9 ± 5.3	0.854
Gender (female/male)	169:107	94:58	28:10	0.326
Pre-range of motion	118.4 ± 7.0°	112.1 ± 10.6°	109.4 ± 8.9°	0.001
Post-range of motion	125.8 ± 6.6°	124.3 ± 5.9°	123.5 ± 6.4°	0.001
Pre-knee alignment (varus)	5.2 ± 2.1°	6.6 ± 2.2°	9.7 ± 2.6°	0.001
Post-knee alignment (varus)	0.6 ± 1.6°	0.8 ± 1.5°	1.2 ± 1.7°	0.222
Pre-KSS	63.7 ± 4.8	60.8 ± 5.9	56.8 ± 6.4	0.001
Post-KSS	89.7 ± 3.4	88.4 ± 4.1	87.5 ± 3.1	0.001
Outliers	10/276	6/152	3/38	0.457

Post- postoperative, *Pre-* preoperative, *KSS* Knee Society Score, *Outliers* deviation beyond 3° of varus or valgus mechanical axis, *Group 1* limited release of capsula and dMCL, *Group 2* release of adhesive medial structure (2–5 cm from the joint line distally), *Group 3* medial soft tissue release combined with tibial reduction osteotomy

Table 2 Gap increases with each procedure in total knee arthroplasty

Surgical step	Extension		Flexion	
	Medial gap increasement (mean ± SD)	Lateral gap increasement (mean ± SD)	Medial gap increasement (mean ± SD)	Lateral gap increasement (mean ± SD)
Release of the dMCL (step 1)	1.6 ± 0.8	0.4 ± 0.2	1.7 ± 0.6	0.5 ± 0.3
Broad medial release (step 2)				
Anterior-medial release (2a)	1.0 ± 0.4 A	0.2 ± 0.2 E	1.6 ± 0.5 a	0.6 ± 0.2 e
Posteromedial release (2b)	1.7 ± 0.6 B	0.4 ± 0.3	1.2 ± 0.5 b	0.5 ± 0.3
Reduction osteotomy (step 3)				
Medial osteotomy (3a)	1.1 ± 0.5 C	0.2 ± 0.3 F	2.0 ± 0.8 c	0.6 ± 0.4 f
Posteromedial osteotomy (3b)	1.5 ± 0.8 D	0.3 ± 0.2	0.8 ± 0.4 d	0.4 ± 0.3

Each value is recorded as the increasement of gap after each surgical step: mean (mm) ± standard deviation (SD). $p < 0.01$ for A versus a, B versus b, C versus c, D versus d, E versus e, and F versus f using paired sample t test
dMCL deep medial collateral ligament

flexion, while posteromedial structure release and posteromedial tibial reduction osteotomy for tightness in extension.

Subperiosteal release of posteromedial corner structures, such as the POL and the SM tendon fibers that merge into the posterior capsule, is often cumbersome in severe varus knee [17]. In the current study, a knee joint position similar to Patrick's sign was used, which was effective for sufficient exposure of the medial structure and reduced the possibility of iatrogenic injury to the saphenous nerve.

Three important ligaments maintain primary medial knee stability: the sMCL, POL, and dMCL [11, 12]. The dMCL, whose attachment is on average about 6 mm distal to the tibial plateau, is often released as the first step of medial release during TKA in terms of efficacy and safety [6]. The POL is a primary restraint to internal rotation and is a secondary restraint to valgus translation

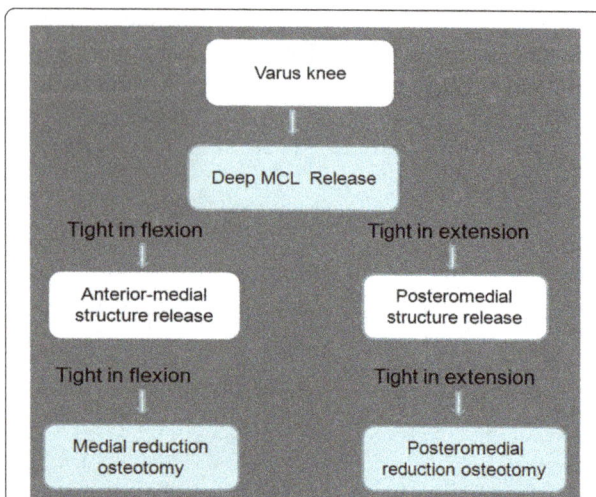

Fig. 4 Algorithmic approach of the medial release based on the principle of selective functional release of the medial soft tissue structure and reduction osteotomy

and external rotation [19]. The POL and sMCL are described as having a complementary relationship in resisting internal rotation torque [20]. Significant increase of rotatory instability is seen on the release of the POL, and thus, retaining the POL has a possibility to improve the outcome after primary TKA [18].

The sMCL plays a consistent role in resisting both the isolated valgus moment and combined valgus and internal rotation moments. Since the proximal division of the sMCL and posterior part of the superficial medial ligament which is attached to the medial meniscus would be released during TKA, the function of the sMCL may be affected [12]. Because the integrity of the sMCL of the knee is crucial to the proper function and longevity of nonconstrained TKA, conservation of sMCL fibers at the tibial insertions, especially on the distal division (62.4 ± 5.5 mm distal to the joint line) is considered to be critical [11–13, 21]. In the current study, the tibial distal division of the sMCL was retained in all cases by using selective medial soft release (less than 5 cm distal to the joint line) combined with selective tibial reduction osteotomy.

It could be argued that the classic extensive medial release associated with iatrogenic injury to the pes anserine and saphenous nerve, instability, and abnormal knee kinematics may be unnecessary [10]. In addition, the concept of constitutionally varus alignment that restores pre-arthritic natural anatomical alignment is emerging in recent years [22–24]. Some studies have reported that kinematically aligned TKA without MCL release and restoration of the limb into patients' natural alignment of slight varus has shown a favorable outcome [6]. Our previous research indicated that a mechanical axis within 3° of varus in the coronal plane remained a satisfactory target in TKA surgery [10]. Thus, mini-invasive release of the medial elements may allow for improved soft tissue balancing leading ultimately to improved functional outcome.

The reduction osteotomy increased component gap width and decreased the varus angle, which might reduce the risk of over release, as well as the amount of medial soft tissue release [25]. It could achieve higher KSS than the TKA series without reduction osteotomy potentially due to reduce medial soft tissue release [15]. There are some tips for tibial reduction osteotomy: firstly, it is important to keep the bone cutting level on the tibia as high as possible, which helps to prevent lateral cortex blowout and maintain the bone quality of the cutting surface [15]. Secondly, in the setting of reduction osteotomy, the tibial base plate is suggested to place along the bony margin of the lateral tibial plateau without downsizing. In the current study, 4-mm reduction osteotomy did not significantly decrease bone quality and a one size smaller tibial component was used in only 2 of 38 knees, where medial osteotomy was used.

Employment of a combined release technique seems to be more effective and minimally invasive than either medial soft structure release or tibial reduction osteotomy alone, since maximal tension exists at the initial phase of each release procedure. For example, 4-mm reduction osteotomy provides approximately 1.7° and 0.7° varus improvement in flexion and extension, respectively, while 8-mm reduction osteotomy only improves 2.8° and 0.9° in flexion and extension, respectively [15]. In addition, employment of a stepwise release technique could avoid unnecessary over release [7, 9].

In the current study, we provide a selective release technique according to extension-flexion gap balance. Release of the anterior-medial soft tissue and medial reduction osteotomy tends to increase the flexion gap more than the extension gap, whereas release of the posteromedial elements and posterior osteotomy tends to affect the extension gap more than the flexion gap. We believe that the results of this study provide valuable information for a TKA procedure to achieve better extension-flexion balancing. Various choices could be selected according to the extension-flexion balancing.

Conclusion
The technique of the tibial reduction osteotomy combined with medial soft structure release using Patrick's sign is effective, safe, and minimally invasive to obtain balanced mediolateral and extension-flexion gaps in primary TKA.

Acknowledgements
Not applicable

Funding
This work was supported by the National Natural Science Foundation of China (nos. 81501869 and .81601983).

Authors' contributions
HXL conceived the study design. QT, HCY, PS, SKT, and HZX performed the study, collected the data, and contributed to the study design. QT and HXL prepared the manuscript. YZ and HXL edited the manuscript. All authors read and approved the final manuscript.

Competing interests
The authors declare that they have no competing interests.

Author details
[1]Department of Orthopaedic Surgery, The Second Affiliated Hospital and Yuying Children's Hospital of Wenzhou Medical University, 109, Xueyuanxi road, 325027 Wenzhou, China. [2]Department of Rehabilitation, The Second Affiliated Hospital and Yuying Children's Hospital of Wenzhou Medical University, 109, Xueyuanxi road, 325027 Wenzhou, China. [3]Department of Clinical Medicine, Second Clinical Medical College, Wenzhou Medical University, 325000 Wenzhou, China.

References
1. Bae DK, Song SJ, Heo DB, Tak DH. Does the severity of preoperative varus deformity influence postoperative alignment in both conventional and computer-assisted total knee arthroplasty? Knee surgery, sports traumatology, arthroscopy : official journal of the ESSKA. 2013;21:2248–54.
2. Fang DM, Ritter MA, Davis KE. Coronal alignment in total knee arthroplasty: just how important is it? J Arthroplast. 2009;24:39–43.
3. Liu HX, Shang P, Ying XZ, Zhang Y. Shorter survival rate in varus-aligned knees after total knee arthroplasty. Knee surgery, sports traumatology, arthroscopy : official journal of the ESSKA. 2016;24:2663–71.
4. Ritter MA, Davis KE, Davis P, Farris A, Malinzak RA, Berend ME, Meding JB. Preoperative malalignment increases risk of failure after total knee arthroplasty. J Bone Joint Surg Am. 2013;95:126–31.
5. Kim MS, Koh IJ, Choi YJ, Kim YD, In Y. Correcting severe varus deformity using trial components during total knee arthroplasty. J Arthroplast. 2017;32:1488–95.
6. Ha CW, Park YB, Lee CH, Awe SI, Park YG. Selective medial release technique using the pie-crusting method for medial tightness during primary total knee arthroplasty. J Arthroplast. 2016;31:1005–10.
7. Kim MW, Koh IJ, Kim JH, Jung JJ, In Y. Efficacy and safety of a novel three-step medial release technique in varus total knee arthroplasty. J Arthroplast. 2015;30:1542–7.
8. Sim JA, Lee YS, Kwak JH, Yang SH, Kim KH, Lee BK. Comparison of complete distal release of the medial collateral ligament and medial epicondylar osteotomy during ligament balancing in varus knee total knee arthroplasty. Clinics in orthopedic surgery. 2013;5:287–91.
9. Verdonk PC, Pernin J, Pinaroli A, Ait Si Selmi T, Neyret P. Soft tissue balancing in varus total knee arthroplasty: an algorithmic approach. Knee surgery, sports traumatology, arthroscopy : official journal of the ESSKA. 2009;17:660–6.
10. Hunt NC, Ghosh KM, Athwal KK, Longstaff LM, Amis AA, Deehan DJ. Lack of evidence to support present medial release methods in total knee arthroplasty. Knee surgery, sports traumatology, arthroscopy : official journal of the ESSKA. 2014;22:3100–12.
11. LaPrade RF, Engebretsen AH, Ly TV, Johansen S, Wentorf FA, Engebretsen L. The anatomy of the medial part of the knee. J Bone Joint Surg Am. 2007;89:2000–10.
12. Liu F, Yue B, Gadikota HR, Kozanek M, Liu W, Gill TJ, Rubash HE, Li G. Morphology of the medial collateral ligament of the knee. J Orthop Surg Res. 2010;5:69.
13. Cho WS, Byun SE, Lee SJ, Yoon J. Laxity after complete release of the medial collateral ligament in primary total knee arthroplasty. Knee surgery, sports traumatology, arthroscopy : official journal of the ESSKA. 2015;23:1816–23.
14. Pedersen RR. The medial and posteromedial ligamentous and capsular structures of the knee: review of anatomy and relevant imaging findings. Semin Musculoskelet Radiol. 2016;20:12–25.
15. Niki Y, Harato K, Nagai K, Suda Y, Nakamura M, Matsumoto M. Effects of reduction osteotomy on gap balancing during total knee arthroplasty for severe varus deformity. J Arthroplast. 2015;30:2116–20.
16. Dorr LD. Bone grafts for bone loss with total knee replacement. Orthop Clin North Am. 1989;20:179.

17. Lavernia C, Contreras JS, Alcerro JC. The peel in total knee revision: exposure in the difficult knee. Clin Orthop Relat Res. 2011;469:146–53.

18. Weimann A, Schatka I, Herbort M, Achtnich A, Zantop T, Raschke M, Petersen W. Reconstruction of the posterior oblique ligament and the posterior cruciate ligament in knees with posteromedial instability. Arthroscopy : the journal of arthroscopic & related surgery : official publication of the Arthroscopy Association of North America and the International Arthroscopy Association. 2012;28:1283–9.

19. Seo JG, Moon YW, Jo BC, Kim YT, Park SH. Soft tissue balancing of varus arthritic knee in minimally invasive surgery total knee arthroplasty: comparison between posterior oblique ligament release and superficial MCL release. Knee surgery & related research. 2013;25:60–4.

20. Elliott M, Johnson DL. Management of medial-sided knee injuries. Orthopedics. 2015;38:180–4.

21. Clizawa N, Mori A, Majima T, Kawaji H, Matsui S, Takai S. Influence of the medial knee structures on valgus and rotatory stability in total knee arthroplasty. J Arthroplast. 2016;31:688–93.

22. Magnussen RA, Weppe F, Demey G, Servien E, Lustig S. Residual varus alignment does not compromise results of TKAs in patients with preoperative varus. Clin Orthop Relat Res. 2011;469:3443–50.

23. Matziolis G, Adam J, Perka C. Varus malalignment has no influence on clinical outcome in midterm follow-up after total knee replacement. Arch Orthop Trauma Surg. 2010;130:1487–91.

24. Parratte S, Pagnano MW, Trousdale RT, Berry DJ. Effect of postoperative mechanical axis alignment on the fifteen-year survival of modern, cemented total knee replacements. J Bone Joint Surg Am. 2010;92:2143–9.

25. Mullaji AB, Shetty GM. Correction of varus deformity during TKA with reduction osteotomy. Clin Orthop Relat Res. 2014;472:126–32.

20

Influence of tourniquet use in primary total knee arthroplasty with drainage: a prospective randomised controlled trial

Kai Zhou, Tingxian Ling, Haoyang Wang, Zongke Zhou*, Bin Shen, Jing Yang, Pengde Kang and Fuxing Pei

Abstract

Background: We aimed to compare the effect of tourniquet use or lack of it on recovery following uncomplicated primary total knee arthroplasty (TKA).

Methods: In a prospective randomised double-blinded study, 150 patients undergoing primary TKA were assigned to either a tourniquet or non-tourniquet group. At the early phase, 3 and 6 months after surgery, an independent observer assessed the primary outcome measure (i.e. total blood loss) and secondary outcome measures (i.e. wound complications, visual analogue scale pain score and knee range of motion).

Results: The tourniquet group exhibited reduced intraoperative blood loss (215.7 ± 113.7 ml vs. 138.6 ± 93.9 ml, $P < 0.001$) and shorter operating time (77.2 ± 14.5 min vs. 82.0 ± 12.7 min, $P = 0.038$). However, the non-tourniquet group showed less postoperative blood loss (180.2 ± 117.0 ml vs. 253.7 ± 144.2 ml, $P = 0.001$) and drainage volume (89.2 ± 66.3 ml vs. 164.5 ± 97.8 ml, $P = 0.004$), less thigh pain (all $P < 0.001$) in the initial 3 weeks, better knee range of motion (ROM) in the initial 3 days (day 1 81.6 ± 17.1 vs. 75.95 ± 14.55, $P = 0.036$; day 3 99.8 ± 13.7 vs. 93.95 ± 11.15, $P = 0.005$) and fewer wound tension vesicles (10.3 vs. 29.2%, $P = 0.005$). Earlier straight-leg raising (4.6 ± 3.8 h vs. 6.4 ± 4.3 h, $P = 0.01$) and shorter length of stay (6.3 ± 1.7 days vs. 7.1 ± 1.9 days, $P = 0.001$) were found in the non-tourniquet group. Similar total blood loss and blood transfusion rate were observed for both groups. All other parameters revealed no significant differences.

Conclusions: Our study suggests that a non-tourniquet TKA would lead to early rehabilitation without increasing side effects.

Trial registration: Chinese Clinical Trials Registry, ChiCTR-IOR-16007851, 1/29/2016

Keywords: Prospective randomised controlled trial, Total knee arthroplasty, Tourniquet

Background

Tourniquets are commonly used in total knee arthroplasty (TKA) to provide better visualisation and facilitate cementing techniques [1]. Although widely accepted, tourniquet-related complications have been reported in the literature, including wound complications, thigh pain, limb swelling, nerve palsy and muscle myofibril injury [2, 3]. In view of the tourniquet-related complications, some surgeons would like to perform TKA without a tourniquet [4, 5].

Several randomised controlled trials (RCTs) have compared the effects of tourniquet and non-tourniquet technique in TKA, but they drew different conclusions, and the sample sizes were small [5–8]. It is not clear whether it is necessary to use a tourniquet during TKA with the advances in surgical techniques and perioperative managements. Moreover, more high-quality research is still needed to identify the effect of the tourniquet in Chinese patients. Therefore, we conducted a randomised, controlled, prospective trial in which the patients receiving primary TKA were divided into two groups according to whether a tourniquet was used or not used. We hypothesised that the tourniquet would decrease intraoperative blood loss and total blood loss, whereas the

* Correspondence: Zhouzongke2016@163.com
Department of Orthopaedics, West China Hospital of Sichuan University, Chengdu 610041, China

non-tourniquet group would experience a decrease in limb swelling and promotion of faster recovery during the early postoperative rehabilitative period.

Methods

The study was approved by the Ethics Committee and Institutional Review Board of West China Hospital, Sichuan University, and informed patient consent was also obtained. The trial was registered in the Chinese Clinical Trials Registry (ChiCTR-IOR-16007851) and conducted at a single centre. One hundred fifty patients who were suffering from end-stage osteoarthritis or rheumatoid arthritis and scheduled for a primary unilateral TKA were recruited. The exclusion criteria were patients with prior surgery involving the femur or tibia, prior lower extremity fracture, coagulopathy and uncontrolled hypertension. Patients were enrolled from January 2016 to May 2016 in our hospital. The patients were randomly divided into a tourniquet group and a non-tourniquet group according to a computerised random sequence generator. The sequence was concealed until the interventions were assigned by a sealed envelope method in the operating room. The observers collecting the data after the surgeries were uninvolved in the experimental operations and were unaware of the intervention assignments.

All the operations were performed by the same surgeon using a Sigma fixed or rotating plant posterior-stabilised total knee prosthesis (PFC, Johnson & Johnson/DePuy, Warsaw, IN, USA). We made an anterior midline skin incision with a medial parapatellar approach, using intramedullary guides for the femur and using extramedullary guides for the tibia. All patients received a general anaesthetic with controlled hypotension [9]. High-pressure pulsatile lavage was used to clean the bone surfaces and soft tissues. We then pressurised the cement into the cancellous bone to ensure better cement interdigitation. At the end of the operation, an intra-articular drain was placed and retained less than 24 h after surgery.

Each patient received the same perioperative treatment strategies: tranexamic acid (TXA), pain control and rehabilitation. TXA was given at the initiation of the surgery and just before closure [10]. Multimodal postoperative pain management and accelerated physical therapy were performed as previously described [11]. For thrombosis prophylaxis, oral rivaroxaban (10 mg per day) was initiated 12 h after the operation and was continued for 2 weeks. After recovery from anaesthesia, quadriceps femoris muscle isometric contraction was immediately started, and rehabilitation began on the first postoperative day, including muscle power training and passive and active range-of-motion (ROM) training.

The primary outcome was perioperative blood loss. The blood volume of each patient was calculated according to a formula that considers patient weight, height and sex [12]. In addition, intraoperative blood loss, postoperative blood loss, hidden blood loss, drainage volume and blood transfusion were also recorded. The increased weight of the gauzes plus the volume in the aspirator bottle excluding rinse represented the intraoperative blood loss. Hidden blood loss was calculated according to a formula published by Gross [13]. The postoperative blood loss was calculated by measuring the drainage volume and by weighing the dressings. The secondary outcome measures were evaluated during hospitalisation (ability to achieve a straight-leg raise; visual analogue scale [VAS] pain score; transfusion requirements; thigh, calf and knee swelling; ROM; hospital for special surgery [HSS] score; length of stay) and 3 weeks to 6 months following surgery (HSS scores, ROM, VAS pain score). Postoperative VAS scores were generated from thigh pain, knee rest and active pain. Thigh circumference (10 cm proximal to the superior border of the patella), knee circumference (midpoint of the patella) and calf circumference (20 cm proximal to the medial malleolus) were recorded to assess the degree of limb swelling. Knee active ROM was measured in a supine position by using a long-arm goniometer. The time to achieve a straight-leg raise after anaesthesia recovery was recorded. The decision to transfuse was based on the clinical symptoms of anaemia and laboratory results. Blood transfusion was given to patients whose postoperative haemoglobin (Hb) was less than 8 or 9 g/dl along with symptoms of anaemia such as tachycardia, dyspnoea, hypotension and light-headedness. Special attention was paid to whether symptomatic pulmonary embolism (PE) or deep vein thrombosis (DVT) occurred. DVT was detected by a regular bilateral lower extremity deep venous colour Doppler ultrasound examination. Other complications, such as erythema/ecchymosis, wound tension vesicle or superficial and deep infection were also recorded.

Statistical analysis

Quantitative data are presented as the mean and standard deviation (SD); categorical variables are reported as proportions. Differences in continuous variables between groups were evaluated with Student's t test or Mann-Whitney U test, depending on the distribution characteristics of the data. A chi-square test or Fisher exact test for difference in proportions was used to estimate the differences between groups in categorical variables. Statistical significance was set at $P < 0.05$. Statistical analysis was completed using SPSS 17.0.

Results

Participant flow and baseline data

One hundred fifty participants were assessed for eligibility. Two were excluded for refusing to participate.

After randomisation, 74 patients did not receive the limb tourniquet and comprised the non-tourniquet group (group A) and 74 patients received the limb tourniquet and constituted the tourniquet group (group B). Six patients in group A and two patients in group B were lost to follow-up, leaving 68 patients in the non-tourniquet group and 72 patients in the tourniquet group (Fig. 1). Baseline demographics, preoperative knee function, preoperative visual analogue scale (VAS) scores and clinical data are presented in Table 1. The two groups were equally matched by age, sex and body mass index (BMI). No significant differences were found between the two groups with regard to preoperative knee HSS scores, ROM, VAS scores and preoperative haemoglobin level.

Haemodynamic changes

The mean operating time in group B (77.2 ± 14.5 min) was significantly shorter than that in group A (82.0 ± 12.7 min) ($P = 0.038$, Table 2). Group A had an increased intraoperative blood loss (215.7 ± 113.7 ml vs. 138.6 ± 93.9 ml, $P < 0.001$), but postoperative blood loss (180.2 ± 117.0 ml vs. 253.7 ± 144.2 ml, $P = 0.001$) and drainage volume (89.2 ± 66.3 ml vs. 164.5 ± 97.8 ml, $P = 0.004$) were reduced when compared to group B. There was no significant difference in total blood loss between the groups (389.2 ± 178.3 ml vs. 374.5 ± 165.3 ml, $P = 0.613$).

Blood transfusion was necessary for three patients in group A (4.4%), whereas eight patients in group B (11.1%) needed it, although the difference was not significant ($P = 0.141$, Table 2).

Clinical outcomes and complications

The differences in VAS score of thigh pain between the groups in the initial 3 weeks were statistically significant (all $P < 0.001$, Fig. 2a). More calf circumference increase was observed in group B at postoperative day 1 (1.87 ± 1.28 vs. 1.03 ± 1.1 cm, $P < 0.001$), day 3 (1.87 ± 1.28 vs. 1.03 ± 1.1 cm, $P < 0.001$) and day 5 (2.24 ± 1.50 vs. 1.5 ± 1.4 cm, $P = 0.007$, Fig. 2b). In the first 3 days after the operation, the patients in group A performed a better knee ROM (day 1 81.6 ± 17.1 vs. 75.95 ± 14.55, $P = 0.036$; day 3 99.8 ± 13.7 vs. 93.95 ± 11.15, $P = 0.005$, Fig. 2c); thereafter, the differences were no longer significant (all $P > 0.05$). A shorter length of stay after surgery (6.3 ± 1.7 days) and an earlier straight-leg raising (4.6 ± 3.8 h) were found in group A ($P = 0.001$, $P = 0.01$, Table 3). Analysis of postoperative knee function did not show any significant differences between the two groups with respect to the knee HSS score (discharge, 3 months, 6 months postoperative). The knee active pain VAS scores and thigh and knee circumference increase of the two groups at all observed time points were also not significantly different

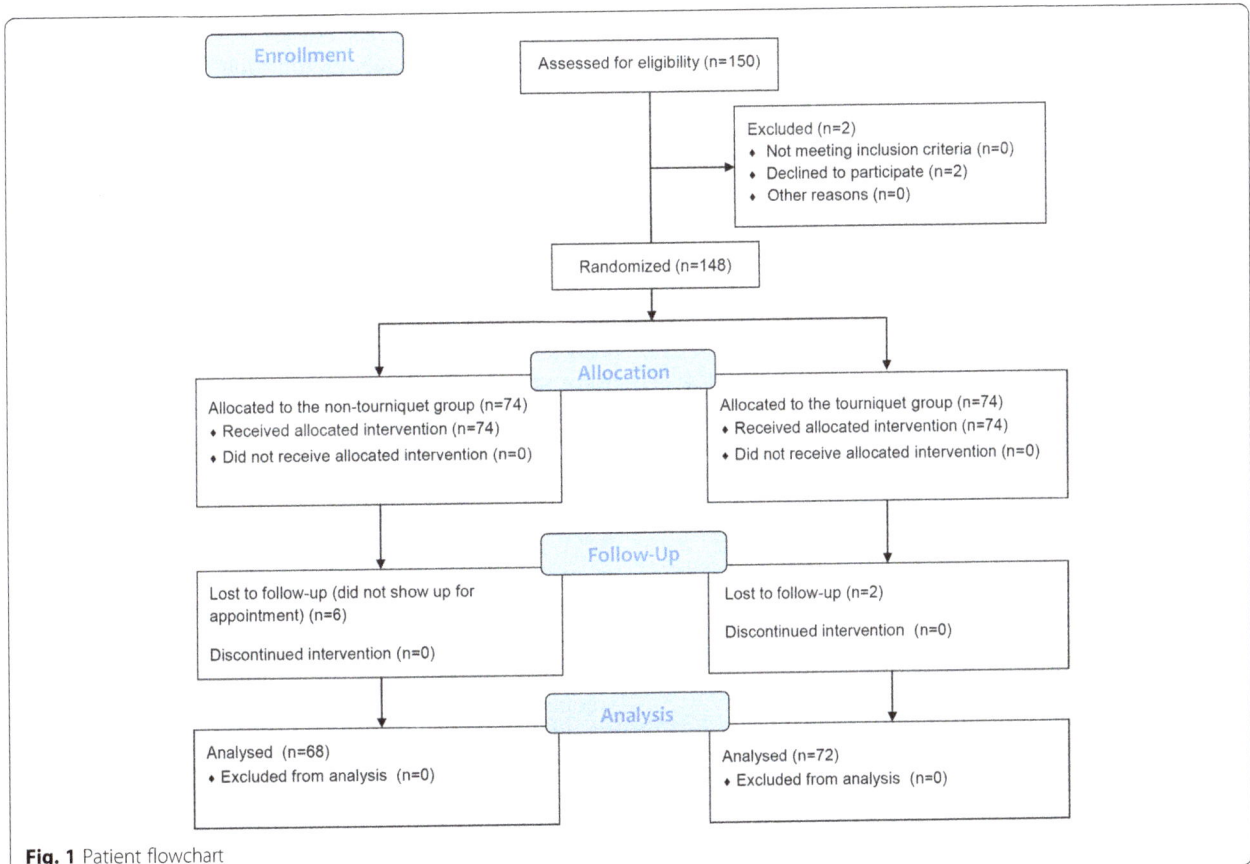

Fig. 1 Patient flowchart

Table 1 Preoperative demographics

Demographics	Non-tourniquet	Tourniquet	P value
Number of patients	68	72	–
Age (years)	69.1 ± 7.6	66.8 ± 8.6	0.095
Gender (female/male)	61/7	59/13	0.19
Diagnosis (OA/RA)	52/16	50/22	0.35
BMI (kg/m^2)	25.7 ± 3.4	26.1 ± 4.1	0.53
Preoperative HSS score	47.7 ± 11.8	49.6 ± 12.3	0.351
Preoperative knee ROM	85.3 ± 27.5	89.5 ± 22.7	0.323
Preoperative haemoglobin (g/dl)	125.1 ± 12.9	123.8 ± 14.9	0.581
Preoperative VAS score			
Thigh pain	0.1 ± 0.6	0.0 ± 0.5	0.284
Knee rest pain	0.7 ± 1.3	0.5 ± 1.5	0.399
Knee active pain	5.5 ± 1.3	5.7 ± 1.6	0.417

Data are shown as mean ± standard deviation or numbers (%). Body mass index (BMI) equals weight in kilogrammes divided by the square of the height in metres

OA osteoarthritis, RA rheumatoid arthritis, ROM range of motion, VAS visual analogue scale, HSS hospital for special surgery

(all P > 0.05). Additional complications and side effects were noted for both groups and are shown in Table 3. Seven patients (10.3%) had wound tension vesicle in group A, and 21 (29.2%) in group B, and the difference was significant (P = 0.005). No significant differences were found in relation to wound erythema/ecchymosis, superficial wound infection or DVT. In addition, no deep prosthesis infection or PE was encountered in our study.

Discussion

The most important finding of the present study is that non-tourniquet TKA with wound drainage could decrease postoperative blood loss, thigh pain, calf swelling and wound tension vesicle. Furthermore, performing TKA without a tourniquet could promote early functional recovery with no additional side effects.

A tourniquet is mainly used to reduce intraoperative blood loss and to achieve better visualisation in TKA. It is reported that 58% of the members of the American Association of Hip and Knee Surgeons (AAHKS) use a tourniquet for TKA [14]. Although widely used, tourniquet-related complications have been reported in

Table 2 Perioperative blood loss and allogeneic blood transfusion

	Non-tourniquet	Tourniquet	P value
Operating time (min)	82.0 ± 12.7	77.2 ± 14.5	0.038
Total blood loss (ml)	389.2 ± 178.3	374.5 ± 165.3	0.613
Intraoperative blood loss (ml)	215.7 ± 113.7	138.6 ± 93.9	< 0.001
Postoperative blood loss (ml)	180.2 ± 117.0	253.7 ± 144.2	0.001
Drainage volume (ml)	89.2 ± 66.3	164.5 ± 97.8	0.004
Blood transfusion (num./%)	3 (4.4%)	8 (11.1%)	0.141

Data are shown as mean ± standard deviation or numbers (%)

the literature, including soft-tissue and muscle damage, injury of calcified vessels, limb swelling, nerve injury and paralysis [15–17].

Notably, the tourniquet controls intraoperative blood loss but cannot stop postoperative blood loss or decrease overall blood loss [5]. Our study also demonstrated that the tourniquet use could decrease operation time and intraoperative blood loss, but there were no benefits in postoperative blood loss or total blood loss. The lost blood could escape into the soft tissue, potentially resulting in limb swelling, which would contribute to thigh pain, and additional swelling may hinder patients' early postoperative function rehabilitation and increase the soft-tissue tension [18]. Similarly, our data suggested a higher level of thigh pain and calf swelling in the initial days after the operation in the tourniquet patients, and the patients without tourniquet presented better clinical outcomes. After the tourniquet was released, the ischemia-reperfusion (I-R) injury would occur when blood perfusion was re-established [19], and it would increase the risk of DVT due to stasis of venous blood in the lower limb and possible damage to blood vessels [17]. In our study, DVT or PE was not detected in either of the two groups. Chemical prophylaxis with rivaroxaban and early physiotherapy may be of great benefit. Two meta-analyses also found no difference in DVT or PE occurrence with the use of the tourniquet application during TKA surgery [16, 17].

Considering these above tourniquet-related complications, much effort has made to optimise tourniquet use by reducing the pressure, changing the cuff size and shortening the time of use. Olivecrona et al. [20] in a randomised study demonstrated that reduced tourniquet cuff pressure would lead to a lower rate of postoperative infections and wound complications. Ejaz et al. reported that the short-duration tourniquet was associated with better clinical outcomes, less pain and less limb swelling during the early stage of rehabilitation. Similar results were reported by Zhang et al. [21]. However, some knee surgeons, considering the side effects, would like to operate without a tourniquet. Especially for patients with popliteal artery calcification, no palpable pedal pulses and known peripheral vascular disease, it is safer to perform TKA without a tourniquet [22]. In addition, numerous studies reported no significant difference in the total blood loss with or without tourniquet [21, 23]. Zhang et al. [21] evaluated 13 RCTs including 698 knees in a meta-analysis. They found a mean 198 ml more intraoperative blood loss without a tourniquet. However, no difference was found in total blood loss. At the same time, postoperative knee ROM in the non-tourniquet group was 10.41° more than that in the tourniquet group at the early stage. These benefits may result from decreasing direct compression on tissue and reperfusion

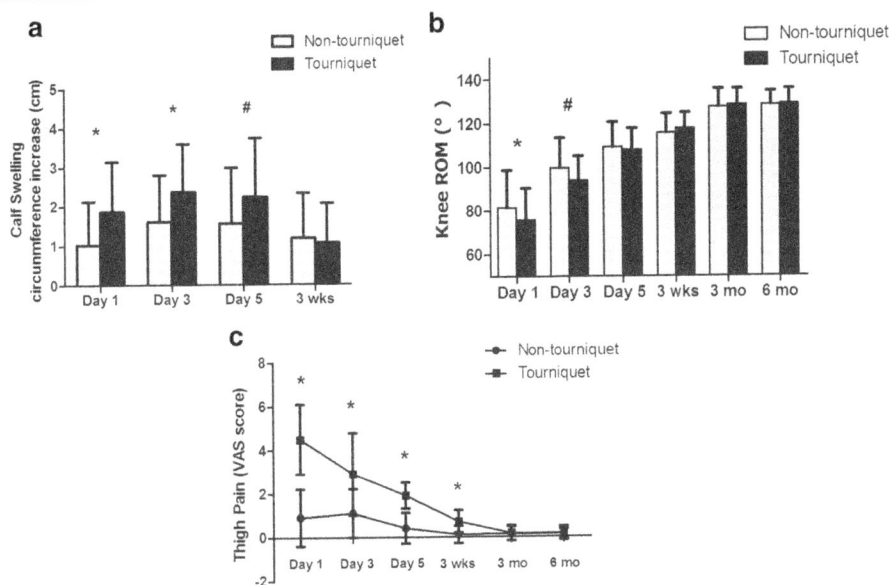

Fig. 2 Difference between the two groups regarding postoperative calf swelling (**a**) and knee ROM (**b**) and knee active pain (**c**)

injury. Moreover, a better surgical haemostasis could be achieved because the bleeding structure is clearly observed without a tourniquet.

Theoretically, however, the absence of a tourniquet does obscure the bloodless surgical field and it requires more meticulous haemostasis during exposure and soft-tissue release because there may be blood, debris and fat on the bone surface, compromising cementation [5].

In our study, the comprehensive bleeding control method was used to minimise soft-tissue and bone surface bleeding to ensure the bone-cement interface fixation. First, our patients received a general anaesthetic with controlled hypotension, and mean arterial pressure was maintained between 60 and 70 mmHg. It helps greatly to reduce intraoperative bleeding without influencing blood supply to important organs [9]. Second, before opening the joint capsule, we injected 40 ml of 0.5% epinephrine along the incision to reduce soft-tissue bleeding. After finishing bone cutting in the non-tourniquet TKAs, hydrogen peroxide was used to remove coagulated blood and fat on the bone surfaces before using high-pressure pulsatile lavage. Our data suggest that the comprehensive bleeding control in non-tourniquet TKAs could lead to acceptable total blood loss.

One of the strengths of our study is that it is a randomised, controlled trial of a non-selected study population with few exclusion criteria. Another is the relatively large sample size we provided to prove that not using a tourniquet during TKA could yield fast recovery without increasing complications. The limitation of our study is the lack of long-term clinical and radiographic results. Future follow-up studies focusing on the clinical and radiographic outcomes might be meaningful.

Conclusion

Based on our data, following the non-tourniquet TKA, postoperative blood loss, calf swelling, wound tension vesicle and thigh pain in the initial postoperative period would be reduced. Moreover, better knee ROM, shorter straight-leg raising time and shorter length of stay could also be attained. Our study suggests that a TKA performed without a tourniquet is safe and would lead to early rehabilitation.

Table 3 Clinical outcomes and complication comparison

Parameters	Non-tourniquet	Tourniquet	P value
Length of stay	6.3 ± 1.7	7.1 ± 1.9	0.001
Straight-leg raising (num./%)	4.6 ± 3.8	6.4 ± 4.3	0.01
HSS score			
Discharge	66.6 ± 8.1	65.4 ± 7.4	0.359
3 months post-op	82.5 ± 4.5	81.6 ± 4.4	0.231
6 months post-op	89.8 ± 4.9	90.7 ± 4.5	0.257
Erythema/ecchymosis (num./%)	9 (13.2%)	15 (20.8%)	0.233
Tension vesicle (num./%)	7 (10.3%)	21(29.2%)	0.005
Superficial infection (num./%)	3 (4.3%)	5 (6.9%)	0.763
DVT (num./%)	0	2	0.497

Data are shown as mean ± standard deviation or numbers (%)
DVT deep vein thrombosis

Abbreviations
BMI: Body mass index; DVT: Deep vein thrombosis; HSS: Hospital for special surgery; PE: Pulmonary embolism; ROM: Range of motion; TKA: Total knee arthroplasty; TXA: Tranexamic acid; VAS: Visual analogue scale

Acknowledgements
Not applicable.

Funding
This study was funded by Health Industry Special Scientific Research Projects of China—the safety and effectiveness evaluation of arthroplasty (grant number 201302007).

Authors' contributions
KZ was a major contributor in writing and revising the manuscript and participated in the design of the study. TXL contributed to the grammar check and performed the statistical analysis. HYW contributed to the data interpretation. BS participated in the design of the study. JY contributed to the revision of the manuscript. PDK participated in the design of the study and contributed to the revision of the manuscript. ZKZ conceived of the study and contributed to the revision the manuscript. FXP participated in the study design and coordination. All authors read and approved the final manuscript.

Competing interests
The authors declare that they have no competing interests.

References

1. Tai TW, Lin CJ, Jou IM, Chang CW, Lai KA, Yang CY. Tourniquet use in total knee arthroplasty: a meta-analysis. Knee Surg Sports Traumatol Arthrosc. 2011;19(7):1121–30.
2. Kato N, Nakanishi K, Yoshino S, Ogawa R. Abnormal echogenic findings detected by transesophageal echocardiography and cardiorespiratory impairment during total knee arthroplasty with tourniquet. Anesthesiology. 2002;97(5):1123–8.
3. Kageyama K, Nakajima Y, Shibasaki M, Hashimoto S, Mizobe T. Increased platelet, leukocyte, and endothelial cell activity are associated with increased coagulability in patients after total knee arthroplasty. J Thromb Haemost. 2007;5(4):738–45.
4. Jawhar A, Hermanns S, Ponelies N, Obertacke U, Roehl H. Tourniquet-induced ischaemia during total knee arthroplasty results in higher proteolytic activities within vastus medialis cells: a randomized clinical trial. Knee Surg Sports Traumatol Arthrosc. 2016;24(10):3313–21.
5. Liu D, Graham D, Gillies K, Gillies RM. Effects of tourniquet use on quadriceps function and pain in total knee arthroplasty. Knee Surg Relat Res. 2014;26(4):207–13.
6. Parvizi J, Diaz-Ledezma C. Total knee replacement with the use of a tourniquet: more pros than cons. Bone Joint J. 2013;95B(11):133–4.
7. Ejaz A, Laursen AC, Kappel A, Laursen MB, Jakobsen T, Rasmussen S, Nielsen PT. Faster recovery without the use of a tourniquet in total knee arthroplasty. Acta Orthop. 2014;85(4):422–6.
8. Li B, Qian QR, Wu HS, Zhao H, Lin XB, Zhu J, Weng WF. The use of a pneumatic tourniquet in total knee arthroplasty: a prospective, randomized study. Zhonghua Wai Ke Za Zhi. 2008;46(14):1054–7.
9. Seruya M, Oh AK, Rogers GF, Boyajian MJ, Myseros JS, Yaun AL, Keating RF. Controlled hypotension and blood loss during frontoorbital advancement. J Neurosurg Pediatr. 2012;9(5):491–6.
10. Yang ZG, Chen WP, Wu LD. Effectiveness and safety of tranexamic acid in reducing blood loss in total knee arthroplasty: a meta-analysis. J Bone Joint Surg Am. 2012;94(13):1153–9.
11. Ranawat AS, Ranawat CS. Pain management and accelerated rehabilitation for total hip and total knee arthroplasty. J Arthroplast. 2007;22(7 Suppl 3):12–5.
12. Nadler SB, Hidalgo JH, Bloch T. Prediction of blood volume in normal human adults. Surgery. 1962;51(2):224–32.
13. Gross JB. Estimating allowable blood loss: corrected for dilution. Anesthesiology. 1983;58(3):277–80.
14. Berry DJ, Bozic KJ. Current practice patterns in primary hip and knee arthroplasty among members of the American Association of Hip and Knee Surgeons. J Arthroplast. 2010;25(6):2–4.
15. Din R, Geddes T. Skin protection beneath the tourniquet. A prospective randomized trial. ANZ J Surg. 2004;74(9):721–2.
16. Tai TW, Chang CW, Lai KA, Lin CJ, Yang CY. Effects of tourniquet use on blood loss and soft-tissue damage in total knee arthroplasty: a randomized controlled trial. J Bone Joint Surg Am. 2012;94(24):2209–15.
17. Alcelik I, Pollock RD, Sukeik M, Bettany-Saltikov J, Armstrong PM, Fismer P. A comparison of outcomes with and without a tourniquet in total knee arthroplasty: a systematic review and meta-analysis of randomized controlled trials. J Arthroplast. 2012;27(3):331–40.
18. Li B, Wen Y, Liu D, Tian L. The effect of knee position on blood loss and range of motion following total knee arthroplasty. Knee Surg Sports Traumatol Arthrosc. 2012;20(3):594–9.
19. Huang ZY, Ma J, Zhu Y, Pei FX, Yang J, Zhou ZK, Kang PD, Shen B. Timing of tourniquet release in total knee arthroplasty. Orthopedics. 2015;38(7):445–51.
20. Olivecrona C, Ponzer S, Hamberg P, Blomfeldt R. Lower tourniquet cuff pressure reduces postoperative wound complications after total knee arthroplasty: a randomized controlled study of 164 patients. J Bone Joint Surg Am. 2012;94(24):2216–21.
21. Zhang W, Li N, Chen SF, Tan Y, Al-Aidaros M, Chen LB. The effects of a tourniquet used in total knee arthroplasty: a meta-analysis. J Orthop Surg Res. 2014;9(1):13.
22. Calligaro KD, DeLaurentis DA, Booth RE, Rothman RH, Savarese RP, Dougherty MJ. Acute arterial thrombosis associated with total knee arthroplasty. J Vasc Surg. 1994;20(6):927–32.
23. Yi SX, Tan JX, Chen C, Chen H, Huang W. The use of pneumatic tourniquet in total knee arthroplasty: a meta-analysis. Arch Orthop Trauma Surg. 2014;134(10):1469–76.

21

Averaging rotational landmarks during total knee arthroplasty reduces component malrotation caused by femoral asymmetry

Tat Woon Chao, Liam Geraghty, Pandelis Dimitriou and Simon Talbot[*] ⓘ

Abstract

Background: Femoral component malrotation is a common cause of patient dissatisfaction after total knee arthroplasty. The sulcus line (SL) is more accurate than Whiteside's line as it corrects for variation in the coronal orientation of the groove. The hypothesis is that averaging the SL and posterior condylar axis (PCA) will reduce femoral malrotation.

Methods: The component was inserted at a position between the SL and PCA in 91 patients. An intraoperative photograph was taken showing the landmarks. These were compared to the component position achieved relative to the surgical epicondylar axis (SEA) on a postoperative CT scan. The component position was compared to the position achieved using the individual landmarks.

Results: Relative to the SEA, the final component position was 0.6° (SD 1.4°, range −3.8° to +4.0°), the coronally corrected SL position was −0.7° (SD 2.3°, −5.5° to +4.6°), the PCA position was 0.9° (SD 1.9°, −6.1° to +5.0°). Averaging the landmarks significantly decreased the variance of the component position compared to using the SL and PCA individually. The number of outliers (>3° from SEA) was also significantly less ($p < 0.05$) for the average position (2/84) when each was compared to the SL (16/84) and PCA (14/84) individually. In 21/84 (25%) of cases, there was more than 4° of divergence between the SL and PCA.

Conclusions: Averaging the SL and the PCA decreases femoral component malrotation. Femora are frequently asymmetrical in the axial plane. Referencing posterior condyles alone to set rotation is likely to cause high rates of patellofemoral malalignment.

Keywords: Knee, Arthroplasty, Malrotation, Prosthesis, Femoral rotation, Whiteside's line, Knee replacement, Trochlear, Asymmetry

Background

Femoral component rotation in total knee arthroplasty (TKA) continues to be a contentious issue. Femoral component malrotation is associated with patella maltracking [1–7], increased patella shear forces [8], flexion instability [9, 10], and soft tissue imbalance. There are several competing theories and techniques described which can be broadly separated into measured resection techniques based on anatomical landmarks and gap-balancing techniques based on ligament tension. The measured resection group can be further divided depending on the particular landmarks referenced. These include the anatomical epicondylar axis (AEA), the surgical epicondylar axis (SEA), the posterior condylar axis (PCA), kinematic alignment (KA) based on the posterior condylar line (PCL), the anteroposterior axis (APA, also known as Whiteside's line) and, more recently, the sulcus line of the trochlear groove (SL).

These landmarks have been extensively studied to determine how they relate to each other and to the flexion-extension axis (FEA) of the knee. The SEA has been recommended as a closer approximation of the FEA of the knee than the AEA [11–15]. However, both landmarks are difficult to reliably isolate intraoperatively [16, 17].

* Correspondence: simontnz@yahoo.com
Department of Orthopaedics, Western Health, 1/210 Burgundy Street, Heidelberg, Victoria 3084, Australia

Referencing the posterior condyles during either mechanical alignment or KA techniques relies on the assumption that the flexion-extension axis of the posterior condyles has a consistent relationship with the axis of rotation of the patella and trochlear groove. There is some research to suggest that on average, the axes are close to parallel [18, 19]. However, the relationship is not consistent, with a wide range of variation [20–24].

A new technique for measuring the rotational alignment of the trochlear groove has recently been developed [25, 26]. The APA has previously been the only technique used to assess the rotation of the trochlear. It has been shown to be unreliable due to parallax error [26]. The sulcus line (SL) technique considers the three-dimensional shape of the trochlear groove. It removes the parallax error by measuring the rotational alignment of the groove after reorienting the femur to look directly along the coronal alignment of the trochlear groove. This coronal direction varies widely between individuals [18, 26]. A simple instrument (Sulcus Line Trochlear Alignment Guide (STAG), (Enztec Ltd, Christchurch, New Zealand) has been developed to allow the SL to be used intraoperatively. The prediction from the previous three-dimensional computed tomography (3DCT) and cadaver studies [25, 26] is that averaging the SL and PCA would decrease the rate of femoral component malrotation.

The aims of this study were to (i) determine the clinical accuracy of the SL and STAG technique, (ii) assess the benefit obtained by averaging the SL and PCA, and (iii) characterise the relationships between the SL, SEA and posterior condyles.

Methods

Approval to conduct the study was gained from the local Human Research Ethics Committee.

A prospective study of a consecutive series of 91 TKAs was conducted. There were no preoperative exclusion criteria. All operations were performed by one surgeon using a standardised technique. Conventional instruments were used. The distal femoral cut was produced at 6° from the anatomical axis of the femur using an intramedullary rod. The tibial cut was produced perpendicular to the long axis of the tibia using an extramedullary jig.

The femoral rotation was determined by averaging the SL and the PCA. The SL was drawn on the distal femur using diathermy after dislocation of the patella and before any bony cuts were made. This was done by carefully palpating the deepest points of the trochlear groove starting at the intercondylar notch and leading anteriorly. The most proximal section of the trochlear groove was not incorporated into the SL as it has been shown to be prone to excessive variability due to arthritic damage, osteophyte formation and anatomical variation [27, 28].

Multiple diathermy marks were made along the groove and then connected to produce a continuous curved line. A drill was then used to open the intramedullary canal in the centre point of the knee.

The STAG intramedullary rod was inserted and the STAG block placed over the rod. The block was then orientated to match both the rotational (Fig. 1) and the coronal (Fig. 2) alignment of the SL. This was checked with an alignment wing in both planes. Care was taken to ensure that the block was perpendicular to the coronal alignment of the SL as viewed on the anterior surface of the femur. This usually left the block sitting off either the medial or lateral femoral condyle. Two smooth 3.2-mm pins were then drilled through parallel holes in the alignment block. The pins, block, and IM rod were then completely removed. The distal femoral cut was then produced using the standard technique described above without any reference to the SL or STAG device. After the distal femoral cut was performed, the holes made from the pin tracks from the STAG pin-holes were then identified on the cut surface.

The PCA was determined with the use of a standard sizing guide. Paddles were placed under the posterior condyles, and an additional 3° of external rotation was added to compensate for the average proximal tibia joint line obliquity. The PCA is defined as 3° of external rotation to the posterior condylar line (PCL). A 3.2-mm drill was used to produce two holes on the distal cut surface which match the rotation of the PCA. In order to report reproducible technique which does not rely on surgeon experience and to allow the calculation of an accurate PCL, no adjustment was made for posterior condylar bone loss.

A sizing guide was used which allowed variation in the rotation from the posterior condyles in 1° increments between 0° and 6° of external rotation. The rotation of the SL (STAG pin-holes) and the PCA (PCL + 3°)

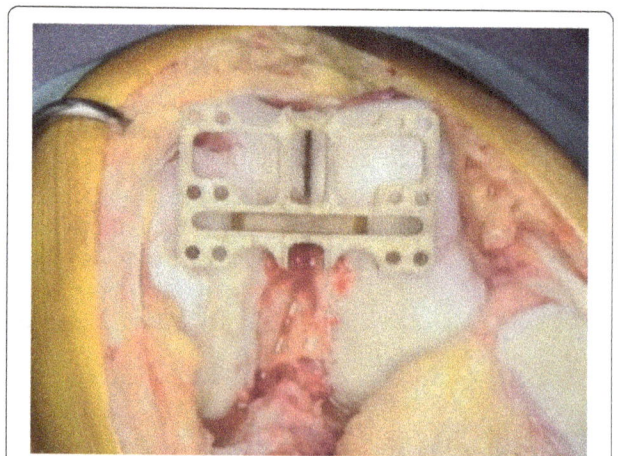

Fig. 1 STAG device (axial view)

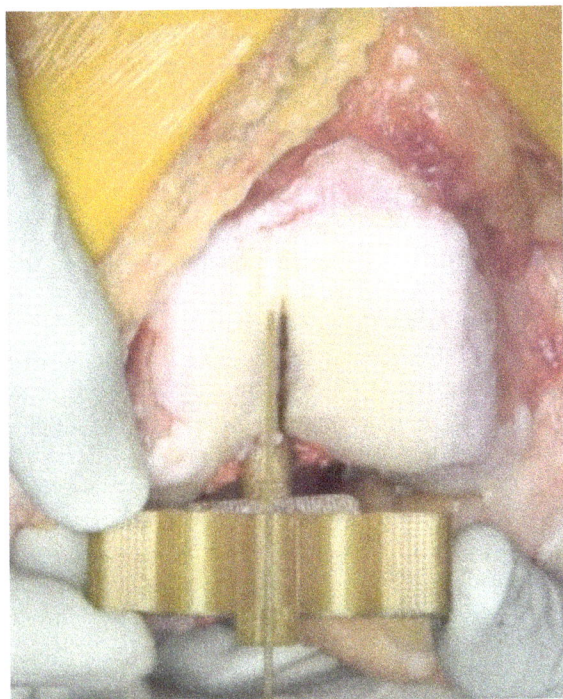

Fig. 2 STAG device (coronal view)

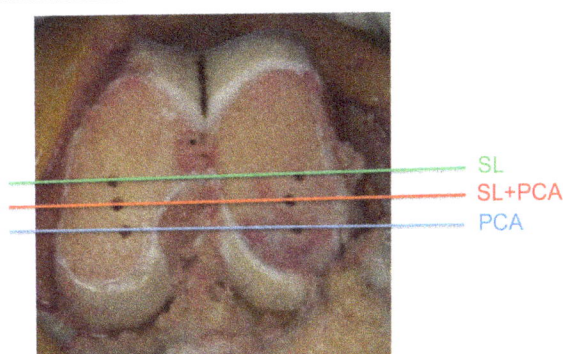

Fig. 3 Pin-holes on distal femur

were compared. These landmarks are able to be accurately compared by placing a sizing guide on the distal cut surface of the femur and dialling the rotation between the two sets of pin-holes. Therefore, the rotational angle between the PCA and SL was able to be accurately determined. When they were different, an average position was produced as accurately as possible by altering the rotation of the sizing guide in 1° increments. This average position was marked with a further set of pin-holes, and the 4-in-1 cutting block was inserted into these pin-holes. The prosthesis was therefore inserted in the average position. Therefore, the relationship between the PCA or SL and the actual component position was able to be determined from the photograph. An intraoperative photograph was taken of the three sets of pin-holes using a camera set in the overhead light (Fig. 3).

The procedure was completed using one of two types of uncemented femoral components (Triathlon CR, Stryker Co., Kalamazoo MI, or Active, Allegra Orthopaedics, Sydney, NSW, Australia). Both components have symmetrical posterior condyles.

A postoperative computed tomography (CT) scan was performed prior to discharge from hospital. A low-dose scanner (GE Optima 660) produced 1.25 mm slices from the proximal end of the femoral component to the tip of the tibial stem.

Measurements were taken of both the intraoperative photographs and the CT scan by two observers (one orthopaedic resident and one orthopaedic surgeon). The first ten cases were measured twice at an interval of 1 week to assess interobserver and intraobserver reliability. Internal rotation was recorded as a negative angle and external rotation as positive. The angles between the three sets of pinholes were measured on the photographs using Adobe Photoshop CS6. The angle between the posterior condyles of the femoral component and the SEA was measured using InteleViewer 4-3-4. The SEA was defined as a line from the most prominent point on the lateral epicondyle to the deepest point of the medial sulcus posterior to the medial epicondyle. Multiple axial slices were referenced when necessary to determine the landmarks. If either observer found that the sulcus was not able to be accurately determined, the scan was excluded. The data was collected using a purpose-designed Excel spreadsheet. Statistical analysis was performed using SPSS (22.0.0.0).

The postoperative component position ("actual component position") (Table 1) was measured on the CT scan relative to the SEA. On the intraoperative photograph, the position in which the component was inserted was determined relative to the SL and PCA. By combining these measurements, the positions of the PCA, PCL, and SL relative to the SEA were calculated. The position

Table 1 Rotational measurements

	Mean	SD	Range
SL to SEA	−0.7°	2.3°	−5.5° to +4.6°*
PCL to SEA	−2.1°	1.9°	−9.1° to +2.0°*
PCA to SEA	+0.9°	1.9°	−6.1° to +5.0°
PCL to SL	−1.4°	3.2°	−10.6° to +6.3°
PCA to SL	+1 6	3.2°	−7.6° to +9.3°
Actual component position	+0.6°	1.4°	−3.8° to +4.0°**
Calculated mean PCA and SL to SEA	+0.1°	1.4°	−3.7° to +2.7°*

Positive measurements are externally rotated
*Decreased variance of *calculated mean PCA and SL to SEA* when compared to either *SL* ($F = 15.805$, $p < 0.001$) or *PCA* ($F = 7.068$, $p < 0.001$) individually
**Decreased variance of *actual component position* when compared to either *SL* ($F = 22.634$, $p < 0.001$) or *PCA* ($F = 4.902$, $p < 0.05$) individually

which would have been achieved if the PCA and SL could be perfectly averaged intraoperatively (*calculated mean PCA and SL to SEA*) (Table 1) was also calculated.

A definition of trochlear condylar divergence (TCD) was developed to identify cases in which the PCL and SL were not perpendicular. This is a measure of femoral rotational asymmetry. A difference of 4° was deemed clinically significant based on the evidence that more than 3° of femoral malrotation is associated with adverse patellofemoral outcomes [2, 3, 6].

Subgroup analysis was performed based on the predominant pattern of arthritis detected on preoperative knee X-rays and intraoperative findings. They were classified as predominantly medial, lateral, patellofemoral or tricompartmental osteoarthritis.

Results

Of the 91 cases, one was excluded as the SL could not be clearly delineated. This patient had a patellectomy 30 years prior to TKA and the groove was grossly deformed. Six cases were excluded due to a poorly visible medial epicondylar sulci on the postoperative CT scans, leaving 84 cases for analysis. Slightly, more female (44, 52%) than male (40, 48%) participants were included in the study. More TKAs were conducted on the right side (46, 55%).

The SL 0.7° internally rotated to the SEA (SD 2.3°, range −5.5° to +4.6°). The PCL was 2.1° internally rotated (SD 1.9°, range −9.1° to +2.0°). The actual component position achieved was 0.6° externally rotated (SD 1.4°, range −3.8° to +4.0°). The calculated mean PCA and SL was 0.1° externally rotated (SD 1.4°, range −3.7° to +2.7°). There was a significant decrease in variance between the calculated mean PCA and SL to SEA to either the *SL* ($F = 15.805$, $p < 0.001$) or the *PCA* ($F = 7.068$, $p < 0.001$) (Table 1). There was also a significant decrease in the variance between the a*ctual component position* to either the SL ($F = 22.634$, $p < 0.001$) or the PCA ($F = 4.902$, $p < 0.05$).

There was a significant difference between the means for both the SL and PCA when compared to either the actual component position or the calculated mean PCA and SL to SEA ($p < 0.05$).

There was a significant difference between the means for the SL, PCA and actual component position

compared to the SEA ($p < 0.05$). There was no significant difference between the SEA and the calculated mean PCA and SL to SEA ($p > 0.05$).

Subgroup analysis did not find any difference in the means or variability of the SL or PCA measurements between patients with predominantly medial, lateral or patellofemoral osteoarthritis (Table 2).

Outliers were considered to be measurements more than 3° from the SEA. By combining the SL and PCA, the rate of outliers decreased from 19% for the SL, 17% for the PCA to 2% for the calculated mean PCA and SL ($p < 0.05$) (Table 3) and 2% for the actual component position ($p < 0.05$).

The rate of femoral rotational asymmetry or trochlear condylar divergence was <25% (21/84).

Interobserver and intraobserver reliability was excellent for all measurements (all Pearson's coefficient >0.95).

Discussion

The STAG device removes parallax errors which occur when referencing APA [26]. These errors occur because the coronal alignment of the trochlear groove is highly variable [18, 26]. Feinstein et al. [29] also reported that the coronal alignment of the groove was highly variable with a range from 6.7° valgus to 7.7° varus to the mechanical axis. These results have been reproduced using 3DCT scan techniques [18, 26]. This coronal variation needs to be considered when measuring the rotational alignment of the groove. By correcting for this variation and looking directly along the coronal direction of the trochlear groove in each individual, the trochlear groove becomes a much more reliable landmark than Whiteside's line. This results in a more accurate landmark which reflects the true rotational alignment of the trochlear groove and which more closely parallels the SEA [26]. This can be achieved by preoperative planning using CT scans, and correcting for the coronal alignment, or intraoperatively with the STAG device. Currently, there are no computer navigation systems which allow for this error to be corrected.

The combination of the SL and PCA produced fewer outliers than predicted by the findings of the 3DCT study suggesting that the intraoperative technique using the STAG is at least as accurate and reproducible as the virtual technique using the CT scans.

Table 2 Subgroup analysis

	Medial	Lateral	Patellofemoral	Tricompartmental
SL to SEA	−0.8° ± 2.2°	−0.7° ± 3.1°	−0.1° ± 1.1°	−0.5° ± 2.8°
PCA to SEA	1.1° ± 1.9°	0.2° ± 1.8°	0.1° ± 1.3°	1.3° ± 1.8°
Calculated mean PCA and SL to SEA	0.1° ± 1.4°	−0.2° ± 1.3°	0.0° ± 1.0°	0.4° ± 1.3°
PCA to SL	1.8° ± 3.0°	0.8° ± 4.4°	0.3° ± 1.4°	1.8° ± 3.8°

Comparative analysis found no significant difference in means or variance amongst any of the subgroups (all $p > 0.05$)

Table 3 Outliers[a] and Trochlear condylar divergence (TCD)[b]

	Medial (n = 59)		Lateral (n = 11)		Patellofemoral (n = 5)		Tricompartmental (n = 9)		Total (n = 84)	
	n	%	n	%	n	%	n	%	n	%
SL	9	15	4	36	0	0	3	33	16	19*
PCA	10	17	2	18	0	0	2	22	14	17*
Combined PCA and SL	2	3	0	0	0	0	0	0	2	2*
Trochlear condylar divergence (TCD)	14	24	4	36	1	20	3	33	21	25

[a]Outliers defined as more than 3° internally or externally rotated to SEA
[b]Trochlear condylar divergence defined as difference between SL and PCL >4°
*Combined PCA and SL vs SL (p < 0.05); combined PCA and SL vs PCA (p < 0.05)

On average, the SL was slightly internally rotated to the PCA and SEA, and externally rotated to the PCL. Referencing the SL using the STAG device produced a landmark with a narrow range and a level of variability which was similar to the PCA. This is an improvement compared with published results using APA [30–32] which have indicated a wide range and high degree of variability.

The comparison of the means revealed that the only technique to produce no statistically significant difference from the SEA was the calculated mean PCA and SL to SEA. While this would support the hypothesis that combining the two landmarks is likely to result in a closer average position relative to the SEA, it is the decrease in variability and outliers which is more important. In addition, the size of the difference in the means relative to the SEA was less than 1° for each of the techniques, which may not be clinically significant. It is the size of the potential variation using each technique which is important. This changes from up to 5.5° for the SL and 6.1° for the PCA down to 4.0° for the actual

component position and 3.7° for the calculated mean PCA and SL to SEA. Averaging the SL and PCA (Fig. 4) produced a significant decrease in both the overall variability and the number of individual outliers. Indeed, the outlier rate achieved was reduced from 18% using PCA alone, or 19% using SL alone, to 2% by combining the landmarks. This compares very favourably with results using other techniques including gap-balancing [33] and measured resection [32, 34–36].

Subgroup analysis showed that the results were equally effective for medial, lateral, tricompartmental and patellofemoral osteoarthritis. The SL was very accurate in cases of predominantly patellofemoral osteoarthritis (mean –0.1°, SD 1.1°). When severe trochlear arthritis is present, there are often parallel grooves in the bone surface which allow easy identification of the SL. In knees with lateral arthritis, there was on average 0.9° of internal rotation of the PCA compared to the medial group. This difference was not significant. There was no difference in the SL between medial and lateral groups.

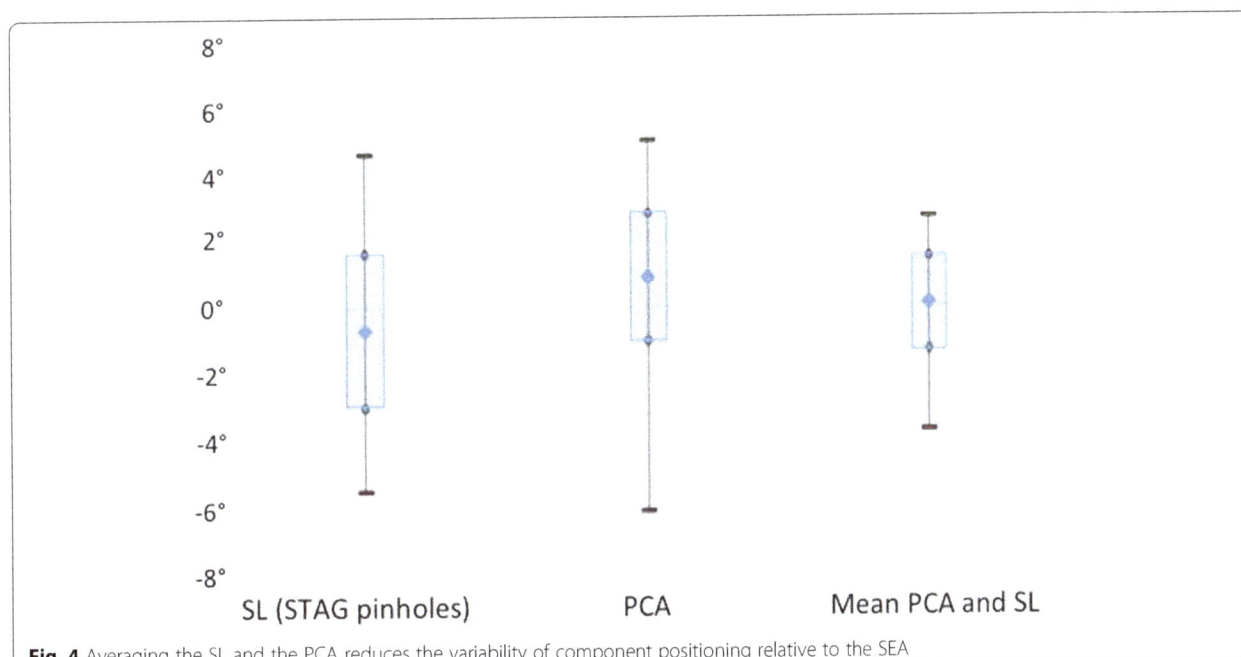

Fig. 4 Averaging the SL and the PCA reduces the variability of component positioning relative to the SEA

Analysis of the relationship between the SL and PCL revealed a high percentage of cases in which the two landmarks were not perpendicular to each other (mean difference 1.4°, SD 3.2°, range −10.6° to 6.3°). Overall, there was only a weak negative correlation between the SL and PCL (Fig. 5). The relationship between the SL and PCL is not predictable and is not correlated with the pattern of arthritis (Table 3).

In 21 of 84 knees, there was more than 4° of difference between the PCL and SL. We have coined the term trochlear condylar divergence to describe this group. In 19 of these 21 knees, the SL shifted, relative to the SEA, in the opposite direction to the PCL. This suggests an anatomical variation in which the rotational alignment of the SL and the PCL may be linked. The direction of this divergence was not influenced by the diagnosis of medial or lateral osteoarthritis. In two of four knees with lateral arthritis and nine of 14 knees with medial arthritis, the divergence occurred in the opposite direction to that anticipated if the variation was due to posterior condylar bone loss. For example, in nine knees with medial arthritis, the PCL was more than 4° internally rotated to the SL. This is despite posterior condylar cartilage and bone loss tending to externally rotate the PCL. Therefore, if the surgeon in these nine cases had internally rotated the femoral component relative to the PCA in order to compensate for posterior medial condylar bone loss the degree of internal malrotation relative to the SEA and SL would have increased. This would indicate that it is a true anatomical variation rather than the effect of arthritic bone loss. Further studies are planned

to assess this variation and determine if it is linked to proximal tibial coronal alignment.

These findings are consistent with the findings of Iranpour et al. [18]. This study used a different technique for measuring the trochlear groove. It also plotted multiple points along the floor of the groove and noted the variation in coronal alignment of the groove. However, they did not remove the parallax error by compensating for this coronal variation. The rotation of the posterior condyles was derived using a sphere-matching technique. The line of the trochlear groove was determined to be "close to parallel" to the transcondylar axis with an average of 1° of external rotation. However, there was a very large degree of variability between the two landmarks, with a standard deviation of 3°. Some of this variability will be due to parallax error, and the remainder will be due to anatomical variation.

Iranpour et al. [19] also published a cadaver study in 2010 which measured variation between the posterior condyles and the path of the patella during flexion. They found that the path of the patella was 88.8° ± 3.8° from their condylar axis. This means that it was on average 1.2° externally rotated to the condyles. This is similar to our finding of the SL being 1.4° externally rotated to the posterior condyles with a SD of 3.2°.

Both studies by Iranpour and colleagues are quoted by proponents of posterior referencing and kinematic alignment as evidence of a consistent rotational relationship between the posterior condyles and the patellofemoral joint [37]. This conclusion ignores the large degree of

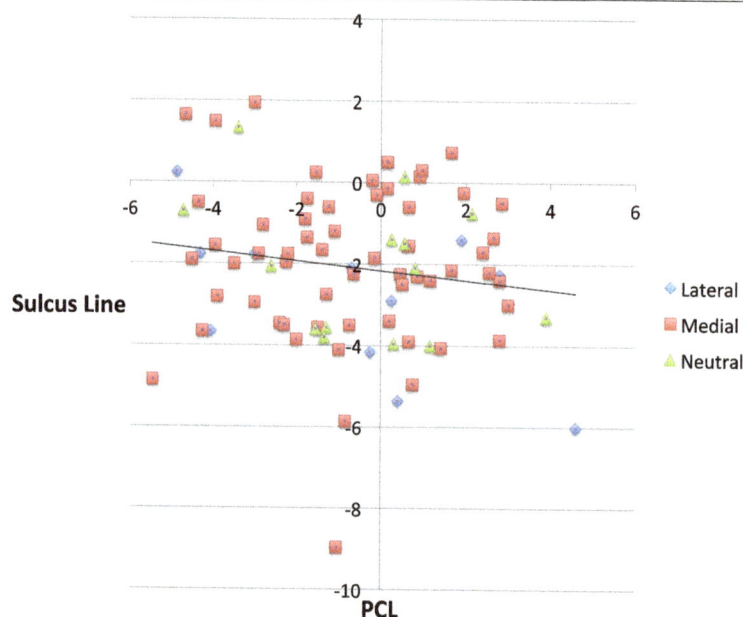

Fig. 5 Graph of data showing the high degree of asymmetry between the posterior condyles and the trochlear groove. The direction of asymmetry is not related to the posterior condylar wear from the medial or lateral location of the arthritis

variability between the landmarks which is reinforced by our findings. A more appropriate conclusion is that femoral axial anatomy is frequently asymmetrical with divergent rotational alignment between the posterior condyles and the patellofemoral joint.

This is also consistent with several recent studies which measured the relationship between the posterior condyles, the epicondyles and the trochlear groove using a variety of techniques. Jones et al. [38] used MRI scans and found that "only 24% had an external rotation angle between 2.5° and 3.5° relative to" the posterior condyles. Loures et al. [24] measured a range of 11.75° for the PCL and 14.29° for the APA on MRI scans. Theinpont et al. [20] looked at 2637 3D reconstructions of preoperative CT scans and predicted a "41% risk of malalignment" from referencing the posterior condyles. Cinotti et al. [39] found that combining the posterior condyles, epicondyles and anteroposterior axis using computer navigation reduced the need for lateral retinacular release over referencing the posterior condyles alone. Several studies have recommended combining the anterior and posterior landmarks [24–26, 39, 40].

The results of this study raise concerns regarding any technique which solely references the posterior condyles to determine rotation. Twenty-five percent of femora have more than 4° of rotational asymmetry, and yet our femoral components are symmetrical. Therefore, referencing solely the posterior condyles may produce a well-balanced tibiofemoral joint but change the rotation of the patellofemoral joint relative to its original position. This may be particularly pertinent in cases of kinematic alignment in which the native knee has a combination of proximal tibial varus and external rotation of the SL relative to the PCL. This combination may lead to an exaggerated internal rotation of the trochlear groove of the femoral component relative to the native position.

One limitation of this study is that we did not attempt to compensate for posterior condylar bone loss when determining the PCA. This was done to maintain a consistent technique and to avoid subjectivity involved in compensating for bone loss intraoperatively. Nam et al. [41] determined that posterior condylar bone loss is a very late event in the arthritic process and that the degree of correction required is small. In addition, our subgroup analysis of outliers demonstrated that compensating for femoral condylar bone loss would have increased the degree of malrotation in 65% of varus knees and 50% of valgus knees. There are likely to be cases with severe posterior condylar bone erosion in which this should be taken into account prior to referencing the posterior condyles, however, relying solely on the posterior condyles to determine femoral component rotation will result in an unacceptable rate of malrotation. Further to this, it is clear that correcting for bone loss

would not improve the consistency of the relationship between the PCL and SL. There clearly will be cases in which either the posterior condyles or trochlear groove are grossly deformed and should not be referenced. However, these cases are rare and in general the concept of averaging landmarks is valid for the vast majority of knees.

Intraoperatively, the ability to perfectly average the SL and PCA was limited by the sizing guide which had 1° or 1.5° rotational increments. In cases where the difference between the SL and PCA was less than the 1° the guide was left at the PCA landmark. Therefore, a measurement based on perfect averaging of the angles from the intraoperative photographs was also calculated. This is why there are "actual" and "calculated" measurements for the average of the SL and PCA. The difference between the two results was minor.

Further limitations of the study involve the exclusion of several cases due to difficulty finding the medial epicondylar sulcus; however, our exclusion rate is similar to other studies [2, 22].

Due to the lack of preoperative long leg X-rays, data on mechanical alignment or severity of deformity was not available. Preoperative knee X-rays and intraoperative assessment of the location of the arthritis were used to produce subgroup data. There are only 11 cases with predominantly lateral compartment osteoarthritis. The results in this group suggest that combining the two landmarks may be a reliable technique; however, the numbers are too small to draw firm conclusions. Further studies assessing non-arthritic knees are planned.

Measurement errors could occur with the identification of the SL and measurement of the intraoperative photographs and the CT scans. However, the very high interobserver and intraobserver reliability makes it unlikely to account for the degree of variation we have identified. Likewise, the measurement error associated with the use of the STAG device was shown to be small (mean 1° for both interobserver and intraobserver measurements) in the previously published cadaver study [25].

Conclusions

A high proportion of femora have axial asymmetry with different rotational alignment of the trochlear groove and posterior condyles. By using a trochlear alignment guide that corrects for the coronal alignment of the trochlear, the rotational alignment of the groove can be more accurately identified during surgery than by using APA. It also allows direct comparison between the anterior and posterior landmarks. Averaging the SL of the trochlear groove and the PCA significantly decreases femoral component malrotation.

Abbreviations
3DCT: Three-dimensional computed tomography; AEA: Anatomical epicondylar axis; APA: Anterior posterior axis; CT: Computed tomography;

FEA: Flexion-extension axis; IM: Intramedullary; KA: Kinematic alignment; MRI: Magnetic resonance imaging; PCA: Posterior condylar axis; PCL: Posterior condylar line; SEA: Surgical epicondylar axis; SL: Sulcus line of the trochlear groove; STAG: Sulcus line Trochlear Alignment Guide; TCD: Trochlear condylar divergence; TKA: Total knee arthroplasty

Acknowledgements
Not applicable.

Funding
Not applicable.

Authors' contributions
TC designed study, collected data and wrote manuscript. LG collected data and wrote manuscript. PD collected intraoperative measurements. ST designed the study, performed the surgery and wrote manuscript. All authors read and approved the final manuscript.

Competing interests
One of the authors holds a patent relating to the content of this manuscript.

References
1. Mochizuki RM, Schurman DJ. Patellar complications following total knee arthroplasty. Journal of Bone & Joint Surgery - American Volume. 1979; 61(6A):879–83.
2. Berger RA, Crossett LS, Jacobs JJ, Rubash HE. Malrotation causing patellofemoral complications after total knee arthroplasty. Clin Orthop. 1998; 356:144–53.
3. Akagi M, Matsusue Y, Mata T, Asada Y, Horiguchi M, Iida H, et al. Effect of rotational alignment on patellar tracking in total knee arthroplasty. Clin Orthop. 1999;366:155–63.
4. Matsuda S, Miura H, Nagamine R, Urabe K, Hirata G, Iwamoto Y. Effect of femoral and tibial component position on patellar tracking following total knee arthroplasty: 10-year follow-up of Miller-Galante I knees. Am J Knee Surg. 2001;14(3):152–6.
5. Rhoads DD, Noble PC, Reuben JD, Mahoney OM, Tullos HS. The effect of femoral component position on patellar tracking after total knee arthroplasty. Clin Orthop. 1990;260:43–51.
6. Fehring TK. Rotational malalignment of the femoral component in total knee arthroplasty. Clin Orthop. 2000;380:72–9.
7. Valkering KP, Breugem SJ, van den Bekerom MP, Tuinebreijer WE, van Geenen RC. Effect of rotational alignment on outcome of total knee arthroplasty. Acta Orthop. 2015;86(4):432–9.
8. Miller MC, Berger RA, Petrella AJ, Karmas A, Rubash HE. Optimizing femoral component rotation in total knee arthroplasty. Clin Orthop. 2001;392:38–45.
9. Olcott CW, Scott RD. The Ranawat Award. Femoral component rotation during total knee arthroplasty. Clin Orthop. 1999;367:39–42.
10. Hanada H, Whiteside LA, Steiger J, Dyer P, Naito M. Bone landmarks are more reliable than tensioned gaps in TKA component alignment. Clin Orthop. 2007;462:137–42.
11. Asano T, Akagi M, Nakamura T. The functional flexion-extension axis of the knee corresponds to the surgical epicondylar axis: in vivo analysis using a biplanar image-matching technique. J Arthroplasty. 2005;20(8):1060–7.
12. Churchill DL, Incavo SJ, Johnson CC, Beynnon BD. The transepicondylar axis approximates the optimal flexion axis of the knee. Clin Orthop. 1998;356:111–8.
13. Hollister AM, Jatana S, Singh AK, Sullivan WW, Lupichuk AG. The axes of rotation of the knee. Clin Orthop. 1993;290:259–68.
14. Kobayashi H, Akamatsu Y, Kumagai K, Kusayama Y, Ishigatsubo R, Muramatsu S, et al. The surgical epicondylar axis is a consistent reference of the distal femur in the coronal and axial planes. Knee Surg Sports Traumatol Arthrosc. 2014;22(12):2947–53.
15. Zambianchi F, Luyckx T, Victor J, Digennaro V, Giorgini A, Catani F. How to improve femoral component rotational alignment in computer-assisted TKA. Knee Surg Sports Traumatol Arthrosc. 2014;22(8):1805–11.
16. Jenny J-Y, Boeri C. Low reproducibility of the intra-operative measurement of the transepicondylar axis during total knee replacement. Acta Orthop Scand. 2004;75(1):74–7.

17. Kinzel V, Ledger M, Shakespeare D. Can the epicondylar axis be defined accurately in total knee arthroplasty? Knee. 2005;12(4):293–6.
18. Iranpour F, Merican A, Dandachli W, Amis A, Cobb J. The geometry of the trochlear groove. Clin Orthop. 2010;468(3):782–8.
19. Iranpour F, Merican AM, Baena FRY, Cobb JP, Amis AA. Patellofemoral joint kinematics: the circular path of the patella around the trochlear axis. J Orthop Res. 2010;28(5):589–94.
20. Thienpont E, Schwab P-E, Paternostre F, Koch P. Rotational alignment of the distal femur: anthropometric measurements with CT-based patient-specific instruments planning show high variability of the posterior condylar angle. Knee surgery, sports traumatology, arthroscopy : official journal of the ESSKA. 2014;22:2995–3002.
21. Mantas JP, Bloebaum RD, Skedros JG, Hofmann AA. Implications of reference axes used for rotational alignment of the femoral component in primary and revision knee arthroplasty. J Arthroplasty. 1992;7(4):531–5.
22. Berger RA, Rubash HE, Seel MJ, Thompson WH, Crossett LS. Determining the rotational alignment of the femoral component in total knee arthroplasty using the epicondylar axis. Clin Orthop. 1993;286:40–7.
23. Matsuda S, Matsuda H, Miyagi T, Sasaki K, Iwamoto Y, Miura H. Femoral condyle geometry in the normal and varus knee. Clin Orthop. 1998;349:183–8.
24. Loures FB, Furtado Neto S, Pinto RL, Kinder A, Labronici PJ, Goes RFA, et al. Rotational assessment of distal femur and its relevance in total knee arthroplasty: analysis by magnetic resonance imaging. Radiologia brasileira. 2015;48:282–6.
25. Talbot S, Dimitriou P, Mullen M, Bartlett J. Referencing the sulcus line of the trochlear groove and removing intraoperative parallax errors improve femoral component rotation in total knee arthroplasty. Knee Surg Sports Traumatol Arthrosc. 2015;1–8.
26. Talbot S, Dimitriou P, Radic R, Zordan R, Bartlett J. The sulcus line of the trochlear groove is more accurate than Whiteside's line in determining femoral component rotation. Knee Surg Sports Traumatol Arthrosc. 2015; 23(11):3306–16.
27. Cerveri P, Marchente M, Manzotti A, Confalonieri N. Determination of the Whiteside line on femur surface models by fitting high-order polynomial functions to cross-section profiles of the intercondylar fossa. Comput Aided Surg. 2011;16(2):71–85.
28. Victor J, Van Doninck D, Labey L, Innocenti B, Parizel PM, Bellemans J. How precise can bony landmarks be determined on a CT scan of the knee? Knee. 2009;16(5):358–65.
29. Feinstein WK, Noble PC, Kamaric E, Tullos HS. Anatomic alignment of the patellar groove. Clin Orthop. 1996;331:64–73.
30. Siston RA, Patel JJ, Goodman SB, Delp SL, Giori NJ. The variability of femoral rotational alignment in total knee arthroplasty. J Bone Joint Surg Am. 2005; 87(10):2276–80.
31. Middleton FR, Palmer SH. How accurate is Whiteside's line as a reference axis in total knee arthroplasty? Knee. 2007;14(3):204–7.
32. Victor J. Rotational alignment of the distal femur: a literature review. Orthop Traumatol Surg Res. 2009;95(5):365–72.
33. Luyckx T, Peeters T, Vandenneucker H, Victor J, Bellemans J. Is adapted measured resection superior to gap-balancing in determining femoral component rotation in total knee replacement? J Bone Joint Surg. 2012;94:1271–6.
34. Poilvache PL, Insall JN, Scuderi GR, Font-Rodriguez DE. Rotational landmarks and sizing of the distal femur in total knee arthroplasty. Clin Orthop. 1996; 331:35–46.
35. Seo J-G, Moon Y-W, Lim J-S, Park S-J, Kim S-M. Mechanical axis-derived femoral component rotation in extramedullary total knee arthroplasty: a comparison between femoral transverse axis and transepicondylar axis. Knee Surg Sports Traumatol Arthrosc. 2012;20(3):538–45.
36. Stockl B, Nogler M, Rosiek R, Fischer M, Krismer M, Kessler O. Navigation improves accuracy of rotational alignment in total knee arthroplasty. Clin Orthop. 2004;426:180–6.
37 Howell SM, Papadopoulos S, Kuznik KT, Hull ML. Accurate alignment and high function after kinematically aligned TKA performed with generic instruments. Knee Surg Sports Traumatol Arthrosc. 2013;21(10):2271–80.
38 Jones C, Nawaz Z, Hassan A, White S, Khaleel A. The variability in the external rotation axis of the distal femur: an MRI-based anatomical study. Eur J Orthop Surg Traumatol. 2016;26(2):199–203.
39 Cinotti G, Ripani FR, Sessa P, Giannicola G. Combining different rotational alignment axes with navigation may reduce the need for lateral retinacular release in total knee arthroplasty. Int Orthop. 2012;36(8):1595–600.

22

The evaluation of the role of medial collateral ligament maintaining knee stability by a finite element analysis

Dong Ren[1,2], Yueju Liu[1,2], Xianchao Zhang[1,2], Zhaohui Song[1,2], Jian Lu[1,2] and Pengcheng Wang[1,2,3*]

Abstract

Background: A three-dimensional finite element model (FEM) of the knee joint was established to analyze the biomechanical functions of the superficial and deep medial collateral ligaments (MCLs) of knee joints and to investigate the treatment of the knee medial collateral ligament injury.

Methods: The right knee joint of a healthy male volunteer was subjected to CT and MRI scans in the extended position. The scanned data were imported into MIMICS, Geomagic, and ANSYS software to establish a three-dimensional FEM of the human knee joint. The anterior-posterior translation, valgus-varus rotation, and internal-external rotation of knee joints were simulated to observe tibial displacement or valgus angle. In addition, the magnitude and distribution of valgus stress in the superficial and deep layers of the intact MCL as well as the superficial, deep, and overall deficiencies of the MCL were investigated.

Results: In the extended position, the superficial medial collateral ligament (SMCL) would withstand maximum stresses of 48.63, 16.08, 17.23, and 16.08 MPa in resisting the valgus of knee joints, tibial forward displacement, internal rotation, and external rotation, respectively. Meanwhile, the maximum stress tolerated by the SMCL in various ranges of motion mainly focused on the femoral end point, which was located at the anterior and posterior parts of the femur in resisting valgus motion and external rotation, respectively. However, the deep medial collateral ligament could tolerate only minimum stress, which was mainly focused at the femoral start and end points.

Conclusions: This model can effectively analyze the biomechanical functions of the superficial and deep layers of the MCLs of knee joints. The results show that the knee MCL II° injury is the indication of surgical repair.

Keywords: Biomechanics, Finite element, Knee joint, Medial collateral ligament, Model

Background

The medial collateral ligament (MCL) plays an important role in limiting and maintaining the movement of the knee joint and protecting its stability [1]. There is a high incidence of injury to the knee MCL in sports activities such as ice hockey, skiing, and soccer [2], accounting for approximately 40% of all severe knee joint injuries, 50% of which involve partial fracture while 30% involve complete fracture and injury of the knee MCL [3]. These injuries may ultimately lead to medial laxity and instability of the knee joints, as well as secondary long-term complications. Most surgeons [4] advocate conservative treatment for the knee MCL I° injury and surgical repair for the knee MCL III° injury, respectively. However, the option to deal with MCL II° injury is controversial. This study is to evaluate the function in detail within MCL maintaining the stability of the knee joint and expects to provide evidence on how to treat the knee MCL II° injury.

Methods

General information

A healthy male volunteer (age, 27 years; height, 177 cm; weight, 75 kg) without any right knee deformity, history

* Correspondence: zhengzainingmeng@163.com
[1]Third Hospital of Hebei Medical University, Shijiazhuang 050051, China
[2]Hebei Provincial Key Laboratory of Orthopaedic Biomechanics, Shijiazhuang 050051, Hebei, China
Full list of author information is available at the end of the article

of trauma, or clinically positive signs was selected for the study. He consented to participate in this test by signing an informed consent.

Acquisition of CT and MR imaging data

The right knee joint of the volunteer was subjected to continuous spiral CT in a relaxation and extended position, from 95 mm above the upper margin of the patella to 110 mm below the knee joint line, i.e., from the middle lower segment of the femur to the middle upper segment of the tibiofibula. The scan parameters were as follows: layer thickness of 0.7 mm, matrix size of 512×512, and pixel size of 0.705 mm; in total, 369 Digital Imaging and Communications in Medicine (DICOM)-format images were acquired.

MR imaging was performed for the same right knee joint in the same position, from 50 mm above the upper margin of the patella to 70 mm below the knee joint line, in which the axial T1W1 sequence was selected. The scan parameters were as follows: TR of 1900 ms, TE of 2.58 ms, layer thickness of 1 mm, matrix size of 256×256, and pixel size of 0.859 mm; a total of 176 DICOM-format images were obtained.

Establishment of bone tissue model of knee joints based on CT images

The obtained CT data were imported into an interactive medical image control system, Materialise Interactive Medical Image Control System (MIMICS) 14.0 (Materialise, Leuven, Belgium). A three-dimensional model of the original bone tissue of the knee joint was obtained using the threshold segmentation and three-dimensional model calculation and was imported into automatic reverse engineering software, Geomagic Studio 12.0 (Geomagic, USA), for optimization, so as to obtain a finer bone tissue model. The model was again imported into MIMICS 14.0 software, which was initially meshed in the 3-matic module, and the 4-node tetrahedral element was transformed into a 10-node tetrahedral element.

Establishment of ligament and meniscus models based on MR images

The method was basically the same as mentioned above, except for the following aspects: (1) Due to the unclear boundary between the soft tissues in the MIMICS 14.0 workspace, individual planes of the meniscus and ligaments were required to be split manually, followed by calculation to obtain the original meniscus and ligament models of the knee joints. (2) In some MCLs, differentiating the superficial and deep layers was difficult; they required to be separated using the trimmer, stretching, Boolean subtraction, and other functions in Geomagic Studio 12.0 according to their length, width [5],

thickness ratio, and differences in their other normal anatomic structures, by obtaining their fine models. (3) Before ligament and meniscus models were initially meshed in the 3-matic module of MIMICS 14.0 software, they were subjected to Boolean subtraction calculation in Geomagic Studio 12.0 software to obtain the three-dimensional models.

Finite element partition and analysis
Model assembly
Bone tissues, ligaments, and meniscus models were saved in cdb format and imported into the workbench of ANSYS 13.0 software (ANSYS, USA). The models were then assembled, and material properties were applied as per the properties reported in the literature [6, 7] (Table 1). Contact of the starting and ending points of each ligament with the bones, and that of the superficial and deep layers of the medial collateral ligament with the meniscus were defined as bonded contact, while contacts at other sites were defined as "no separation contacts." The models were remeshed using an interactive mesh of pentahedral and hexahedral elements, and a total of 877,070 nodes and 354,003 elements were obtained, as shown in Fig. 1.

Loads and boundaries
The upper femur was fixed in 6 degrees of freedom (DOF), and 134-N forward force, 134-N backward force, 10-N m valgus torque, and 10-N m external rotation torque and internal rotation torque were applied to the femur.

Table 1 Material parameters of the normal finite element model

Structure	E (MPa)	V
Femur	3883.4	0.3
Tibia	4184.6	0.3
Fibula	–	0.3
Patella	–	0.3
Menisci	59	0.3
ACL	1.046	0.4
PCL	1.035	0.4
SMCL	1.063	0.4
DMCL	1.063	0.4
LCL	1.063	0.4
PL	1.035	0.4

ACL anterior cruciate ligament, *DMCL* deep medial collateral ligament, *E* Young's modulus, *LCL* lateral collateral ligament, *PCL* posterior cruciate ligament, *PL* patellar ligament, *SMCL* superficial medial collateral ligament, *V* Poisson's ratio

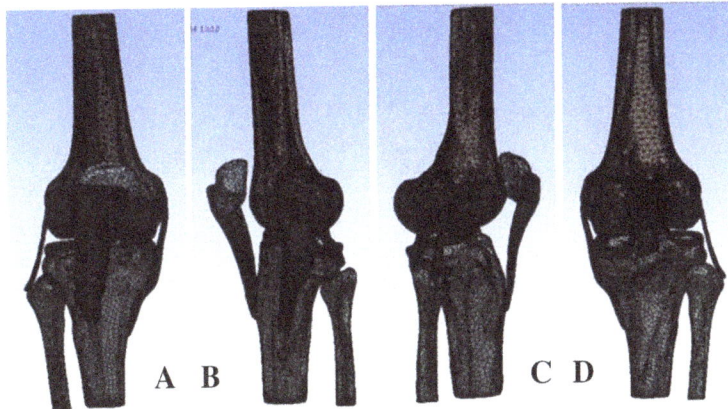

Fig. 1 Mesh generation in ANSYS Workbench. **a** Anterior view. **b** Medial view. **c** Lateral view. **d** Posterior view

Calculation and post processing

The tibial displacement or valgus angle as well as the stress magnitude and distribution in the superficial and deep layers of medial collateral ligaments under conditions of intact MCL (case 1) as well as superficial MCL (SMCL) deficiency (case 2), deep MCL (DMCL) deficiency (case 3), and overall deficiencies of the MCL (case 4) is described in Fig. 2.

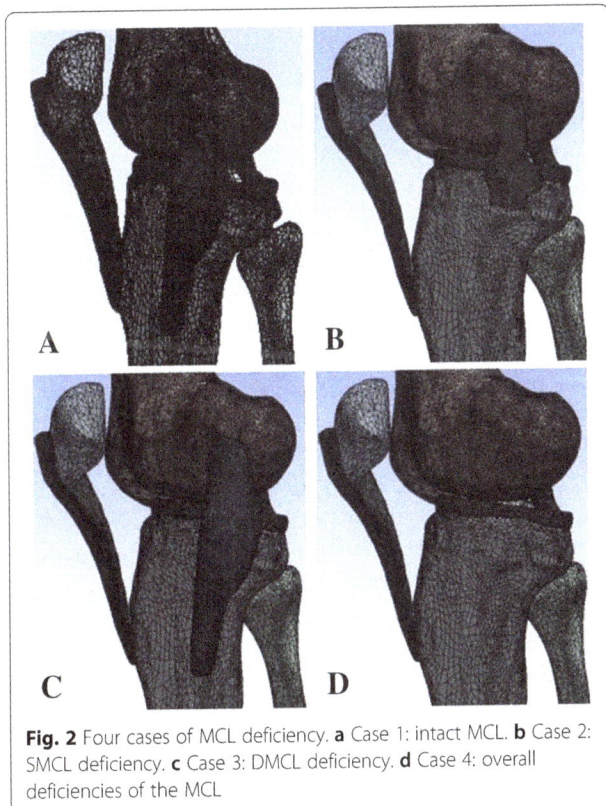

Fig. 2 Four cases of MCL deficiency. **a** Case 1: intact MCL. **b** Case 2: SMCL deficiency. **c** Case 3: DMCL deficiency. **d** Case 4: overall deficiencies of the MCL

Model validation

The tibial anterior translation was observed to be 4.89 mm when constraining the 6 DOF in the upper femur and applying a forward force of 134 N to the tibia in an extension position of the knee joint; the translation was reported to be 4.6–5.0 mm using the same load in previous studies [8]. Thus, our results were consistent with the previously reported results on FEM studies, suggesting the effectiveness of our model.

Results

Under the load of the 134-N forward force, the tibial displacement changed from 4.89 mm at intact MCL to 5.17, 5.04, and 5.17 mm at SMCL deficiency, DMCL deficiency, and overall MCL deficiency, respectively. The peak stress was maximum at the anterior cruciate ligament (ACL), lower at SMCL, and minimum at DMCL (Table 2) and was mainly located at the femoral end point at both ACL and SMCL and at the start and end points at DMCL (Fig. 3).

Under the load of the 134-N backward force, the tibial displacement changed from 4.98 mm at intact MCL to 4.99, 4.92, and 5.02 mm at SMCL deficiency, DMCL deficiency, and overall MCL deficiency, respectively. The

Table 2 Response parameters of the knee joint under a force of 134 N in anterior translation

	Tibial displacement (mm)	Peak stress (MPa)			
		ACL	PCL	SMCL	DMCL
Case 1	4.89	23.31	14.70	15.18	7.95
Case 2	5.17	26.60	14.40	–	8.73
Case 3	5.04	24.84	14.83	16.08	–
Case 4	5.27	27.38	14.83	–	–

ACL anterior cruciate ligament, *DMCL* deep medial collateral ligament, *PCL* posterior cruciate ligament, *SMCL* superficial medial collateral ligament

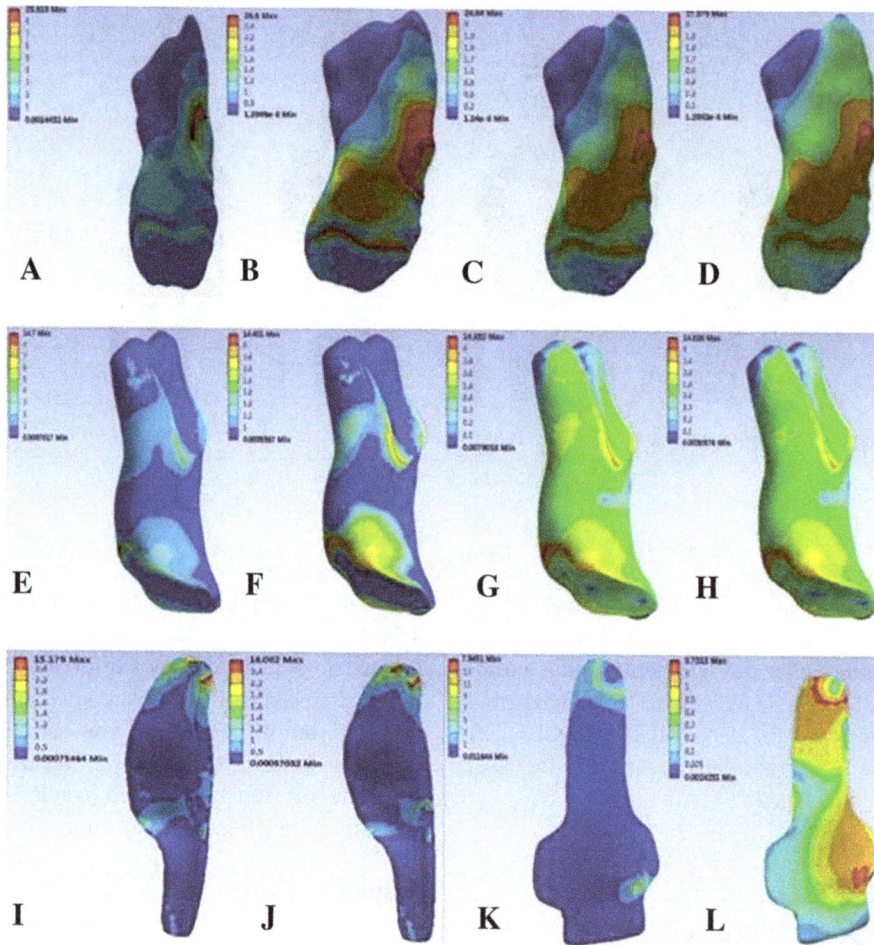

Fig. 3 von Mises stress distribution of the ACL, PCL, SMCL, and DMCL under a force of 134 N in anterior translation. **a** ACL in case 1. **b** ACL in case 2. **c** ACL in case 3. **d** ACL in case 4. **e** PCL in case 1. **f** PCL in case 2. **g** PCL in case 3. **h** PCL in case 4. **i** SMCL in case 1. **j** SMCL in case 3. **k** DMCL in case 1. **l** DMCL in case 2

peak stress was maximum at the posterior cruciate ligament (PCL), lower at SMCL, and very low at DMCL (Table 3) and was mainly located at the femoral start and end points at PCL and DMCL and only at the femoral end point at SMCL (Fig. 4).

Under the load of the 10-N m valgus torque, the tibial valgus angle changed from 4.06° at intact MCL to 6.08°,

Table 3 Response parameters of the knee joint under a force of 134 N in posterior translation

	Tibial displacement (mm)	Peak stress (MPa)			
		ACL	PCL	SMCL	DMCL
Case 1	4.98	10.68	26.32	7.26	3.44
Case 2	4.99	12.62	26.32	–	6.78
Case 3	4.92	11.90	26.32	8.40	–
Case 4	5.02	12.72	26.32	–	–

ACL anterior cruciate ligament, *DMCL* deep medial collateral ligament, *PCL* posterior cruciate ligament, *SMCL* superficial medial collateral ligament

4.86°, and 6.22° at SMCL deficiency, MCL deficiency and overall MCL deficiency, respectively. The peak stress was maximum at SMCL and gradually decreased at DMCL, ACL, and PCL (Table 4); it was mainly located at the femoral end point and anterior part at SMCL and at the femoral start and end points at DMCL (Fig. 5).

Under the load of the 10-N m external rotation torque, the tibial external rotation angle changed from 5.92° at intact MCL to 5.95°, 5.94°, and 6.10° at SMCL deficiency, DMCL deficiency, and overall MCL deficiency, respectively. The peak stress was maximum at SMCL, relatively lower at ACL and PCL, and the lowest at DMCL (Table 5). The peak stress at SMCL was mainly located at the end point and posterior part of the femur, and that at DMCL was located at the start and end points (Fig. 6).

Under the load of the 10-N m internal rotation torque, the tibial internal rotation angle changed from 6.64° at intact MCL to 7.48°, 6.72°, and 7.57° at SMCL deficiency,

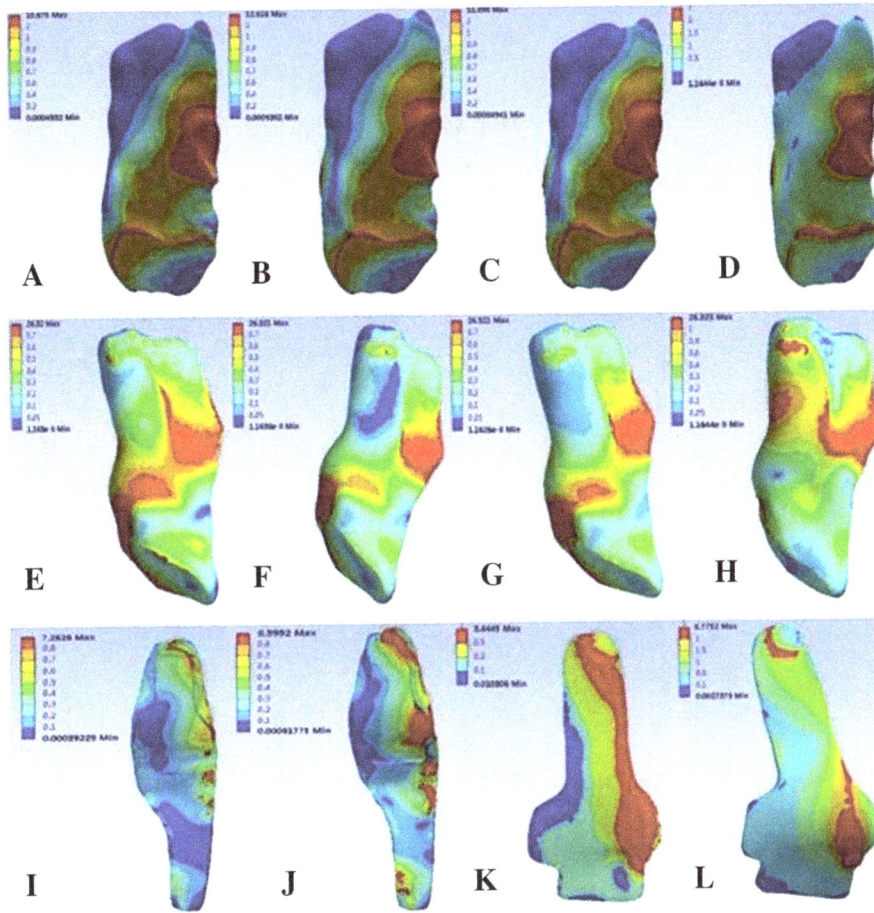

Fig. 4 von Mises stress distribution of ACL, PCL, SMCL, and DMCL under a force of 134 N in posterior translation. **a** ACL in case 1. **b** ACL in case 2. **c** ACL in case 3. **d** ACL in case 4. **e** PCL in case 1. **f** PCL in case 2. **g** PCL in case 3. **h** PCL in case 4. **i** SMCL in case 1. **j** SMCL in case 3. **k** DMCL in case 1. **l** DMCL in case 2

DMCL deficiency, and overall MCL deficiency, respectively. Meanwhile, the peak stress was maximum at SMCL, relatively lower at ACL and PCL, and minimum at DMCL (Table 6) and was mainly located at the femoral end point at SMCL and at the femoral start and end points at DMCL (Fig. 7).

Table 4 Response parameters of the knee joint under 10 N m of valgus moment

	Tibial valgus angle (°)	Peak stress (MPa)			
		ACL	PCL	SMCL	DMCL
Case 1	4.06	6.77	4.88	30.17	9.49
Case 2	6.08	12.01	10.14	–	16.11
Case 3	4.86	9.40	8.40	48.63	–
Case 4	6.22	20.22	20.22	–	–

ACL anterior cruciate ligament, *DMCL* deep medial collateral ligament, *PCL* posterior cruciate ligament, *SMCL* superficial medial collateral ligament

Discussion

Establishment of the knee joint model

The knee joint is one of the most complex joints in the human body, with a complex anatomic structure and biomechanical properties. The traditional mechanical method to study its biomechanical functions usually involves the application of extra-articular loads and use of mechanical measuring instruments [9], and it is difficult to investigate the stress distribution within the joints and other issues using this method. Therefore, establishing knee joint models such as the crossed four-link physical model and the two-dimensional mathematical model of the sagittal knee joint as well as the three-dimensional model of dynamic response of the knee joint has become an important measure for further studying the biomechanical characteristics of knee joints [10]. Since its first application in orthopedic biomechanics by Brekelmans et al. [11] in 1972, the FEM has been widely used in modeling teeth, artificial limbs,

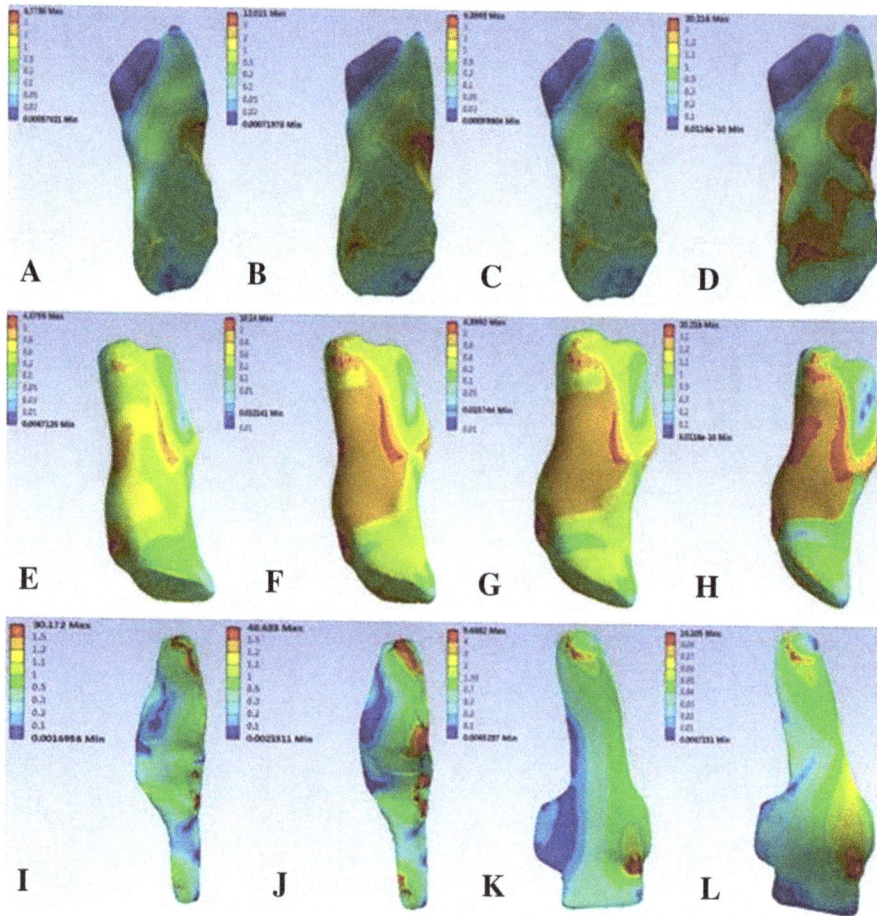

Fig. 5 von Mises stress distribution of ACL, PCL, SMCL, and DMCL under 10 N m of valgus moment. **a** ACL in case 1. **b** ACL in case 2. **c** ACL in case 3. **d** ACL in case 4. **e** PCL in case 1. **f** PCL in case 2. **g** PCL in case 3. **h** PCL in case 4. **i** SMCL in case 1. **j** SMCL in case 3. **k** DMCL in case 1. **l** DMCL in case 2

spine, etc. [12] and has been gradually applied to the biomechanics of ankles, knees, wrists, and other joints [13, 14].

Single-mode CT or MR images are typically unable to provide a clear contrast for intact knee joints, leading to difficulty in accurately constructing an FEM of knee joints containing multiple anatomic structures. Studies have found that although CT

Table 5 Response parameters of the knee joint under 10 N m of external rotation moment

	Tibial external rotation angle (°)	Peak stress (MPa)			
		ACL	PCL	SMCL	DMCL
Case 1	5.92	8.45	6.79	13.76	4.39
Case 2	5.95	9.66	7.67	–	4.45
Case 3	5.94	10.69	8.96	16.08	–
Case 4	6.10	11.35	9.67	–	–

ACL anterior cruciate ligament, *DMCL* deep medial collateral ligament, *PCL* posterior cruciate ligament, *SMCL* superficial medial collateral ligament

image data alone can be used to accurately construct bone structure models, it cannot be used to accurately simulate the cartilage, ligament, meniscus, and other soft tissues [15]. In contrast, MR imaging data alone can be used to accurately construct the anatomic structure models of various soft tissues including knee joints, while it cannot be used to accurately simulate bone structures [16]. Thus, using CT or MR imaging alone will significantly decrease the accuracy of these models, leading to inaccurate mechanical analysis of the knee joints.

Yao et al. [17] accurately constructed FEMs of the femoral cartilage, tibial cartilage, and medial meniscus using MATLAB and Hypermesh software, but not of other structures of knee joints. Therefore, a single software often has some limitations, and the constructed FEM fails to truly represent the anatomic characteristics of knee joints; thus, the FEMs of knee joints can be accurately constructed only by collaborative application of a variety of modeling software.

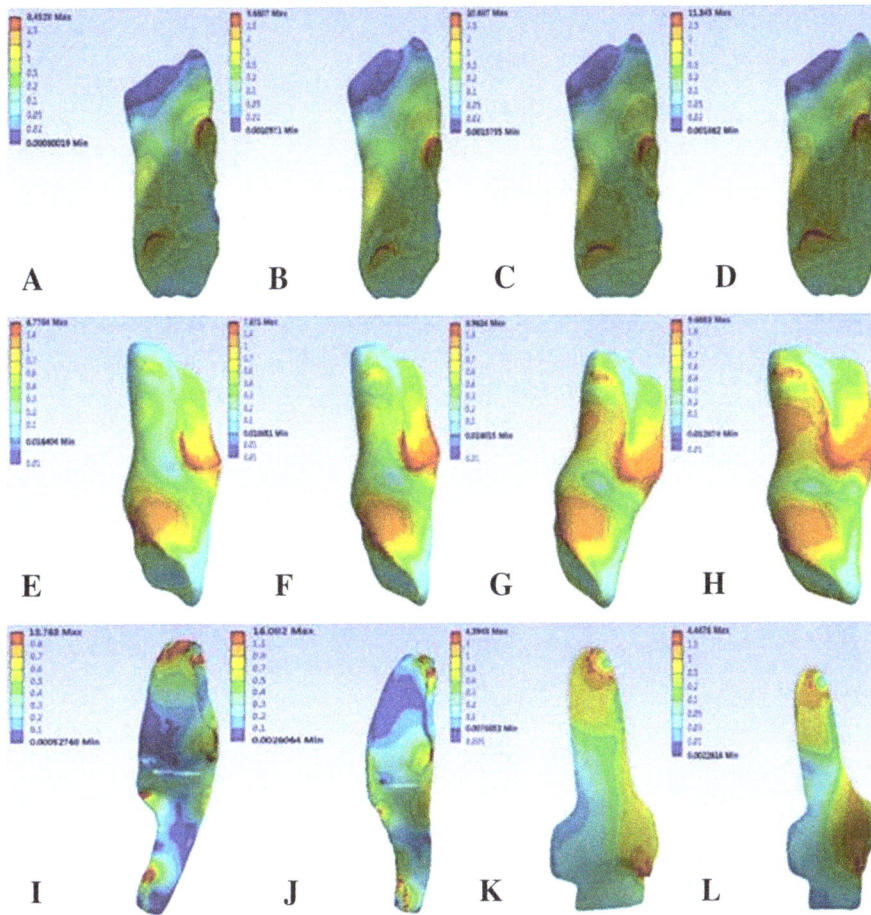

Fig. 6 von Mises stress distribution of the ACL, PCL, SMCL, and DMCL under 10 N m of external rotation moment. **a** ACL in case 1. **b** ACL in case 2. **c** ACL in case 3. **d** ACL in case 4. **e** PCL in case 1. **f** PCL in case 2. **g** PCL in case 3. **h** PCL in case 4. **i** SMCL in case 1. **j** SMCL in case 3. **k** DMCL in case 1. **l** DMCL in case 2

In this study, a variety of modes of CT and MR imaging as well as MIMICS 14.0, Geomagic Studio 12.0, and ANSYS modeling software were applied to construct a three-dimensional FEM of knee joints using the reverse engineering (RE) principle. In the MIMICS software, the structures in CT and MR images were assembled according to the human anatomy. However,

Table 6 Response parameters of the knee joint under 10 N m of internal rotation moment

	Tibial internal rotation angle (°)	Peak stress (MPa)			
		ACL	PCL	SMCL	DMCL
Case 1	6.64	9.06	7.26	14.75	4.71
Case 2	7.48	10.35	8.22	–	4.77
Case 3	6.72	11.45	9.60	17.23	–
Case 4	7.57	12.16	10.36	–	–

ACL anterior cruciate ligament, *DMCL* deep medial collateral ligament, *PCL* posterior cruciate ligament, *SMCL* superficial medial collateral ligament

this assembled model was very coarse due to the presence of interference surfaces. This issue could be addressed using Geomagic Studio 12.0, in which the interference surfaces in the model were removed. However, this software was not able to generate ANSYS preprocessing files; therefore, the repaired models were imported again into the 3-matic module of MIMICS software for initial meshing before being imported into ANSYS for finite element analysis (FEA). In addition, since this study focused on the mechanical analyses of the ligaments, their mesh size was refined at 1 mm, and the bone structures were set as a solid body with a mesh size of 4 mm, reflecting the different focuses of subjects in FEA. Because the meshing quality determined the accuracy of the FEA results, an even finer mesh would be required to analyze non-linear contacts. Local meshes with poor quality were optimized, and interactive meshes with satisfactory 6-node pentahedrons and 8-node hexahedrons were obtained based on the high-

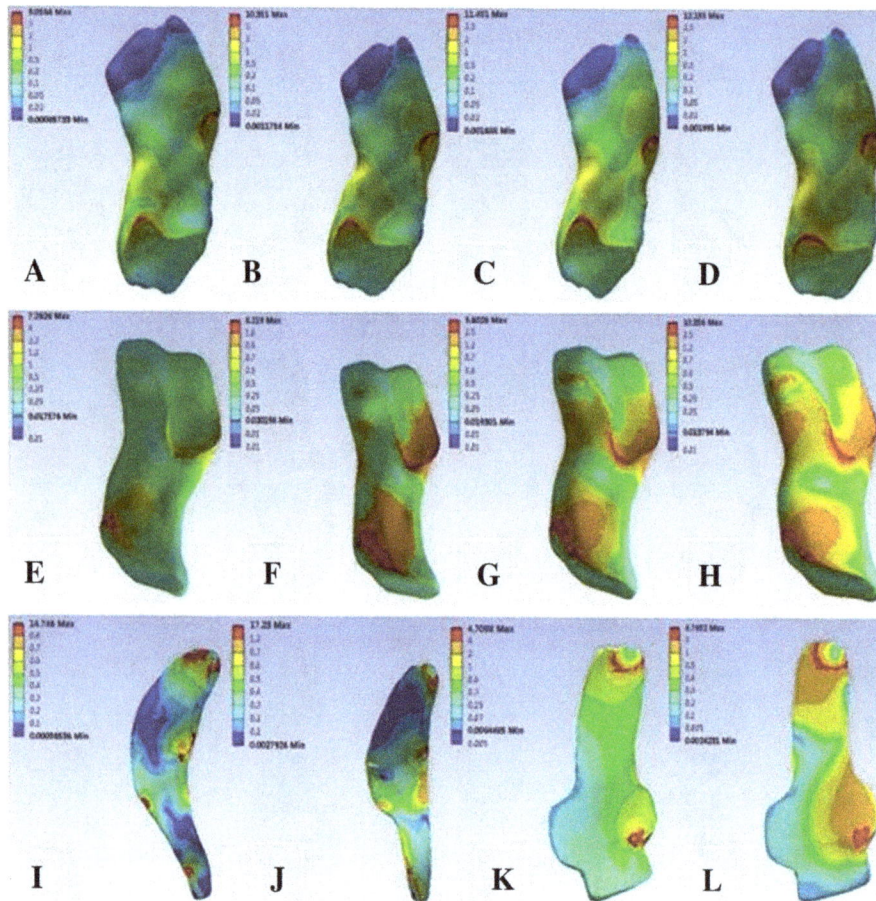

Fig. 7 von Mises stress distribution of the ACL, PCL, SMCL, and DMCL under 10 N m of internal rotation moment. **a** ACL in case 1. **b** ACL in case 2. **c** ACL in case 3. **d** ACL in case 4. **e** PCL in case 1. **f** PCL in case 2. **g** PCL in case 3. **h** PCL in case 4. **i** SMCL in case 1. **j** SMCL in case 3. **k** DMCL in case 1. **l** DMCL in case 2

quality area meshes, in order to achieve more accurate results compared to those obtained using meshes with 10-node tetrahedron elements. Ultimately, a three-dimensional model of the human right knee joint containing a variety of anatomic structures, such as the middle and upper segments of the femur, middle and upper segments of the tibia, fibula, patella, meniscus, ACL, PCL, MCL, lateral collateral ligament, and patellar ligament, was constructed. Meanwhile, high-quality volume meshes were developed, satisfying the requirements for FEA of biomechanics of knee joints. This FEM can be used to analyze the stress distribution of ligaments, contacts of tibiofemoral joints, stress distribution on articular surface, changes of stress distribution under different ligament deficiencies, and other biomechanical studies, as well as to simulate the effects of surgical results on the biomechanics of knee joints under different surgical conditions, and conduct biomechanical analyses of surgical fixations.

Biomechanical analyses of medial collateral ligament of the knee joint

The anatomy of MCL has been extensively studied [5]. In this experiment, based on the human anatomy, an FEM of the knee joint was established to simulate the anterior-posterior translation, valgus-varus rotation, and internal-external rotation of the knee joint, so as to study the biomechanical functions of its superficial and deep MCLs, in which the knee joint varus was excluded because the knee MCL is completely relaxed in this condition. In the experiment, a gradually increasing color grading from blue to red color indicated gradually increasing von Mises stress, which represented a greater load on the ligament and a greater role of the site and likelihood of damage.

Under the load of the 134-N forward force, the tibial displacement changed from 4.89 mm at intact MCL to 5.17, 5.04, and 5.17 mm at SMCL deficiency, DMCL deficiency, and overall MCL deficiency, respectively. A greater variation of tibial displacement at overall MCL deficiency indicated that MCL plays a role in limiting the forward translation of the tibia. Meanwhile, the tibial displacement showed a greater variation at SMCL deficiency compared with that at DMCL deficiency, suggesting that SMCL has a greater effect than the DMCL. During this process, the stress at ACL maintained a maximum value, suggesting that ACL plays the most important role in limiting the tibial anterior translation. Moreover, a greater stress at SMCL than that at DMCL indicated that the SMCL has a greater effect. The stress nephogram showed that the peak stresses at ACL and SMCL were mainly located at the femoral end point, indicating that during tibial anterior translation, injury to the femoral end point is most likely to occur at ACL and SMCL, and less likely to occur at DMCL.

Under the load of the 134-N backward force, the tibial translation showed a very small variation with MCL deficiency, during which the stress at PCL maintained a maximum value, while the stresses at SMCL and DMCL were relatively small, suggesting that PCL plays the most important role in constraining the tibial posterior translation, while the effects of SMCL and DMCL are very small. Meanwhile, the peak stress at PCL occurred at the tibial start and end points, suggesting that in tibial posterior translation, injury is most likely to occur at the femoral start and end points at PCL, while the risk of injury at SMCL and DMCL is small.

Under the load of the 10-N m valgus torque, the tibial valgus angle showed a large variation with MCL deficiency, which changed from 4.06° at intact MCL to 6.08°, 4.86°, and 6.22° at SMCL deficiency, MCL deficiency, and overall MCL deficiency, respectively, suggesting that MCL tends to resist the valgus motion of knee joints. Meanwhile, the stress was the largest at SMCL followed by that at DMCL, indicating that SMCL plays the most important role in limiting the valgus motion and the effect of DMCL is relatively smaller. As evident in the stress nephogram, the peak stress at SMCL occurred at the end point and anterior part of the femur, indicating that injury is most likely to occur at the end point and anterior part of the femur in valgus motion of knee joints at SMCL. In contrast, the peak stress at DMCL occurred at the femoral start and end points, suggesting that they are prone to injury at DMCL.

Under the load of the 10-N m external rotation torque, the tibial external rotation angle changed from 5.92° at intact MCL to 5.95°, 5.94°, and 6.10° at SMCL deficiency, DMCL deficiency, and overall MCL deficiency, respectively. The tibial external rotation angle showed a large variation at overall MCL deficiency, suggesting that MCL tends to resist the external rotation of the knee joints. Although the tibial external rotation angle did not show significant difference between SMCL

and DMCL deficiencies, the stress at SMCL was larger than that at DMCL, indicating that SMCL plays a more significant role in limiting the external rotation of the knee joint than the DMCL. As observed in the stress nephogram, the peak stress at SMCL was mainly located at the femoral end point and posterior part, indicating that they are prone to injury at SMCL during external rotation of knee joints, while the injury at DMCL was smaller.

Under the load of the 10-N m internal rotation torque, the tibial internal rotation angle changed from 6.64° at intact MCL to 7.48°, 6.72°, and 7.57° at SMCL deficiency, DMCL deficiency, and overall MCL deficiency, respectively. The tibial internal rotation angle showed a larger variation than the tibial external rotation angle with MCL deficiency, suggesting that knee joint MCL has a greater effect on limiting the internal rotation than the external rotation. Similarly, greater stress at SMCL than that at DMCL indicated that the SMCL has a greater effect on limiting the internal rotation of knee joints than the DMCL. As observed in the stress nephogram, the peak stress at SMCL occurred at the femoral end point, indicating that the femoral end point was prone to injury at SMCL during internal rotation of knee joints, while the injury at DMCL was smaller.

The above analyses show that in the extended position of knee joints, the main effect of MCL is to resist the valgus motion of knee joints, along with limiting the tibial forward displacement as well as the internal and external rotations of knee joints. The SMCL plays the most important role in the structure of the MCL of knee joints, while the effects of DMCL are relatively lesser. In various motions of knee joints, the femoral end point at SMCL is the most prone to injury. The anterior part of the femur is more prone to injury in resisting valgus motion, and the posterior part in resisting external rotation at SMCL. However, injury is less likely to occur at DMCL, and when it does occur, it occurs at the femoral start and end points.

Conclusions

In summary, this model to evaluate the function of the MCL by FEA is reliable [18–20]. The results indicate that the knee MCL II° injury should be repaired by surgery. However, the shortcoming of this study is the lack of clinical evidence. We hope to achieve a further investigation in the clinic.

Abbreviations

ACL: Anterior cruciate ligament; CT: Computed tomography; DICOM: Digital Imaging and Communications in Medicine; DMCL: Deep medial collateral ligament; E: Young's modulus; FEA: Finite element analysis; FEM: Finite element model; LCL: Lateral collateral ligament; MCL: Medial collateral ligament; MIMICS: Materialise Interactive Medical Image Control System; MRI: Magnetic resonance imaging; PCL: Posterior cruciate ligament; PL: Patellar ligament; RE: Reverse engineering; SMCL: Superficial medial collateral ligament; V: Poisson's ratio

Acknowledgements
We thank MedSci who provided medical writing services.

Funding
No authors received any funding.

Authors' contributions
DR contributed to this article by making substantial contributions to the conception and design of the study. XZ and DR contributed equally to this paper. YL contributed to the acquisition, analysis, and interpretation of the data. PW performed the operations. ZS, and JL were involved in drafting the manuscript. All authors read and approved the final manuscript.

Competing interests
The authors declare that they have no competing interests.

Author details
[1]Third Hospital of Hebei Medical University, Shijiazhuang 050051, China. [2]Hebei Provincial Key Laboratory of Orthopaedic Biomechanics, Shijiazhuang 050051, Hebei, China. [3]Department of Orthopedic Center, Third Hospital of Hebei Medical University, 139 Zi Qiang Road, Shijiazhuang 050051, Hebei, China.

References
1. Hetsroni I, Mann G. Combined reconstruction of the medial collateral ligament and anterior cruciate ligament using ipsilateral quadriceps tendon-bone and bone-patellar tendon-bone autografts. Arthrosc Tech. 2016;5(3): e579–87.
2. Najibi S, Albright JP. The use of knee braces, part 1: prophylactic knee braces in contact sports. Am J Sports Med. 2005;33(4):602–11.
3. Hamilton TW, Strickland LH, Pandit HG. A meta-analysis on the use of gabapentinoids for the treatment of acute postoperative pain following total knee arthroplasty. J Bone Joint Surg Am. 2016;98(16):1340–50.
4. Yenchak AJ, et al. Criteria-based management of an acute multistructure knee injury in a professional football player: a case report. J Orthop Sports Phys Ther. 2011;41(9):675–86.
5. Liu F, et al. Morphology of the medial collateral ligament of the knee. J Orthop Surg Res. 2010;5(1):69.
6. Pena E, et al. A finite element simulation of the effect of graft stiffness and graft tensioning in ACL reconstruction. Clin Biomech (Bristol, Avon). 2005; 20(6):636–44.
7. Shirazi R, Shirazi-Adl A. Computational biomechanics of articular cartilage of human knee joint: effect of osteochondral defects. J Biomech. 2009;42(15): 2458–65.
8. Gabriel MT, et al. Distribution of in situ forces in the anterior cruciate ligament in response to rotatory loads. J Orthop Res. 2004;22(1):85–9.
9. Hinterwimmer S, Baumgart R, Plitz W. Tension changes in the collateral ligaments of a cruciate ligament-deficient knee joint: an experimental biomechanical study. Arch Orthop Trauma Surg. 2002;122(8):454–8.
10. Abdel-Rahman EM, Hefzy MS. Three-dimensional dynamic behaviour of the human knee joint under impact loading. Med Eng Phys. 1998;20(4):276–90.
11. Brekelmans WA, Poort HW, Slooff TJ. A new method to analyse the mechanical behaviour of skeletal parts. Acta Orthop Scand. 1972;43(5):301–17.
12. Silva MJ, Keaveny TM, Hayes WC. Load sharing between the shell and centrum in the lumbar vertebral body. Spine (Phila Pa 1976). 1997;22(2): 140–50.
13. Li G, et al. A validated three-dimensional computational model of a human knee joint. J Biomech Eng. 1999;121(6):657–62.
14. LeRoux MA, Setton LA. Experimental and biphasic FEM determinations of the material properties and hydraulic permeability of the meniscus in tension. J Biomech Eng. 2002;124(3):315–21.
15. Chantarapanich N, et al. A finite element study of stress distributions in normal and osteoarthritic knee joints. J Med Assoc Thai. 2009;92 Suppl 6: S97–103.
16. Donahue TL, et al. A finite element model of the human knee joint for the study of tibio-femoral contact. J Biomech Eng. 2002;124(3):273–80.
17. Yao J, et al. Stresses and strains in the medial meniscus of an ACL deficient knee under anterior loading: a finite element analysis with image-based experimental validation. J Biomech Eng. 2006;128(1):135–41.
18. Liu F, et al. In vivo length patterns of the medial collateral ligament during the stance phase of gait. Knee Surg Sports Traumatol Arthrosc. 2011;19(5): 719–27.
19. Ellis BJ, et al. Medial collateral ligament insertion site and contact forces in the ACL-deficient knee. J Orthop Res. 2006;24(4):800–10.
20. Hosseini A, et al. In vivo length change patterns of the medial and lateral collateral ligaments along the flexion path of the knee. Knee Surg Sports Traumatol Arthrosc. 2015;23(10):3055–61.

Permissions

The contributors of this book come from diverse backgrounds, making this book a truly international effort. This book will bring forth new frontiers with its revolutionizing research information and detailed analysis of the nascent developments around the world.

We would like to thank all the contributing authors for lending their expertise to make the book truly unique. They have played a crucial role in the development of this book. Without their invaluable contributions this book wouldn't have been possible. They have made vital efforts to compile up to date information on the varied aspects of this subject to make this book a valuable addition to the collection of many professionals and students.

This book was conceptualized with the vision of imparting up-to-date information and advanced data in this field. To ensure the same, a matchless editorial board was set up. Every individual on the board went through rigorous rounds of assessment to prove their worth. After which they invested a large part of their time researching and compiling the most relevant data for our readers.

The editorial board has been involved in producing this book since its inception. They have spent rigorous hours researching and exploring the diverse topics which have resulted in the successful publishing of this book. They have passed on their knowledge of decades through this book. To expedite this challenging task, the publisher supported the team at every step. A small team of assistant editors was also appointed to further simplify the editing procedure and attain best results for the readers.

Apart from the editorial board, the designing team has also invested a significant amount of their time in understanding the subject and creating the most relevant covers. They scrutinized every image to scout for the most suitable representation of the subject and create an appropriate cover for the book.

The publishing team has been an ardent support to the editorial, designing and production team. Their endless efforts to recruit the best for this project, has resulted in the accomplishment of this book. They are a veteran in the field of academics and their pool of knowledge is as vast as their experience in printing. Their expertise and guidance has proved useful at every step. Their uncompromising quality standards have made this book an exceptional effort. Their encouragement from time to time has been an inspiration for everyone.

The publisher and the editorial board hope that this book will prove to be a valuable piece of knowledge for researchers, students, practitioners and scholars across the globe.

List of Contributors

Bobin Mi, Guohui Liu, Yi Liu, Kun Zha, Qipeng Wu and Jing Liu
Department of Orthopedics, Union Hospital, Tongji Medical College, Huazhong University of Science and Technology, 1277, Jiefang Avenue, Wuhan, China

Huijuan Lv
Department of Rheumatology, Tangdu Hospital, The Fourth Military Medical University, 1, Xinsi Avenue, Xi'an, China

Melissa D. Gaillard and Thomas P. Gross
Midlands Orthopaedics & Neurosurgery, 1910 Blanding Street, Columbia, SC 29201, USA

Qian Tang, Gang Zheng, Hua-Zi Xu, Hua-chen Yu, Yu Zhang and Hai-Xiao Li
Department of Orthopaedic Surgery, The Second Affiliated Hospital and Yuying Children's Hospital of Wenzhou Medical University, 109, Xueyuanxi road, 325027 Wenzhou, China.

Ping Shang
Department of Rehabilitation, The Second Affiliated Hospital and Yuying Children's Hospital of Wenzhou Medical University, 109 Xueyuanxi road, Wenzhou 325027, China

Li-ping Ma and Ying-mei Qi
China-Japan Union Hospital of Jilin University, Changchun, People's Republic of China

Dong-xu Zhao
Department of Orthopedics, China-Japan Union Hospital of Jilin University, 126 Xiantai Street, Changchun, Jilin, People's Republic of China

Ye-Ran Li, Yu-Hang Gao, Xin Qi, Jian-Guo Liu, Lu Ding, Chen Yang, Zheng Zhang and Shu-Qiang Li
Department of Orthopaedic Surgery, The First Hospital of Jilin University, Jilin University, Xinmin St 71, Chang Chun, China

Michael Ulrich Jensen and Mogens Berg Laursen
Department of Orthopaedic Surgery, Aalborg University Hospital, Hobrovej 18-22, 9000 Aalborg, Denmark

Christian Lund Petersen, Jonas Bruun Kjærsgaard and Nicolai Kjærgaard
School of Medicine and Health, Aalborg University, Niels Jernes Vej 12 A5, 9220 Aalborg Ø, Denmark

Zheng Hao and Baocheng Zhao
Center of Diagnosis and Treatment for Developmental Dysplasia of the Hip, Nanjing Zhongyangmen Community Health Service Center, Kang'ai Hospital, Nanjing 210037, Jiangsu, People's Republic of China

Xin Li
Department of HIV/ AIDS/STI Prevention and Control, Nanjing Municipal Center for Diseases Control and Prevention, Nanjing 210009, Jiangsu, People's Republic of China

Jin Dai and Qing Jiang
Department of Sports Medicine and Adult Reconstructive Surgery, Drum Tower Hospital, School of Medicine, Nanjing University, 321 Zhongshan Road, Nanjing 210008, Jiangsu, People's Republic of China. Laboratory for Bone and Joint Disease, Model Animal Research Center (MARC), Nanjing University, Nanjing 210093, Jiangsu, China

Tsuneo Kawahara
Graduate School of Engineering, Chiba University, 1-33 Yayoi-cho, Inage-ku, Chiba 263-8522, Japan Medical Corporation Jinseikai, Togane, Japan

Takahisa Sasho
Center for Preventive Medicine, Musculoskeletal disease and pain, Chiba University, Chiba, Japan Department of Orthopaedic Surgery, School of Medicine, Chiba University, Chiba, Japan

Joe Katsuragi
Department of Orthopaedic Surgery, Local Incorporated Administrative Agency, Sanmu Medical Center, Sanmu, Japan

Takashi Ohnishi and Hideaki Haneishi
Center for Frontier Medical Engineering, Chiba University, Chiba, Japan

Kadir Oznam
Department of Orthopaedic and Traumatology, Istanbul Medipol University School of Medicine, 34214 Istanbul, Turkey

Duygu Yasar Sirin
Department of Molecular Biology and Genetic, Namik Kemal University Faculty of Arts and Sciences, 59100 Tekirdag, Turkey

Ibrahim Yilmaz and Hanefi Ozbek
Department of Medical Pharmacology, Istanbul Medipol University School of Medicine, 34810 Istanbul, Turkey

Yasin Emre Kaya
Republic of Turkey, Ministry of Health, Department of Orthopaedic and Traumatology, Corlu State Hospital, 59100 Tekirdag, Turkey

Mehmet Isyar
Department of Orthopaedic and Traumatology, Acibadem Hospitals Group, 34180 Istanbul, Turkey

Seyit Ali Gumustas
Republic of Turkey, Ministry of Health, Dr. Lutfi Kirdar Research and Training Hospital, 34890 Istanbul, Turkey

Semih Akkaya
Department of Orthopaedic and Traumatology, Denizli Private Surgery Hospital, 20070 Denizli, Turkey

Arda Kayhan
Department of Radiology, Istanbul Kanuni Sultan Suleyman Training and Research Hospital, 34303 Istanbul, Turkey

Mahir Mahirogullari
Department of Orthopaedic and Traumatology, Memorial Health Group, 34384 Istanbul, Turkey

Amir A. Jamali
Joint Preservation Institute, 2825 J Street, Suite 440, Sacramento, CA 95816, USA

John P. Meehan
UC Davis Medical Center, 4860 Y St., #4800, Sacramento, CA 95817, USA

Nathan M. Moroski
Department of Orthopaedic Surgery, University of California, Irvine, 101 The City Drive South, Pavillion III, Building 29A, Orange, CA 92868, USA

Matthew J. Anderson
UC Davis Department of Orthopaedics, 4635 2nd Ave, Research 1 Room 2000, Sacramento, CA 95817, USA

Ramit Lamba
UC Davis Department of Radiology, 4860 Y St., #3100, Sacramento, CA 95817, USA

Arol Parise
Sutter Institute for Medical Research, 2801 Capitol Ave Suite 400, Sacramento 95816, USA

Hidenori Tanikawa and So Nomoto
Department of Orthopaedic Surgery, Saiseikai Yokohamashi Tobu Hospital, 3-6-1 Shimosueyoshi, Tsurumi, Yokohama, Kanagawa, Japan

Kengo Harato, Shu Kobayashi and Yasuo Niki
Department of Orthopaedic Surgery, Keio University School of Medicine, Shinjyuku, Tokyo, Japan

Ryo Ogawa
Department of Orthopaedic Surgery, Kitasato University Kitasato Institute Hospital, Minato-ku, Tokyo, Japan

Tomoyuki Sato
Department of Anesthesiology, Saiseikai Yokohamashi Tobu Hospital, Yokohama, Kanagawa, Japan

Kazunari Okuma
Department of Orthopaedic Surgery, Saitama City Hospital, Saitama-shi, Saitama, Japan

Alexandra Nowak and Adrien Jean-Pierre Schwitzguebel
Division of Orthopaedics and Trauma Surgery, La Tour Hospital, Rue J.-D Maillard 3, 1217 Meyrin, Switzerland

Alexandre Lädermann
Division of Orthopaedics and Trauma Surgery, La Tour Hospital, Rue J.-D Maillard 3, 1217 Meyrin, Switzerland
Faculty of Medicine, University of Geneva, Rue Michel-Servet 1, 1211 Geneva 4, Switzerland
Division of Orthopaedics and Trauma Surgery, Department of Surgery, Geneva University Hospitals, Rue Gabrielle-Perret-Gentil 4, CH-1211 Geneva 14, Switzerland

Jérome Tirefort
Division of Orthopaedics and Trauma Surgery, Department of Surgery, Geneva University Hospitals, Rue Gabrielle-Perret-Gentil 4, CH-1211 Geneva 14, Switzerland

Patrick Joel Denard
Southern Oregon Orthopedics, Medford, Oregon, USA
Department of Orthopaedics and Rehabilitation, Oregon Health & Science University, Portland, Oregon, USA

Philippe Collin
Saint-Grégoire Private Hospital Center, Boulevard Boutière 6, 35768 Saint-Grégoire cedex, France

Yi Tang, Xu Tang, Qinghua Wei and Hui Zhang
Department of Orthopedics, People's Hospital of JianYang, No. 180, Yiyuan Road, Jiancheng zhen, Jianyang, Sichuan Province, China

Feng-Jen Tseng
Department of Life Science and the Institute of Biotechnology, National Dong Hwa University, Hualien 974, Taiwan, Republic of China
Department of Orthopedics, Hualien Armed Force General Hospital, Hualien 971, Taiwan, Republic of China

Wei-Tso Chia
Department of Health, Hsin Chu General Hospital, Hsinchu 300, Taiwan, Republic of China

Ru-Yu Pan, Leou-Chyr Lin and Hsian-Chung Shen
Department of Orthopaedics, Tri-Service General Hospital, National Defense Medical Center, Neihu 114, Taipei, Taiwan, Republic of China

Chih-Hung Wang
Graduate Institute of Medical Science,National Defense Medical Center, Neihu 114, Taipei, Taiwan, Republic of China

Jia-Fwu Shyu
Department of Biology and Anatomy, National Defense Medical Center, Neihu 114, Taipei, Taiwan, Republic of China

Hai Ding, Jian Yao, Wenju Chang and Fendou Liu
Department of Orthopedics, The First Affiliated Hospital of Bengbu Medical College, No. 287 Changhuai Road, Bengbu, Anhui 233004, People's Republic of China

Yingchun Zhang, Caishan Wang and Pan Mao
Department of Ultrasound, The Second Affiliated Hospital of Soochow University, San Xiang Road 1055, Suzhou 215004, China

Huajun Xu
Department of Ultrasound, The Second Affiliated Hospital of Soochow University, San Xiang Road 1055, Suzhou 215004, China
Department of Ultrasound, Huzhou Central Hospital, Hong Qi Road 198, Huzhou 313000, China

Huimei Zhang
Department of Radiology, Huzhou Central Hospital, Hong Qi Road 198, Huzhou 313000, China

Wei-Bin Hsu and Shr-Hsin Chang
Sports Medicine Center, Chang Gung Memorial Hospital, No. 6, West Section, Chia-Pu Road, Putz City 61363, Chiayi Country, Taiwan, Republic of China

Wei-Hsiu Hsu and Robert Wen-Wei Hsu
Sports Medicine Center, Chang Gung Memorial Hospital, No. 6, West Section, Chia-Pu Road, Putz City 61363, Chiayi Country, Taiwan, Republic of China
Department of Orthopaedic Surgery, Chang Gung Memorial Hospital, No. 6, West Section, Chia-Pu Road, Putz City 61363, Chiayi Country, Taiwan, Republic of China

Wun-Jer Shen
PO CHENG Orthopedic Institute, No. 100, Bo-ai 2nd Road, Kaohsiung 81357, Zuoying District, Taiwan, Republic of China

Zin-Rong Lin
Department of Athletic Sports, National Chung Cheng University, No.168, University Road, Minhsiung Township 62102, Chiayi Country, Taiwan, Republic of China

Jian-xiong Ma, Ming-jie Kuang, Jie Zhao, Bin Lu, Ying Wang and Zheng-rui Fan
Biomechanics Labs of Orthopaedics Institute, Tianjin Hospital, No. 155, Munan Road, Heping District, Tianjin 300050, People's Republic of China

Lu-kai Zhang
Biomechanics Labs of Orthopaedics Institute, Tianjin Hospital, No. 155, Munan Road, Heping District, Tianjin 300050, People's Republic of China

Graduate School of Tianjin University of Traditional Chinese Medicine, Tianjin 300193, People's Republic of China

Xin-long Ma
Biomechanics Labs of Orthopaedics Institute, Tianjin Hospital, No. 155, Munan Road, Heping District, Tianjin 300050, People's Republic of China Department of Orthopedics, Tianjin Hospital, Tianjin 300211, People's Republic of China

Shang-kun Tang
Department of Clinical Medicine, Second Clinical Medical College, Wenzhou Medical University, 325000 Wenzhou, China

Kai Zhou, Tingxian Ling, Haoyang Wang, Zongke Zhou, Bin Shen, Jing Yang, Pengde Kang and Fuxing Pei
Department of Orthopaedics, West China Hospital of Sichuan University, Chengdu 610041, China

Tat Woon Chao, Liam Geraghty, Pandelis Dimitriou and Simon Talbot
Department of Orthopaedics, Western Health, 1/210 Burgundy Street, Heidelberg, Victoria 3084, Australia

Dong Ren, Yueju Liu, Xianchao Zhang, Zhaohui Song and Jian Lu
Third Hospital of Hebei Medical University, Shijiazhuang 050051, China
Hebei Provincial Key Laboratory of Orthopaedic Biomechanics, Shijiazhuang 050051, Hebei, China

Pengcheng Wang
Third Hospital of Hebei Medical University, Shijiazhuang 050051, China
Hebei Provincial Key Laboratory of Orthopaedic Biomechanics, Shijiazhuang 050051, Hebei, China
Department of Orthopedic Center, Third Hospital of Hebei Medical University, 139 Zi Qiang Road, Shijiazhuang 050051, Hebei, China

Index

www.ingramcontent.com/pod-product-compliance
Lightning Source LLC
Chambersburg PA
CBHW082014190326
41458CB00010B/3183